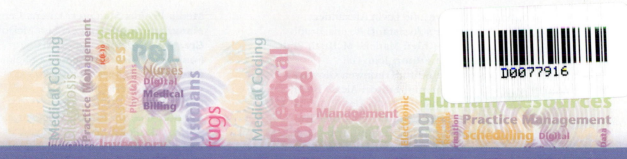

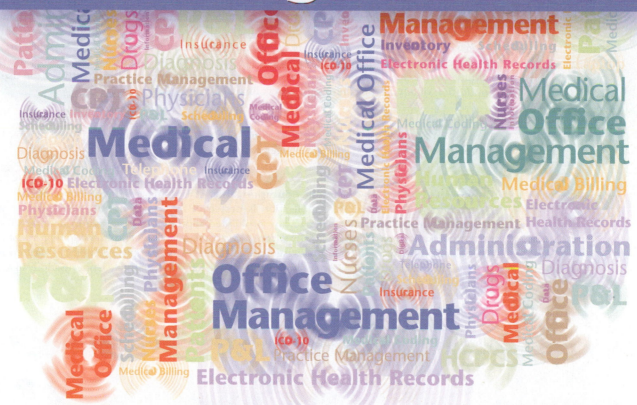

Medical Office Management

Christine Malone

PEARSON

Boston   Columbus   Indianapolis   New York   San Francisco   Upper Saddle River   Amsterdam   Cape Town
Dubai   London   Madrid   Milan   Munich   Paris   Montreal   Toronto   Delhi   Mexico City
São Paulo   Sydney   Hong Kong   Seoul   Singapore   Taipei   Tokyo

Publisher: Julie Levin Alexander
Publisher's Assistant: Regina Bruno
Editor-in-Chief: Marlene McHugh Pratt
Executive Editor: Joan Gill
Associate Editor: Bronwen Glowacki
Developmental Editor: Alexis Breen Ferraro,
  iD8-TripleSSS Media Development, LLC
Editorial Assistant: Stephanie Kiel
Director of Marketing: David Gesell
Marketing Manager: Katrin Beacom
Senior Marketing Coordinator: Alicia Wozniak
Managing Production Editor: Patrick Walsh
Production Liaison: Julie Boddorf
Production Editor: Peggy Kellar
Senior Media Editor: Matt Norris

Media Project Manager: Lorena Cerisano
Manufacturing Manager: Lisa McDowell
Creative Director: Andrea Nix
Senior Art Director: Maria Guglielmo
Interior Designer: Dina Curro
Cover Designer: Ilze Lemesis
Cover Image: Ilze Lemesis
Chapter Opener Photo: Volodymyr
  Krasyuk/ Fotolia.com
Composition: Aptara®, Inc.
Printing and Binding: Courier/Kendallville
Cover Printer: Lehigh-Phoenix Color/
  Hagerstown
Text Font: ITC Garamond Std

Notice: The authors and the publisher of this volume have taken care that the information and technical recommendations contained herein are based on research and expert consultation, and are accurate and compatible with the standards generally accepted at the time of publication. Nevertheless, as new information becomes available, changes in clinical and technical practices become necessary. The reader is advised to carefully consult manufacturers' instructions and information material for all supplies and equipment before use, and to consult with a healthcare professional as necessary. This advice is especially important when using new supplies or equipment for clinical purposes. The author[s] and publisher disclaim all responsibility for any liability, loss, injury, or damage incurred as a consequence, directly or indirectly, of the use and application of any of the contents of this volume.

Credits and acknowledgments borrowed from other sources and reproduced, with permission, in this textbook appear on appropriate pages within text.

Library of Congress Cataloging-in-Publication Data available upon request.

10 9 8 7 6 5 4 3 2 1

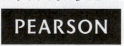

ISBN-13: 978-0-13-506067-4
ISBN-10: 0-13-506067-2

DEDICATION

To my mentor, Jude Bulman, who possesses so many of the virtues I most admire in a manager, leader, and professional woman.

Brief Contents

Contents

CHAPTER 9 Duties of the Medical Office Manager 186

CHAPTER 10 Use of Computers in the Medical Office 204

CHAPTER 11 Office Policies and Procedures 220

CHAPTER 12 Accounting and Payroll in the Medical Office 234

CHAPTER 13 Billing and Collections   260

CHAPTER 14 Health Insurance   282

The Development of This Text

As someone who has spent over 25 years in medical office management, I have seen many changes to the way medicine is practiced and the way medical offices are managed. In developing this text, it has been my goal to present material in an easy-to-understand format, providing benefit both to the new medical office manager or the student intent on entering the field, as well as to the established manager who may be looking for tips and insights to make his or her job easier.

This text contains information that addresses the specific needs of the medical office manager, from hiring and retaining the right personnel, to researching, developing, and marketing new product lines. A thorough review of the competition showed numerous areas where other texts were lacking. With information included on the development of staffing models, proper coding techniques, and tips for coaching and mentoring of staff, this text is robust in all areas of the medical office manager's job.

Organization of the Text

The material in *Medical Office Management* is presented in a way that provides the reader with a natural flow, from information on why a person might choose to work in the field of medical office management to how to actually perform the job. This text presents a unique approach to teaching medical office management and includes specific procedures and techniques that have proven effective in the management of the medical office. The text's inclusion of the Registered Medical Assistant (RMA) Task List and the Occupational Analysis of the CMA (AAMA) (see Appendices F and G, respectively) make this book a useful tool for medical office management in medical assisting programs.

The material in this text is divided into 17 chapters that include the latest information on the design and management of the medical office. From developing the skills needed to succeed as a medical office manager, to attracting and keeping the best staff, the material in this text is presented in a way such that a beginning office manager or student might use the text as a how-to guide. At the same time, an experienced office manager might use the text as a guide for perfecting the art of managing the medical office.

Chapter 1 contains information on today's healthcare environment. This chapter outlines the type of practice settings a manager may encounter and includes information on the traits of the medical office manager.

Chapter 2 addresses communications in the medical office, including both verbal and nonverbal communication. This chapter includes information on written communication, including the components to writing a business letter.

Chapter 3 contains in-depth information on the legal and ethical issues involved in managing the medical office. This chapter outlines the process of maintaining professional files for physicians and the legal obligations associated with mandatory reporting in healthcare.

Chapter 4 describes the steps to successfully managing the personnel in the medical office. This chapter contains information on how to perform a staffing model profile as well as advertising for, interviewing, and hiring the right candidate for a particular job.

Chapter 5 discusses the steps for managing the front office in a medical clinic. The use of telephones, including features of various telephone systems, and the greeting of patients in the front office are covered in this chapter.

Chapter 6 goes into detail about appointment scheduling and the process of triaging and screening callers to the medical office.

Chapter 7 includes information on the management of medical records in the medical office. This chapter contains current information on the use of electronic medical records, as well as the use of paper records, for those offices that are not yet using an electronic system for medical records management.

Chapter 8 contains important information on the regulatory requirements of the medical office manager, including recently passed legislation, such as the Red Flags rule.

Chapter 9 contains information on the duties of the medical office manager, including conducting staff meetings, coaching and motivating employees to higher performance, and dealing with suppliers and service contracts.

Chapter 10 details the use of computers in the medical office, including the design of training programs for new employees.

Chapter 11 outlines the use and creation of office policies and procedures in the medical office, including policies that apply to the administrative, as well as clinical areas of the office. (Appendix B includes a sample policy and procedure manual.)

Chapter 12 addresses the function of accounting and payroll in the medical office. This chapter has great detail on the use of various IRS forms as well as details on managing accounts payable.

Chapter 13 describes the function of billing and collecting in the medical office. From creating a fee schedule to managing the accounts receivables, this chapter provides a lot of detail for the management of finances in the medical office.

Chapter 14 has current information on health insurance and the processing of medical claims.

Chapter 15 contains information on the use of procedural and diagnostic coding in the medical office.

Chapter 16 outlines the use of quality improvement and risk management programs in the medical office, an important area to concentrate on in order to reduce patient and employee injuries and increase patient satisfaction.

Chapter 17 describes the function of marketing in the medical office, including details on creating a robust website and the use of social media in advertising.

Unique Features of the Text

- **Learning Objectives:** Specific learning objectives appear at the beginning of each chapter, stating what will be achieved upon successful completion of the chapter.

- **Key Terminology:** Key term definitions appear in the margins where the terms are first introduced. Key terms are also defined in the comprehensive glossary.

- **Chapter Outline:** A list of major chapter topics appears at the beginning of each chapter to highlight key areas of study.

- **Case Studies:** A thought-provoking case study is presented at the beginning of each chapter, and case-specific questions appear at the end of each chapter. Answers to the case study questions are provided in Appendix D.

- **Introduction:** The introduction presents the main concepts discussed in each chapter.

- **Critical Thinking Questions:** Critical thinking questions are interspersed throughout the chapter. Students must rely on the content in the text and their own critical thinking skills to answer the questions.

- **Photos and Illustrations:** These support the textual material presented and reinforce key concepts.

- **Informational Tables:** These tables appear throughout the text and summarize pertinent information for the reader. They provide students with visuals and comparisons to reinforce the lesson.

- **Chapter Summary:** The chapter summary is a brief restatement of key points in the chapter.

- **Chapter Review Questions:** End-of-chapter questions are provided in multiple-choice, true/false, and matching format, and are designed to help reinforce learning. The review questions measure the students' understanding of the material presented in the chapter, and are available for use by the student or by the instructor as an outcomes assessment.

- **Chapter Resources:** A list of related books and websites appears at the end of each chapter. In addition, Appendix A lists valuable Internet resources for healthcare professionals.

- **Appendices:** Many useful appendices appear at the end of the book, including Internet websites for healthcare professionals, a sample medical office policy and procedure manual, guidelines for documenting in the medical record to ensure proper coding, answers to chapter case study questions, the Registered Medical Assisting (RMA) Task List, the Occupational Analysis of the CMA (AAMA), and medical terminology word parts.

The Learning Package

THE STUDENT PACKAGE

- Textbook
- MyHealthProfessionsKit™

THE INSTRUCTIONAL PACKAGE

- Instructor's resource manual with lesson plans
- PowerPoint™ lecture slides
- MyTest™

About the Author

Christine Malone, MHA, CMPE, CPHRM, FACHE, studied management practice and theory at Henry Cogswell College, receiving her bachelor of science in professional management. She continued her education at the University of Washington, obtaining her master's degree in health administration.

Christine has over 25 years of experience in the healthcare field, having spent time working as a dental assistant, medical receptionist, x-ray technician, medical clinic director, and as a consultant to healthcare providers, focusing on strategic management, efficient office flow, and human resource management. Since 2004, Christine has been teaching within the Health Professions Department at Everett Community College in Washington State. There she teaches Medical Office Management, Computer Applications in the Medical Office, Medical Practice Finances, Intercultural Communication in Healthcare, and Medical Law and Ethics. Christine is the author of *Administrative Medical Assisting: Foundations and Practice* and the coauthor of *Comprehensive Medical Assisting: Foundations and Practice*.

In 2006 Christine researched and developed a certificate program in healthcare risk management. This series of three courses is offered via distance learning and provides the student who successfully completes the three courses with a certificate in healthcare risk management.

Christine was elected to the Snohomish County Charter Review Commission, a one-year position during 2005–2006. She has served as the chair of the Young Careerists Group within the Business and Professional Women's Association of Greater Everett, she is a member of the Northwest Partnership for Palliative Care, and she is active in volunteer work with Planned Parenthood of the Northwest.

Christine has achieved certifications in numerous professional groups, including the American College of Healthcare Executives, the American Society for Healthcare Risk Management, and the American College of Medical Practice Executives. She is also a member of many other professional associations, including the Washington State Healthcare Executive Forum. Christine has been the guest speaker at various events on healthcare issues and in continuing education meetings across the country and has received her certification in vocational teaching, as well as in pediatric palliative care training.

Christine and her husband have five children and live in a 100-year-old home in Everett, Washington. In 1999, their third child, Ian, was injured due to medical negligence during his birth. Ian lived four and a half years before succumbing to his injuries in 2004. This was the genesis of Christine's work toward improving patient safety in healthcare. Her input has been sought by legislative committees, editorial boards, and many policymakers. A nationally recognized healthcare reform advocate, Christine has appeared on the *Today Show, NBC Nightly News, ABC Nightly News,* the CBC's *The National, in The New York Times, The Los Angeles Times,* and on *Salon.com*.

Acknowledgments

The author would like to extend a thank you to executive editor Joan Gill and to Alexis Breen Ferraro, developmental editor, for their experienced management and oversight with this project.

I would also like to thank my husband Dylan and children Corey, Mallory, Molly, and Riley—I appreciate your patience while this project was completed.

Reviewers

The author and publisher wish to thank the following reviewers, all of whom provided valuable feedback and helped shape the final text:

Brian Dickens, MBA, RMA, CHI
Regional Medical Assistant Program Director
Keiser Career College and Southeastern Institute, Florida

Kathryn M. Foit, CMA (AAMA), AAS, MSEd, CPC
Associate Professor
Erie Community College, New York

Melissa D. Hibbard, CEHRS, CMRS, CPC, CPhT
Program Director, Medical Business
Miami Jacobs Career College, Ohio

Olivia Kerr, MBA
Coordinator, Professor of Business Office Systems and Support Program
El Centro College, Texas

Joann Monks, RN, BSN, BC, MBA, RMA
Program Director of Medical Assistant Program
Salter College, Massachusetts

Traci Strobel, BC, CBCS, CCS-P
Oakton Community College, Illinois

Medical Office Management

CHAPTER 1

Today's Healthcare Environment

LEARNING OBJECTIVES

Upon completion of this chapter, you should be able to:

- Spell and define the key terms in this chapter.
- Describe the different backgrounds of those who choose to go into the field of medical office management.
- List and describe the types of medical practice ownership.
- Discuss the various types of medical practice settings.
- Discuss the educational requirements and roles of various members of the healthcare team.
- Describe various specialty care practices.
- Discuss the educational background and role of the medical office manager.
- Describe the different types of continuing education opportunities available for the medical office manager.
- Discuss the future of healthcare management.

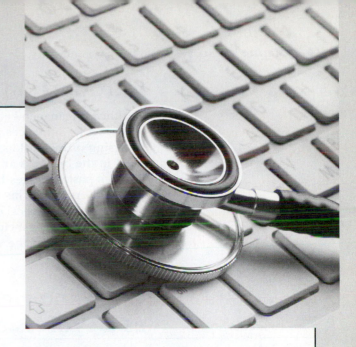

Get to know

advanced registered nurse practitioner (ARNP)
allergist
anesthesiologist
autocratic leadership style
cardiologist
democratic leadership style
dermatologist
emergency physician
family practice physician
gastroenterologist
general partnership
gerontologist
gynecologist
hematologist
hepatologist
infectious disease physician

internist
laissez-faire leader
licensed practical nurse (LPN)
licensed vocational nurse (LVN)
limited liability partnership
medical assistant (MA)
nephrologist
neurologist
nutritionist
obstetrician
oncologist
ophthalmologist
optometrist
orthopedist
otolaryngologist
pathologist
pediatrician

phlebotomist
physiatrist
physician assistant (PA)
podiatrist
primary care practice
professional corporation
psychiatrist
pulmonologist
radiologist
registered nurse (RN)
retail clinic
rheumatologist
sleep medicine physician
sole proprietorship
specialty care practice
surgeon
urologist

Case Study

Take note of the following scenario and answer the case study questions that appear at the end of this chapter.

Steve Magnus has recently begun taking classes in healthcare management. He believes he would like working in the medical field and he wonders if this is a field that will be challenging to him. Steve enjoys working closely with others and he has always had a strong desire to help people. He has found that he does well at organizing tasks and supervising others.

Introduction

Healthcare management is a field that attracts a diverse population of people. Although some medical practices prefer to hire medically trained managers, such as a person with a nursing or medical assisting background, other practices look for a manager who has skills in the business area. The healthcare field today is far different from what it was in decades past. Changes have occurred on many levels, from the way physicians are paid for their services by insurance companies to the scope of practice of the various medical personnel. The medical office manager needs to stay current with the changes in the field as they occur. This includes changes on the federal, state, and local levels, where laws passed may impact the way healthcare is delivered.

Choosing Healthcare Management as a Profession

The healthcare field attracts people who care about others. Healthcare is a diverse environment, with many different cultures and skill sets represented in its workforce. The vast majority of those who work in the healthcare field do so because they want to help others. Some are in clinical positions, such as nurses and medical assistants, who enjoy hands-on care of patients. Others, such as receptionists and billing office staff, enjoy a more administrative role. Those who choose to work in health administration, such as medical office managers (Figure ■ 1-1), may hold a role that is purely administrative, or one that includes some clinical work as well.

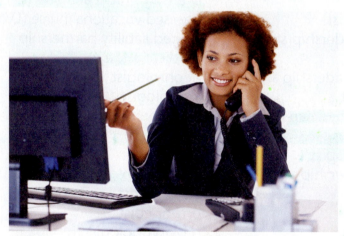

FIGURE ■ 1-1 The professional medical office manager.
Source: © Yuri Arcurs/Fotolia.com.

It is not uncommon for a medical office manager to come from a clinical or administrative background, such as a medical assistant, nurse, or a receptionist. In these cases, the manager typically works for a number of years in his or her clinical or administrative role before moving into the management arena. In years past, medical office managers were often clinically trained as nurses or medical assistants who aspired to be involved in the management of the medical practice. In some practices today, physicians prefer a clinically trained manager to oversee the clinical functions of the practice and to direct staff in their clinical care of patients.

In some cases, the medical office manager may be someone who has little or no healthcare experience, but has been to school to earn a degree in health administration or medical office management. These managers may have some background in management, and coupled with their education in the healthcare field, they are prepared to enter the medical office management workforce.

Many medical facilities and practices today look for a manager who has a background in both the clinical area and the administrative area. Typically, this is accomplished by a clinically trained person (nurse or medical assistant, for example) returning to school in order to obtain a degree in business or health administration. This often takes the form of a bachelor's or master's degree.

For medical office managers who come from a clinical background, the education may consist of an RN degree or a medical assisting certificate. For those who come from a business background, it is not uncommon to see managers with business or health administration degrees. Although having a clinical background is not required for a medical office manager to succeed in a managerial position, it is helpful to have some understanding of healthcare delivery, and the roles and responsibilities of the medical staff members. Many nonclinically trained medical office managers use other resources in order to address clinical questions or concerns. An example would be a patient who complains about the quality of care a physician has rendered. A nonmedically trained manager may ask another physician or clinical member of the staff to offer a clinical opinion on the quality of the care the patient received.

Critical Thinking 1.1 **?**

What are some examples of the skills and education required of a medical office manager? Suppose an individual has a background in nursing. How might that individual's skills and education help him in the role of a medical office manager?

Types of Medical Practice Ownership

Medical practices differ in a variety of ways, from the size of the practice to the type of specialties represented, to the management structure. Although many medical practices in past decades were **sole proprietorships**, that type of practice is not as common today, according to the IRS. Table ■ 1-1 compares the different types of medical practice ownership.

A sole proprietorship (Figure ■ 1-2) typically consists of a physician who practices alone, with a staff that may include nurses, medical assistants, and receptionists. Within this structure, a physician is solely responsible for the expenses incurred in his or her practice, including those associated with liability from negligence claims. One of the main drawbacks of the sole proprietorship is the lack of a partner physician to cover the practice's patients in the event the owner-physician is on vacation or unable to see patients for

sole proprietorship
physician who practices alone, with support staff, and is entirely responsible for all costs associated with maintaining his or her practice

TABLE ■ 1-1   Comparison of Medical Practice Ownership

Ownership Model	Description
Sole proprietorship	■ Physician practices alone. ■ All costs and liability risks associated with operating the practice are borne by the sole physician.
General partnership or group practice	■ Physicians partner to share in expenses of running the practice. ■ Physicians share liability risks with each other.
Limited liability partnership	■ Physicians partner and share in costs. ■ In this type of legal arrangement, physicians do not share liability risks.
Professional corporation	■ Legally, this business is an individual entity. ■ Physicians are shielded from liability risks. ■ Physicians are typically paid a salary, similar to an employee.
Retail clinic	■ Operates in a retail setting. ■ Typically see a small number of conditions—nothing urgent. ■ May operate with an ARNP, rather than a physician. ■ Most take cash only—no insurance billing offered.

FIGURE ■ **1-2** Sole proprietor physicians often practice in freestanding buildings.
Source: © Lbarn/Dreamstime.com.

a period of time. For those physicians who see patients both in the medical office as well as the hospital setting, operating within a sole proprietorship is time consuming in that one physician must care for the needs of patients in multiple settings.

A **general partnership**, or group practice (Figure ■ 1-3), is a type of medical practice with two or more physicians partnering to work together. In this structure, the physicians will typically share in the expenses of the medical practice, including the costs associated with staffing, building costs, and supplies. With a general partnership, each physician is open to liability should one of his or her partners be sued for medical malpractice. Within this type of practice structure, physicians will typically cover their partners' patients for vacations or extended leaves.

general partnership
a type of medical practice with more than one physician partnering to work together; also referred to as *group practice*

FIGURE ■ **1-3** In a group practice setting, physicians typically share reception staff and a common reception area.
Source: Andy Crawford © Dorling Kindersley.

For physicians who see patients in the hospital setting, a partnership or group practice design will often have one physician who sees all of the partners' patients at the hospital on any given day or week, rather than each individual physician seeing his or her own patients. This rotation of hospital coverage is not only time-saving for the physicians, it also provides better coverage of the appointments in the medical office. Physicians operating within a group practice will often see physician-partners' patients in the medical office setting as well. This is particularly helpful to patients who wish to be seen for an appointment soon, yet their own physician's schedule is fully booked.

A **limited liability partnership (LLP)** is a type of practice in which the physician partners have registered with their state in order to obtain limited liability for all of the partners. The limited liability pertains to the liability for debts, such as staffing, equipment, and building costs, but does not include sharing in the liability should one of the physician partners be sued for medical malpractice. This type of medical practice structure is typically set up in concert with legal counsel. From the patients' perspectives, a limited liability partnership does not look any different than a group practice. Within this partnership, physicians will cover for one another, just as in a group practice setting.

A **professional corporation** is a medical practice structure in which the physicians have filed paperwork with the state where the practice resides in order to obtain corporation status. As a corporation, the business is treated as its own entity, and taxes are filed on behalf of the corporation as if it were an individual. In a professional corporation, physicians are protected from liability should one or the other be sued for medical malpractice or in cases of fraud or contract dispute.

Many physicians today accept employment with larger healthcare organizations. In this type of structure, physicians are typically paid a salary and are contracted for the services they provide. As employees of the organization, physicians are not liable for the medical malpractice claims of their physician colleagues. In some of these settings, physicians are paid according to the services they provide. In other words, the more services they provide (or patients they see), the more money the physician may earn.

Physicians who are employed are often given paid vacation time, medical insurance, and disability coverage, similar to the benefits given to other employees. Physicians in these settings also will often have their medical malpractice insurance covered by the employer. Because malpractice insurance premiums may be costly, especially to a new physician or a physician in a high-risk specialty such as obstetrics or neurosurgery, this is one benefit that steers many new physicians to accept an employment contract.

Retail clinics are those settings where healthcare providers offer services in a retail setting (Figure ■ 1-4). These types of clinics may be found in retail pharmacies or department store chains. Typically, a provider operating in such a setting accepts a limited number of conditions or patients, and all care is cash based, with no insurance billing offered. The fees charged in these settings are typically lower than those charged in a traditional medical office setting. Most retail clinics are staffed with advance care practitioners, such as an advanced registered nurse practitioner (ARNP). Retail clinics offer quick, walk-up care, without an appointment necessary. Patients without health insurance may appreciate the quick access and lower fees, as well as the easy access to the retail pharmacy. The retail store finds this partnership with providers to be beneficial

limited liability partnership
type of practice where the physician partners have registered with their state in order to obtain limited liability for their partners

professional corporation
a medical practice structure in which the physicians have filed paperwork with the state where the practice resides in order to obtain corporation status

retail clinic
healthcare setting where providers offer services in a retail setting

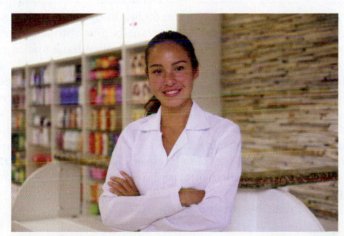

FIGURE ■ 1-4 Retail clinics are typically found in pharmacies or other retail locations.
Source: © Mangostock/Dreamstime.com.

because patients will commonly shop while waiting for their time with the healthcare provider, as well as fill prescriptions and purchase over-the-counter items in the retail location.

Patients who have health insurance are able to submit the receipt for the paid medical care to their insurance carrier for reimbursement. For those patients with high insurance copays, treatment at the retail clinic may cost less than what would be reimbursed by the insurance company. As an example, imagine a patient has a $50 copay that must be paid by the patient before costs for an individual medical visit are covered. If the cost of a visit to the retail clinic is $40, the patient in this situation will save money by going to the retail clinic instead of a traditional medical clinic setting.

> **Critical Thinking 1.2 ?**
>
> Why might a physician choose to practice in a limited liability partnership as opposed to a group practice? What are some of the advantages, as well as drawbacks, of operating a retail clinic?

Types of Healthcare Settings

Medical practices vary in size from small offices with a small number of physicians and support staff, to large practices with multiple physicians of varying specialties and a large number of support staff. In addition to the size of the practice, the location will also vary. Medical practices may be located in rural or urban settings or they may be located within a hospital setting.

primary care practice
practice where providers offer services that are primary care in nature

Primary care practices are those where the services provided are primary in nature. Physicians in these settings are typically family practice physicians, pediatricians, and internists. Services provided in this type of practice will vary, from physical exams and immunizations to minor surgical procedures that can be done in the ambulatory setting. Although patients may present to a primary care office with a variety of health concerns, the primary care provider may not treat all conditions. For example, a family practice physician will see patients with a condition such as high blood pressure, but if a patient presents with a condition that is more complicated, such as a need for cardiac surgery, the family practice physician will refer the patient to a specialist.

Types of Physicians

All physicians who are licensed to practice medicine in the United States must undergo a lengthy education process. Education of physicians begins with a 4-year undergraduate degree at a college or university. Most premedical students pursue undergraduate degrees in the sciences, such as biology, chemistry, or physics.

After obtaining a bachelor's degree, medical students then enter a medical school for an additional 4 years of education. After completing training in an accredited medical school, students earn the degree of MD (medical doctor) or DO (doctor of osteopathy). After obtaining this degree, physicians must then enter a residency program, which consists of 3 to 7 years of additional training. It is within their residency program that physicians choose their specialty. Some specialties require a longer residency than others. For example, family practice, internal medicine, and pediatric specialties require a residency of 3 years in length. General surgery specialty requires a residency of 5 years. The more specialized the field of medicine, the longer the residency period.

Some physicians choose to go into a medical field that is highly specialized, such as pediatric cardiology or adolescent psychiatry. For those fields, physicians will perform an additional 1 to 3 years of training after their residency. This additional training is referred to as a fellowship.

After completing all training for their desired field, physicians will then apply for a license to practice medicine in the state where they wish to practice. Many physicians also choose to become board certified. Board certification is an optional process physicians may pursue in order to indicate their proficiency in a field of medicine.

FAMILY PRACTICE PHYSICIANS

Family practice physicians treat patients of all ages, from newborns to geriatric patients. Some family practice physicians treat pregnant woman and deliver babies. Family practice physicians will often perform minor surgery in the medical office for conditions that require only local anesthetic. For more advanced surgical needs, the physician will refer the patient to a surgeon for treatment.

family practice physician
physician who treats patients of all ages for a variety of conditions

PEDIATRICIANS

Pediatricians limit their patients to children, typically up to the age of 16 to 18 years. Many pediatricians (Figure ■ 1-5) see patients from birth to adulthood, when the patient transitions to an adult care provider, such as a family practice provider or internist. Similar to adult patients, some pediatric patients may present to the pediatrician with a condition that requires the attention of a specialist. When this occurs, the pediatrician will refer the patient to the specialist for treatment of that particular condition, but will continue to see the patient for any other general health concerns.

pediatrician
physician who limits care to that of children

INTERNISTS

Internal medical providers, also referred to as **internists**, are those who treat adult patients, typically those over the age of 16 years (Figure ■ 1-6). Internists treat many of the same conditions and symptoms as those treated by family practice physicians. Because their practices are limited to adults, internists may see a larger proportion of elderly patients.

internist
physician who treats conditions in adult patients

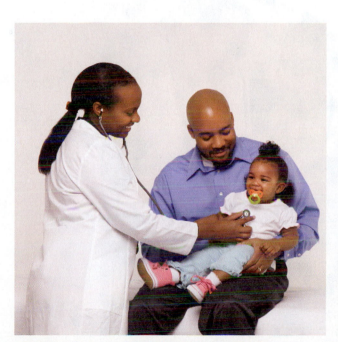

FIGURE ■ 1-5 A pediatrician treating a child.
Source: © lofoto/Dreamstime.com.

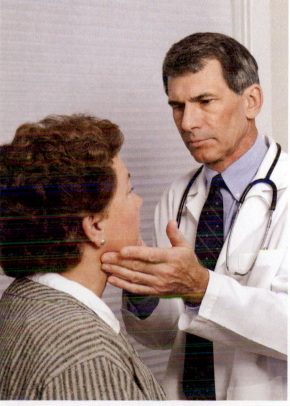

FIGURE ■ 1-6 An internist examines his patient.
Source: © Forestpath/Dreamstime.com.

Specialty Care Practices

specialty care practice
practice where providers offer care that is specialty related

Specialty care practices may exist apart from primary care, or specialists may practice in the same setting with primary care providers. Patients are typically referred to a specialist by their primary care provider when a condition warrants such a referral. This is done when the primary care provider feels the patient requires care that is somewhat beyond the scope of the primary care provider's training. In these situations, patients will see the specialist for a particular condition, while continuing to see their primary care physician for other general medical care. Some patients, especially those who have multiple healthcare conditions, see a large number of specialists, in addition to their primary care provider. In these cases, the primary care provider will typically coordinate the patient's care, keeping track of the various specialists the patient is seeing and the medications the patient may be taking for her or his health conditions.

ALLERGISTS

allergist
physician who treats allergic conditions

Allergists are physicians who treat allergic conditions, including food and environmental allergies. Patients may be referred to an allergist for allergies ranging from seasonal pollen allergies to sensitivity to foods or inhalants. The allergist may order skin or blood tests to determine the source of a patient's allergies, as well as medications to treat those conditions. Allergists will generally see patients of all ages. While some patients may see an allergist only a handful of times, patients with more severe allergies may see an allergist their entire life.

CARDIOLOGISTS

cardiologist
physician who treats conditions associated with the cardiovascular system

Cardiologists are physicians who treat conditions of the heart and cardiovascular system (Figure ■ 1-7). These conditions range from heart attacks to heart defects and irregularities of the heartbeat. Within the cardiology profession, cardiologists may be subspecialists and concentrate their practice solely on patients with arrhythmias or on those patients who have internal devices to regulate their heartbeat. Some cardiologists limit their practices to only adults, whereas others may specialize in cardiac conditions experienced by children.

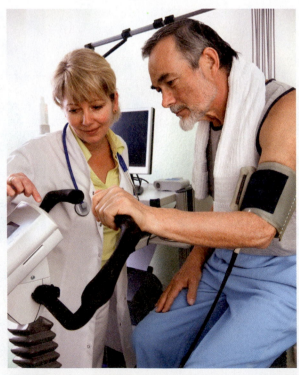

FIGURE ■ 1-7   Cardiologists focus on the patient's heart.
Source: © Alexraths/Dreamstime.com.

DERMATOLOGISTS

Dermatologists are physicians who treat disorders of the skin. As the largest organ in the body, the skin has a wide variety of conditions that may need to be treated. These range from rashes to viral conditions, such as warts, to skin cancer. Dermatologists will generally see patients of all ages. Some dermatologists specialize in certain conditions, whereas others will see a wide variety of patients.

dermatologist
physician who diagnoses and treats skin conditions

GASTROENTEROLOGISTS

Gastroenterologists are physicians who treat conditions of the esophagus, gallbladder, stomach, liver, pancreas, intestines, and rectum. These physicians treat patients with conditions such as ulcers, hepatitis, and inflammatory bowel disease. Within the gastroenterology profession, some physicians choose to focus on a particular condition, such as irritable bowel disease or hepatitis. Gastroenterologists are often referred to as GI physicians, where GI means *gastrointestinal*.

gastroenterologist
physician who specializes in the diagnosis and treatment of conditions associated with the digestive system

GERONTOLOGISTS

Gerontologists are physicians who specialize in conditions associated with aging. Patients seeking care from these physicians are typically elderly, and the conditions treated may be either physical or mental conditions. These physicians will often see patients in nursing homes or assisted living centers.

gerontologist
physician who specializes in the treatment of conditions associated with aging

GYNECOLOGISTS

Gynecologists treat women for female-related conditions, such as hormone imbalances or uterine disorders. These physicians offer preventive screening tests, such as Pap smears and breast exams, as well as surgeries to correct disorders of the female reproductive system. Some gynecologists also practice as obstetricians; obstetrics is the practice of treating pregnant women and delivering babies.

gynecologist
physician who diagnoses and treats conditions associated with the female anatomy

HEMATOLOGISTS

A **hematologist** is a physician who treats disorders of the blood. These physicians specialize in conditions ranging from leukemia to sickle cell anemia.

hematologist
physician who diagnoses and treats conditions of the blood

HEPATOLOGISTS

Hepatologists are physicians who specialize in the treatment of the liver. This physician is a subspecialist, because gastroenterologists also treat liver disorders. Hepatologists may specialize in one type of liver disorder, or they may concentrate on the treatment of liver transplant patients.

hepatologist
physician who diagnoses and treats conditions of the liver

INFECTIOUS DISEASE PHYSICIANS

Infectious disease physicians are those who specialize in the treatment of infectious diseases, such as *E. coli* or HIV. These specialists have special training in understanding how the body fights disease.

infectious disease physician
physician who specializes in the treatment of infectious disease

NEPHROLOGISTS

Nephrologists are physicians who specialize in the treatment of the kidneys. This physician may treat patients with a variety of conditions, such as diabetes or kidney failure. Nephrologists may be involved in kidney transplants or the treatment of kidney stones.

nephrologist
physician who specializes in the treatment of kidney disorders

NEUROLOGISTS

Neurologists are physicians who treat conditions associated with the nervous system. These may include seizure disorders or other conditions, such as stroke or dizziness.

neurologist
physician who specializes in the treatment of conditions associated with the nervous system

OBSTETRICIANS

Obstetricians are physicians who specialize in the treatment of pregnant women and the delivery of babies (Figure ■ 1-8). Physicians in this area typically treat both gynecology and obstetric patients. Obstetricians monitor women throughout pregnancy, diagnosing possible adverse conditions in the unborn fetus.

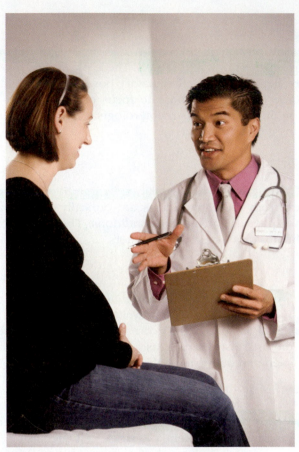

FIGURE ■ 1-8   Obstetricians see patients for pregnancy and delivery.
Source: © lofoto/Dreamstime.com.

ONCOLOGISTS

Oncologists are physicians who diagnose and treat conditions associated with cancer. Many oncologists specialize in certain types of cancers, such as bladder cancer or lung cancer. Other oncologists may practice general oncology, seeing patients with any cancerous condition.

OPHTHALMOLOGISTS AND OPTOMETRISTS

Ophthalmologists treat conditions associated with the eye. **Optometrists** are providers who specialize in treating some conditions of the eye and can perform routine eye exams and prescribe corrective lenses for patients. Ophthalmologists are able to perform eye surgery for conditions such as cataracts or glaucoma.

ORTHOPEDISTS

Orthopedists are physicians who specialize in the treatment of the bones and joints. These specialists treat conditions ranging from sprained ankles to the treatment of complex fractures. Orthopedists may specialize in the area of joint replacements, such as the knees or hips. Within the field of orthopedics, some physicians choose to focus on one part of the body, such as the hands or knees, whereas other orthopedists see a wide range of patients with orthopedic conditions.

OTOLARYNGOLOGISTS

Otolaryngologists are physicians who diagnose and treat conditions associated with the ears, nose, and throat. These physicians may perform surgical interventions such as removing the tonsils or installation of ear tubes. These physicians are commonly referred to as ENT, or ears, nose, and throat, physicians.

otolaryngologist
physician who specializes in the treatment of conditions associated with the ears, nose, and throat

PHYSIATRISTS

Physiatrists are physicians who diagnose and treat conditions associated with the musculoskeletal system. These physicians use treatments such as heat and cold therapy, massage, ultrasound, and electrical stimulation to treat pain, swelling, and dysfunction in the musculoskeletal system. Some physiatrists provide procedures, such as injections into the spine or joints, for patients with pain in those areas.

physiatrist
physician who specializes in the diagnosis of musculoskeletal conditions and their treatment by use of therapeutic means

PODIATRISTS

Podiatrists are physicians who treat patients for conditions associated with the feet (Figure ■ 1-9). These patients may present with conditions such as warts or ingrown toenails or for treatment of the feet due to other disease, such as diabetes.

podiatrist
physician who specializes in the treatment of the feet

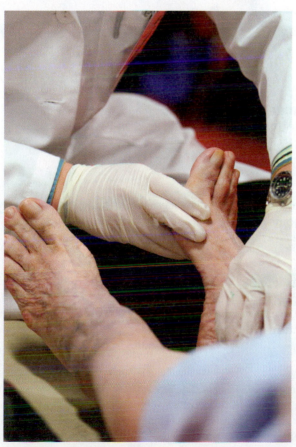

FIGURE ■ 1-9   Podiatrists focus on conditions of the feet.
Source: © Joregeantonio/Dreamstime.com.

psychiatrist
physician who specializes in the diagnosis and treatment of mental disorders

pulmonologist
physician who specializes in the diagnosis and treatment of lung conditions

radiologist
physician who specializes in the diagnosis and treatment of patients via the use of x-rays, magnetic resonance imaging, computed tomography scans, and radioactive materials

PSYCHIATRISTS

Psychiatrists are physicians who treat patients who suffer from mental and emotional disorders. These physicians see patients with conditions ranging from severe depression to personality disorders. Psychiatrists may treat their patients with counseling as well as medications.

PULMONOLOGISTS

Pulmonologists are physicians who treat patients for conditions associated with the lungs. These patients may have a short-term illness, such as pneumonia, or a chronic disease, such as emphysema or cystic fibrosis.

RADIOLOGISTS

Radiologists are physicians who specialize in the diagnosis and treatment of patients via the use of x-rays, magnetic resonance imaging (MRI), computed tomography (CT) scans, and radioactive materials (Figure ■ 1-10). Radiologists read the images taken by technicians in these areas and diagnose conditions seen on the images.

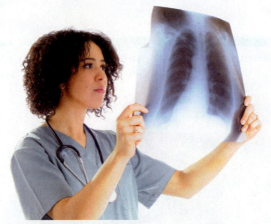

FIGURE ■ 1-10   Radiologists read x-ray images in order to diagnose patients.
Source: © Pichunter/Dreamstime.com.

RHEUMATOLOGISTS

Rheumatologists are physicians who diagnose and treat disorders related to the joints, such as arthritis or joint inflammation.

SLEEP MEDICINE PHYSICIANS

Sleep medicine physicians are often pulmonologists who specialize in the diagnosis and treatment of sleep disorders. These physicians will typically order sleep studies for patients who have conditions such as sleep apnea, a condition where the patient stops breathing at times during the sleep cycle.

SURGEONS

Surgeons are physicians who specialize in performing surgery. Most surgeons limit their practice to a certain portion of the body, such as the chest, brain, or reproductive system. Some surgeons may treat a variety of surgical conditions, whereas others may focus on a more specialized field, such as tumor removal for patients with cancer. Surgeons may see patients for procedures in the medical office, in an ambulatory surgery center (or outpatient center), or in the hospital with the patient as an inpatient.

rheumatologist
physician who specializes in the treatment of conditions associated with arthritis

sleep medicine physician
physician who specializes in treating conditions associated with sleep disorders

surgeon
physician who specializes in surgical interventions

UROLOGISTS

Urologists are physicians who specialize in treatment of the urinary system of both male and female patients. These physicians treat patients for conditions such as urinary tract infections or bladder retention.

urologist
physician who specializes in the treatment of conditions associated with the urinary system

Medical Practice Settings

Some physicians are located mainly in the hospital setting and others in the ambulatory setting (Figure ■ 1-11). Physicians who are typically found in the hospital setting are **emergency physicians**, those who have specialized training in emergency conditions; **pathologists**, physicians who supervise the clinical laboratory and the tests that are performed there; and **anesthesiologists**, physicians who perform and oversee anesthesia for surgical cases.

emergency physician
physician who has specialized training in emergency medicine

pathologist
physician who supervises the clinical laboratory and the tests performed there

anesthesiologist
physician who performs and oversees anesthesia for surgical cases

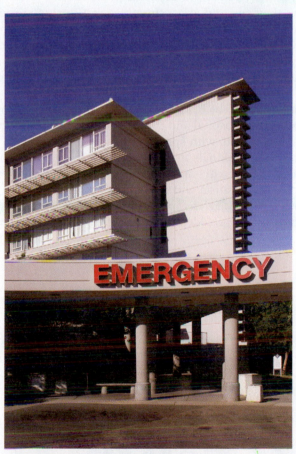

FIGURE ■ 1-11 Emergency room entrance at a hospital.
Source: © Photoroller/Dreamstime.com.

Critical Thinking 1.3 ?

When a patient is referred to a specialist by the primary care provider, how might this benefit the patient? If the patient asks the medical office manager why his primary care physician cannot address the condition for which the patient is being referred, what answer could the medical office manager provide?

Types of Healthcare Professionals

Aside from the physician, a number of other healthcare professionals are involved in the care of patients. The type of healthcare professional working in any given setting depends on the size and location of the facility, as well as the type of patients treated there. In most healthcare organizations, physicians work with a variety of allied healthcare professionals as well.

An **advanced registered nurse practitioner (ARNP)** is a healthcare professional who has pursued additional education beyond a nursing degree. In many states, an ARNP is allowed to treat his or her own panel of patients as a primary care provider. ARNPs are also used in conjunction with physicians in both the hospital and clinic settings and do not require direct supervision by the physician. In many cases, ARNPs have become specialized and will focus on a particular segment of the population for care, such as women's health, cardiology, or orthopedics. An ARNP is a registered nurse (RN) with a graduate degree in nursing.

Physician assistants (PAs) are healthcare providers who work under the direct supervision of a physician. In most states, these providers are able to prescribe medications for the patients they see and assist the physician during surgery. Physician assistants must complete an accredited physician assistant education program and maintain certification by receiving continued medical education every 2 years and becoming recertified every 6 years. Similar to the ARNP, a PA may work in a specialized setting, such as family practice, or cardiology, where he or she is assisting physicians in the care of patients.

A **nutritionist** is a healthcare professional who specializes in the field of nutrition. Nutritionists are found in the hospital and clinic settings, performing tasks such as designing specialized diets for patients with special needs or consulting on food allergy conditions. These healthcare professionals may also specialize in the dietary needs of certain populations, such as patients with diabetes or gastrointestinal problems. Nutritionists have received specialized education and degrees in nutrition.

A **registered nurse (RN)** (Figure ■ 1-12) may work in the hospital or clinic setting. These healthcare professionals provide direct patient care and may administer medications

advanced registered nurse practitioner (ARNP)
registered nurse who has pursued additional education beyond a nursing degree

physician assistant (PA)
healthcare provider who works under the supervision of a physician. In most states, PAs are able to prescribe medications and assist during surgeries

nutritionist
a healthcare professional who specializes in the field of nutrition

registered nurse (RN)
healthcare professional who provides direct patient care, including administering medications and treatments under a physician's orders

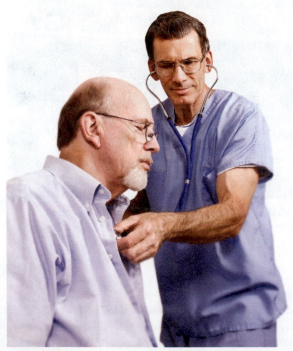

FIGURE ■ 1-12 Nurses carry out many tasks in the medical office.
Source: © Forestpath/Dreamstime.com.

and treatments to patients under a physician's orders. Registered nurses may not practice alone; they must be supervised by a physician. Educational requirements for registered nurses vary from a 2-year associate degree to a 4-year bachelor's degree.

A **licensed practical nurse (LPN)** or **licensed vocational nurse (LVN)** is a nurse who has had less training than an RN. The scope of practice of an LPN/LVN varies from one state to another; however, the scope is generally less than what an RN is able to provide. LPNs and LVNs have completed nursing programs that last about 1 year and are offered by vocational or technical schools or community colleges. In many healthcare settings, LPNs report directly to an RN.

A **medical assistant (MA)** is a healthcare professional who assists the physician or nurse, typically in the ambulatory clinic setting. MAs may have gone through an accredited program, or they may have been trained on the job. In many states, medical assistants must have achieved certification status in order to administer injections to patients. Medical assistants may perform such functions as EKGs and take vital signs, such as blood pressure, weight, and height. The scope of practice of the medical assistant has grown during the past decade, mainly due to the shortage of nurses. This trend is likely to continue in the future.

Phlebotomists are healthcare professionals trained to draw blood for physician-ordered laboratory work (Figure ■ 1-13). This training includes blood draws from a variety of veins in the body, as well as capillary draws, such as fingersticks. Phlebotomists are trained in educational programs that typically take no more than two to three courses to complete. This professional is also trained to perform EKGs and to process certain types of blood and urine lab samples.

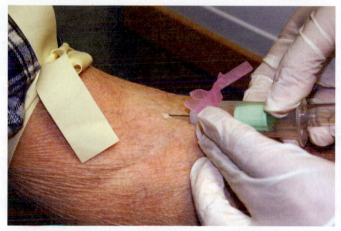

FIGURE ■ **1-13** Phlebotomists perform blood draws in the medical office.
Source: © Susy56/Dreamstime.com.

Aside from the clinical staff in the medical office setting, a variety of administrative staff work there as well. This staff consists of receptionists, billing and coding staff, and medical records personnel. The number and type of staff will depend on the setting and size of the practice or facility, as well as the specialization of the physicians.

licensed practical nurse (LPN)
nurse who has less training than an RN. The scope of practice for an LPN is generally more limited than that of an RN, and an LPN may be overseen by an RN

licensed vocational nurse (LVN)
nurse who has less training than an RN. The scope of practice is generally more limited than that of an RN

medical assistant (MA)
allied healthcare professional who assists the physician or nurse, typically in the ambulatory clinic setting

phlebotomist
healthcare professional trained to draw blood for physician-ordered laboratory work

Critical Thinking 1.4 ?

If a physician were to employ an ARNP in her practice, what might be the benefit over hiring a PA for the same position? Where would the medical practice manager look for information on the scope of practice for the ARNP or PA?

The Medical Office Manager

Medical office managers are responsible for managing the day-to-day functions of the medical practice. Healthcare is a business and, like any business, it needs proper management in order to run smoothly. The medical office manager may manage an entire facility or department, or may co-manage with other managers. The type and size of the medical facility dictates the management structure.

Larger facilities may have several assistant administrators who provide assistance to the top administrator or manager. In such an arrangement, each of the assistant managers may manage a particular department, such as cardiology or radiology. In smaller facilities, the medical office manager may control all functions, from management of staff to financial operations, such as payroll and billing.

In a group medical practice, the office administrator will typically work closely with the physicians on issues relating to strategic planning. The day-to-day functions, including personnel matters and patient flow are typically left to the medical office manager(s) to manage.

In some healthcare organizations, physicians practice both in the clinic and hospital settings. These organizations may employ a medical office manager who oversees the functions of the physicians both in the clinic and hospital environments. The medical office manager may work in a private office, whereas others may share space with other staff. Most medical office managers work long hours, and those who oversee more than one location will need to travel from one facility to another. Hours worked may depend on the hours the facility is open as well; some healthcare facilities are open 24 hours per day, 7 days per week. For the medical office manager who responds to urgent issues at any time of the day or night, this may involve disruptions to the manager's schedule after hours.

Educational requirements of the medical office manager vary from one organization to another. Some medical office managers have achieved a master's degree in health or business administration (MHA or MBA). Other managers may have been trained on the job and have very little formal education.

Critical Thinking 1.5 ?

What are some examples of urgent issues that a medical office manager may need to respond to after hours? What kind of resources would the medical office manager need to have available for responding to those after-hours emergencies?

TRAITS OF THE SUCCESSFUL MEDICAL OFFICE MANAGER

To be successful, a medical office manager must have excellent communication and organizational skills. These skills will be used with the staff, with the providers, and with the patients. The medical office manager must deal with a variety of issues, from hiring the best staff, to disciplinary actions, to dealing with angry patients. Proper communication, geared for the professional medical setting, is imperative.

Good organizational skills are also important for the medical office manager. Often, the medical office manager will need to juggle multiple things at the same time. The job can be stressful at times, and the manager must be able to remain calm. The staff in the medical office will look to their manager for direction in times of crisis. The medical office manager needs to be prepared for anything that may happen throughout the day. Being organized is the first step toward being properly prepared to handle any situation that may arise.

Because part of the job of managing the medical office is to understand and be involved in the budgeting process, the medical office manager should have a good grasp on how to read and understand financial reports and also be able to predict costs associated with supplies and staffing.

The medical office manager must possess good leadership skills. Leadership takes on one of three basic styles. In an **autocratic leadership style**, the leader makes all of the decisions for the group. Although this style works well in emergent situations where someone needs to take charge right away, working under such a management style on a regular basis can be overwhelming. The **democratic leadership style** is one in which the leader seeks input from others before making final decisions. Although this style does not work well in emergent situations, it is a successful style to use when attempting to reach a decision based on consensus of the group. Leaders who use this style will find that, in many cases, employees are more engaged in the work and loyal to the employer. The **laissez-faire leader** is one who sits back and allows others to make decisions. This style works well when the leader has a strong group, or one that has worked together as a team for a long time. Within such a group, the leader may have a high level of trust that the employees will make the right decision; therefore, the leader takes a more hands-off approach.

Successful managers know when to shift into the leadership style that is best for any particular situation. Staying within only one leadership style is a common reason for failure as a medical office manager. For example, managers who stay within the autocratic style all of the time will likely find that their staff members are not willing or able to make their own decisions.

> **autocratic leadership style**
> style where the leader makes all of the decisions for the group
>
> **democratic leadership style**
> style where the leader seeks input from others before making final decisions
>
> **laissez-faire leader**
> leader who sits back and allows others to make decisions within the group

Continuing Education Opportunities for the Medical Office Manager

As in all professions, medical office managers will find that continuing their education via conferences and seminars keeps them informed of changes occurring in their profession. Medical office managers may find continuing education opportunities in the form of seminars or conferences. For those managers working in specialty settings, continuing education opportunities may take the form of courses in managing that type of specialty practice.

Other medical office managers may choose to pursue certification with a professional organization, such as the Medical Group Management Association (MGMA) or the American College of Healthcare Executives (ACHE). These organizations offer continuing education courses on a variety of medical office management topics, as well as courses that prepare the medical office manager to sit for a national certification exam. Successful completion of the exam earns the manager the designation of Certified Medical Practice Executive (CMPE) with the MGMA, or Fellow (FACHE) with the ACHE. Achieving certification status is a sign that the manager has demonstrated a firm grasp of healthcare management knowledge.

Critical Thinking 1.6 ❓

Why might a medical office manager working with a cardiology group find it helpful to go to a conference focusing on the management of the cardiology practice? Where would the medical office manager look for information on conferences?

The Future of Healthcare Management

With the advancement of technology in healthcare, the services and procedures offered to patients will likely continue to change in the coming years. With the move toward evidence-based medicine, and the goal of lowering the costs associated with providing healthcare, more and more services will be provided in the ambulatory setting, rather than the hospital. With the passage of healthcare reform, more focus will be on containing costs, and the expectation is that reimbursement for healthcare providers will decrease. As the U.S. population grows older, more healthcare will be needed. The continued shortage of highly trained healthcare professionals will pose a further strain on the system as the aging population of healthcare workers begins to retire.

All of these areas create the need for highly trained medical office managers. The need for managers who can focus both on cost containment, as well as efficient management of the office flow, will cause this profession to become more in demand. The U.S. Department of Labor projects demand for healthcare managers to grow faster than the average rate of growth for jobs.

One of the biggest issues facing the future of healthcare is access. With more patients entering the healthcare system, access to care will become problematic, especially in areas where recruiting healthcare professionals is difficult. With reimbursements to healthcare providers continuing to decrease, the need for shorter appointment times, and more efficient processes for getting patients through the system will be required. All of these concerns must be balanced with the concern for quality and patient safety.

Critical Thinking 1.7 ?

Why does the aging of the American population pose the need for more healthcare in this country? If the physicians the medical office manager works with asked him to design a program to educate patients about preventive medicine, do you think this would help decrease the need for more acute care?

Case Study Questions

Refer to the case study presented at the beginning of this chapter to answer the following questions:

1. After reading about the various members of the healthcare team, and the characteristics of the medical office manager, how do you think someone like Steve would do in this job?

2. With Steve's desire to have a job that is challenging, do you believe this job would provide a challenge for him?

Chapter Review

Summary

- Medical office managers are skilled in the area of practice management. Though training and experience may differ, managers are responsible for a variety of tasks.

- Training and formal education may vary from one manager to another. Clinically trained managers are common, though medical offices managed by business-trained managers are just as well run.

- The medical practice manager must be able to remain calm and handle a variety of situations in the clinic setting. This includes keeping the staff and patients calm and directing people as needed during an emergency.

- The medical office manager must work with physicians, as well as various allied healthcare professionals. Each of these professionals plays an important part on the healthcare team.

- In overseeing the staff, the medical office manager must be comfortable dealing with performance and personality issues in the workplace. These issues must be addressed in a professional way, with the goal of coaching staff members to alter their behavior when needed.

- The advancement of technology in healthcare, the move toward evidence-based medicine, the lowering of costs associated with providing healthcare, the passage of healthcare reform, and the growing U.S. population will result in the need for more healthcare. All of these issues create the need for highly trained medical office managers.

Multiple Choice

Choose the letter that best answers each question or completes each statement.

1. Which of the following physicians focuses on treating conditions of the feet?
   a. Pulmonologist
   b. Radiologist
   c. Gerontologist
   d. Podiatrist

2. A physician who practices alone is practicing within which of the following?
   a. Sole proprietorship
   b. Limited liability corporation
   c. Group practice
   d. Group partnership

3. Which of the following is **not** a trait of a successful medical office manager?
   a. Appropriate communication skills
   b. Ability to multitask
   c. Ability to move into different leadership styles
   d. Leads only in an autocratic style

4. Which of the following is an example of the educational requirements for a medical office manager?
   a. Master's degree
   b. No formal training
   c. Trained on the job
   d. All of the above

5. Which of the following is a healthcare professional who is trained to draw blood per physician orders?
   a. Physician assistant
   b. Registered nurse
   c. Phlebotomist
   d. Receptionist

6. A physician who oversees the clinical laboratory and the tests that are performed there is a:
   a. pathologist.
   b. anesthesiologist.
   c. gastroenterologist.
   d. cardiologist.

7. A physician who diagnoses and treats conditions related to the stomach is a:
   a. pathologist.
   b. anesthesiologist.
   c. gastroenterologist.
   d. cardiologist.

8. Which of the following is a physician who diagnoses and treats conditions related to the heart and vascular system?
   a. Pathologist
   b. Anesthesiologist
   c. Gastroenterologist
   d. Cardiologist

9. A healthcare professional who specializes in designing dietary plans for patients is a:
   a. pathologist.
   b. nutritionist.
   c. medical assistant.
   d. registered nurse.

10. Which of the following is a physician who specializes in the treatment of the liver?
   a. Nephrologist
   b. Neurologist
   c. Obstetrician
   d. Hepatologist

True/False

Determine if each of the following statements is true or false.

_____ 1. The medical office manager must be able to switch management styles based on the situation.

_____ 2. A licensed practical nurse may also be called a licensed vocational nurse.

_____ 3. A retail clinic is one where physicians will see all kinds of patients, for any kind of condition.

_____ 4. Medical office managers may find continuing education opportunities that cater to the type or specialty of practice where they work.

_____ 5. A rheumatologist is a physician who specializes in surgical interventions.

_____ 6. A sole proprietorship is the most common type of practice setting today.

_____ 7. An internist is a physician who treats only patients under the age of 18.

_____ 8. One of the biggest issues facing the future of healthcare is access.

_____ 9. An optometrist treats more complicated surgical cases than an ophthalmologist can treat.

_____ 10. Some family practice physicians deliver babies.

Matching

Match each of the following medical specialists to the type of condition each treats.

a. urologist

b. anesthesiologist

c. obstetrician

d. orthopedist

e. pediatrician

f. gerontologist

g. dermatologist

h. gastroenterologist

i. neurologist

j. emergency physician

1. Patients who require emergency care

2. A 2-month-old infant who requires a well-child check

3. An 85-year-old patient who has a variety of conditions related to aging

4. A patient who requires anesthesia for a surgery

5. A patient who requires surgery for a severely broken leg

6. A patient who has a recurring rash on her forearm

7. A patient who has had trouble urinating

8. A patient who suffers from dizzy spells

9. A patient who has a stomach ulcer

10. A patient who is pregnant

Chapter Resources

American College of Healthcare Executives: www.ache.org

Medical Group Management Association: www.mgma.com

PEARSON myhealthprofessionskit™ ————————

Additional interactive resources for this chapter can be found at **www.myhealthprofessionskit. com.** Choose "Medical Assisting" from the discipline menu and then click on the book cover for *Medical Office Management.*

CHAPTER 2

Communications in the Medical Office

CHAPTER OUTLINE

- Verbal Communication
- Active Listening
- Written Communication
- Components of the Business Letter
- Sending Letters to Patients
- Proofreading
- Accepted Abbreviations
- Memos within the Office
- Mailing Written Communications

- Communicating with Patients via E-mail
- Managing Incoming Mail and Correspondence
- Reading Body Language
- Therapeutic Touch
- Communicating with Physicians
- Communicating with Peers and Direct Reports
- Communicating with Patients
- Communicating across Cultures

LEARNING OBJECTIVES

Upon completion of this chapter, you should be able to:

- Spell and define the key terms in this chapter.
- Describe the nuances of verbal communication.
- Define active listening.
- Discuss the importance of proper grammar and punctuation in written communication.
- Discuss how to compose a patient letter.
- List the reasons why letters are sent to patients.
- Proofread a business letter.
- List accepted healthcare abbreviations.
- Describe appropriate memo use within the medical office.
- Describe the process of mailing written communication.
- Classify mail, including its size and postage requirements.
- Develop a policy for incoming and outgoing e-mail to patients.
- Manage incoming mail and correspondence.

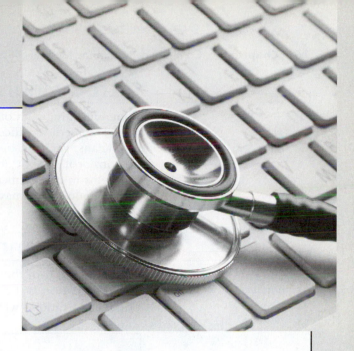

- Describe the interpretation of various forms of body language.
- Describe the purpose of therapeutic touch.
- Describe proper communication with physicians, coworkers, patients, and service providers.
- Discuss communication across different cultures.

KEY TERMS

active listening
body language
Daily Management System (DMS)

direct reports
huddles
Lean process

therapeutic touch
verbal communication
written communication

Case Study

Take note of the following scenario and answer the case study questions that appear at the end of this chapter.

Sylvia Lang is the medical office manager of a busy orthopedic practice. She manages 25 people in the office and she uses various methods to communicate with her team. There are times when Sylvia communicates with an individual member, and times when she needs to communicate with the entire group. One challenge Sylvia faces is that the staff members work varying schedules, and their lunch and break times overlap. There is no single time of the day when all members of the department are available to meet in person.

Introduction

Communicating with others is vital in any workplace, and the medical office is no exception. The medical office manager must be proficient at communicating with employees, physicians, vendors, insurance companies, and patients. This communication may be in person, or it may be in written form—either via a mailed letter or via electronic mail. Problems in communication may lead to misunderstandings and, in the healthcare field, miscommunication may lead to errors or injuries.

Verbal Communication

verbal communication
communication in spoken words

Communication in the medical office is vital to the proper care of the patient. **Verbal communication** is the use of spoken words. Proper communication follows the "five Cs of communication," which are outlined in Figure ■ 2-1.

Content – communication must include all pertinent facts needed to fully understand what is being said.
Concise – communication must get to the point and avoid including extra content that may confuse or distract the listener.
Clarity – communication must be clear, with words used that accurately convey the meaning.
Coherence – communication must be in a logical format.
Check – the communicator must ask for feedback in order to be sure the communication has been properly understood.

FIGURE ■ 2-1   The five Cs of communication.

Like any other form of communication in the medical office, verbal communication must be professional. The medical office manager must exhibit behavior and language that is the model for the employees in the office. Professional communication includes using proper grammar and speaking in a courteous and respectful manner.

Critical Thinking 2.1 ?

Imagine the medical office manager is in a conversation with the front desk receptionist. The two are joking and laughing about a patient who just left the office. How might this interaction be viewed by a patient who can witness this conversation from the waiting room?

When speaking with another person, it is important to note the mannerisms of the other party. If the other person is speaking slowly, it is important to match the tempo of his or her speech. It is also important to observe the facial expressions of the other person to whom you are speaking. In the event the person appears confused, this is the time to ask for feedback to determine the level of understanding.

By using the five Cs of communication, the medical office manager is able to get to the point in the most efficient manner, while still covering all important points in the conversation. Asking for feedback is especially important when discussing something that may be new information for the receiver (Figure ■ 2-2).

Follow these guidelines for effective verbal communication:

- Do not chew gum or eat food while speaking. This is distracting to the listener.
- Be sure to speak loud enough to be heard by the listener. If the conversation is personal in nature, move to a private area within the office.
- Pronounce all words correctly. This is especially important when speaking to a person who speaks English as a second language.
- Use a respectful tone of voice. Tone of voice conveys whether the speaker is frustrated or irritated, even if the words are professional.

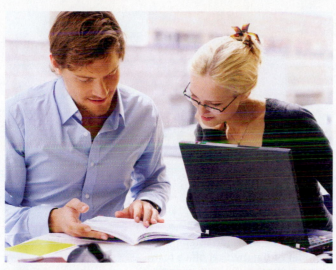

FIGURE ■ 2-2   The medical office manager will need to communicate with physicians and staff on a regular basis.
Source: © Yuri Arcurs.

- Match the tempo of speech to that of the listener. Speaking too fast or too slow may cause a misunderstanding.
- Speak directly to the person to whom the conversation is directed. Not doing so is a common mistake made when speaking via a language interpreter.
- Do not interrupt others when they are speaking. Interrupting another person conveys the message that what the person is saying is not important.
- Be sure to use terminology that is appropriate for the conversation. In particular, medical terminology may be confusing when speaking with patients.
- Be aware that any conversation made within patient hearing range must be compliant with the Health Insurance Portability and Accountability Act (HIPAA) in terms of keeping private information confidential.
- Ask for feedback to ensure the message was properly received.

Active Listening

Active listening requires more listening than talking. To actively listen to another person, one must pay complete attention to not only what is being verbally communicated, but also the body language and tone of voice of the speaker. This is especially important when dealing with an angry employee or patient. Active listening means not interrupting the speaker and using facial expressions, including direct eye contact, that convey concern for the person speaking (Figure ■ 2-3).

Active listening also means devoting all of one's attention to the speaker. This means minimizing distractions, or taking the speaker to a quiet, private location for the conversation. Distractions, such as telephone calls or other people interrupting the conversation, detract from the ability to truly listen to what the speaker is saying. These types of distractions may send the message to the speaker that the distraction is more important to the listener than what the speaker is saying.

active listening
listening as well as observing behaviors during a conversation

Critical Thinking 2.2 ?

What are some ways you can think of to minimize distractions when speaking with another person? How might the medical office manager prepare for a conversation ahead of time?

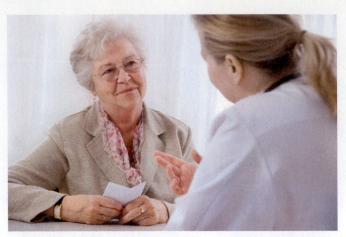

FIGURE ■ 2-3 Good listening skills are essential for every member of the medical office team.
Source: © Alexraths/Dreamstime.com.

Written Communication

written communication
communication in written form

Any **written communication** that comes out of the medical office is a direct reflection of the physicians and the entire practice. When typographical, grammatical, or punctuation errors occur, this sends the message that the office is disorganized or that no importance is placed on details.

The medical office manager will commonly send written communications to patients, employees, other medical facilities, or insurance companies. Just as with verbal communication, written communication should conform to the five Cs (see Figure ■ 2-1). Words used should be professional, yet not beyond the comprehension of the receiver.

In a professionally written letter, each paragraph should address one topic and contain between three and six sentences. Professional letters should contain the date the letter was written, the name and address of the person to whom the letter is being sent, a topic section, and the name and signature of the sender. See Figure ■ 2-4 for an example of a professional letter from a medical office manager.

USE OF THE SPELL CHECK FEATURE

Most computer software programs have built-in spell check ability. Use of a spell check program, however, is not a fail-safe way to verify that words are spelled correctly. Some words may be spelled correctly, but may not have been the word the physician wishes to use. For example, the words *two, to,* or *too* will all pass a spell check within the software program, but each of the words means something different, and it is important to know which one the physician meant to use. Also, many spelling verification programs are not able to check the spelling of many medical terms, creating the need for a medical dictionary to be on hand in the medical office. Though using the computer software to check spelling is handy, the staff member typing the document should also take the time to read the document to verify the spelling is correct before giving the document to the physician to sign.

GRAMMAR, SPELLING, AND PUNCTUATION USE

The English language contains many words that are commonly misspelled. This is especially true of many medical terms. When a staff member is unsure of the correct spelling of a medical term, she should refer to a comprehensive medical dictionary. See Table ■ 2-1 for a list of commonly misspelled words.

Margaret Thompson, MHA
Modern Way Family Practice
6645 Seaview Lane
Portage, MI 12345

July 18, 2013

Marty Prince, RN
Midway Pediatric Clinic
3901 Loyers Lane
Ft. Lauderdale, FL 12345

RE: Gail Smalls, CMA

Dear Marty:

I am writing to convey my experience in working with Gail Smalls, CMA in our family practice clinic. Gail worked for us for just over four years before relocating to the Ft. Lauderdale area. She worked mainly with our pediatric patients; administering vaccinations and updating health profiles.

Gail possesses an outstanding work ethic. In her four years with our practice, she was not late for her shifts, and she always arranged time off in advance. Gail is one to quickly volunteer to work on projects in the office and she was well liked by her co-workers.

I highly recommend Gail for employment with your clinic. She is a valuable asset to any practice, and her attention to detail and concern for patient comfort and safety will be valuable to the patients she works with.

Please let me know if you have any further questions.

Sincerely,

Margaret Thompson, MHA

FIGURE ■ 2-4 Sample letter from a medical office manager regarding an employee reference.

Proper grammar is essential when composing a letter in the medical office. Because the letter is a reflection of the physician, poor grammar will be seen as unprofessional. In the event the physician uses improper grammar in the document they have given a staff member to type, the staff member should correct the grammar prior to printing the document. It is important, however, for the intent of the letter to not be changed when correcting the grammar. See Table ■ 2-2 for a list of common grammatical errors.

TABLE ■ 2-1 Commonly Misspelled Words

acceptable	column	inoculate	privilege
accidentally	conscience	judgment	publicly
accommodate	conscientious	leisure	questionnaire
acquire	conscious	liaison	receive
a lot	discipline	maintenance	recommend
apparent	embarrass	maneuver	referred
believe	foreign	miniature	relevant
calendar	gauge	minuscule	schedule
category	guarantee	noticeable	threshold
cemetery	harass	occurrence	
changeable	height	personnel	
collectible	immediate	possession	

TABLE ■ 2-2 Common Grammatical Errors

Error	Example
Noun/verb mismatch	"The office feels that this is a bad idea." (The office cannot feel, only people can.)
Adjective used as an adverb	"I did good on that exam." (Should use "well" instead of "good."
Ending a sentence with a preposition.	"This is something we need to work on."
Run-on sentences.	"This lab is a dangerous place, patients shouldn't be back here." (Should use a semicolon instead of a comma.)
Mixing up words that sound alike but have different spellings and meanings.	their/there/they're or to/two/too

Proper punctuation is another vital area to focus on when composing written documentation. Table ■ 2-3 contains a description of common punctuation and the rules for their use.

WRITING NUMBERS IN CORRESPONDENCE

As a general rule, numbers from one to ten should be written out when writing letters, rather than written as numerals (i.e., 1 or 10). Numbers larger than ten are commonly written in their numerical form, such as 24 or 876. There are exceptions to this rule, some of which are very common in healthcare correspondence. When writing any unit of measurement, such as dosages of medications, or weight or height, those numbers should be in their numerical form. For example, "The patient is taking 5 milligrams of the medication every hour." Another exception is when writing the time of day, such as "1 p.m.," rather than "one p.m."

RULES FOR PLURALS OF MEDICAL TERMS

The rules to use for plurals of medical terms can create confusion in the medical office. See Table ■ 2-4 for the rules for plurals of medical terms.

TABLE ■ 2-3 Punctuation Rules

Period (.) – Used to indicate the end of a sentence and following some abbreviations.

Comma (,) – Used to separate words or phrases, to separate two independent clauses, and to set off elements that interrupt or add information in a sentence.

Semicolon (;) – Used to separate a long list of items in a series that contains commas and independent clauses.

Colon (:) – Used following a salutation in a business letter, before a list, before quotations, to separate independent clauses, and for numerical expressions of time.

Apostrophe (') – Used to indicate a missing or omitted letter from a word, and to indicate the possessive case of nouns.

Diagonal (/) – Used in some abbreviations (w/o), dates (6/1/07), and fractions (1/2).

Parentheses ( ) – Used to set off a part of a sentence that is not part of the main thought.

Quotation marks (" ") – Used to indicate a direct quote.

Ellipsis (...) – Used to indicate a thought that trails off, or to connect two parts of a quoted sentence when the middle section is left out (John was driving to work . . . before his medical appointment).

TABLE ■ 2-4   Punctuation Rules

Singular form ends in	Rule	Example
a	ae	bulla to bullae
ax	aces	thorax to thoraces
ex or ix	ices	appendix to appendices
on	a	ganglion to ganglia
um	a	ilium to ilia
us	i	mellitus to melliti
y	ies	idiosyncrasy to idiosyncrasies
nx	ges	phalanx to phalanges

Components of the Business Letter

All business letters contain the same basic components; this rule holds true with medical office correspondence as well. Each letter should begin with a letterhead. Most medical offices will have professionally printed letterhead stationary to use for composing letters. This letterhead typically consists of the clinic name and address, telephone and fax numbers, and e-mail address. The physicians' names will also typically be printed on the letterhead. The letterhead may contain a logo—some form of artwork that indicates the type of practice or other item of significance. For example, a pediatric office might have a logo that has something to do with children; a chiropractic office might have a logo that includes a spine.

Every correspondence composed in the medical office must contain the date. Normally, the date printed on the letter is the date the letter was written or dictated by the physician—even if the letter is not typed by the medical staff member until the next day. The date on professional correspondence is not abbreviated. Instead, it is written out; for example, May 26, 2013. The date is normally placed three lines down from the letterhead and is typically followed by an additional three to six lines before the inside address. The inside address includes the name, title, company name, and address of the person to whom the letter is intended. This information is typed at the left margin and should not include abbreviations, except for the name of the state (Figure ■ 2-5). See Table ■ 2-5 for the proper two-letter abbreviation for each state.

Marnie Logan, MD

1904 Wilbur Lake Road

Vincent, WA 99201

FIGURE ■ 2-5   Example of an inside address.

The salutation is the greeting that begins the business letter. It is typically placed two lines down from the inside address and should be the same name as the name in the inside address. If the medical staff member typing the letter is unsure of the spelling of a person's name, he or she should call to ask for the correct spelling. If the letter is a formal one, the salutation should include the person's proper name and courtesy title, such as "Dear Dr. Hagen." If the letter is informal, as in between two physicians who are well known to one another, the salutation may begin "Dear Shawn." See Table ■ 2-6 for guidelines on using courtesy titles.

TABLE ■ 2-5 Two-Letter Abbreviations for Each State (Source: USPS)

State	Abbreviation	State	Abbreviation
Alaska	AK	North Carolina	NC
Alabama	AL	North Dakota	ND
Arkansas	AR	Nebraska	NE
Arizona	AZ	New Hampshire	NH
California	CA	New Jersey	NJ
Colorado	CO	New Mexico	NM
Connecticut	CT	Nevada	NV
Delaware	DE	New York	NY
Florida	FL	Ohio	OH
Georgia	GA	Oklahoma	OK
Hawaii	HI	Oregon	OR
Iowa	IA	Pennsylvania	PA
Idaho	ID	Rhode Island	RI
Illinois	IL	South Carolina	SC
Indiana	IN	South Dakota	SD
Kansas	KS	Tennessee	TN
Kentucky	KY	Texas	TX
Louisiana	LA	Utah	UT
Massachusetts	MA	Virginia	VA
Maryland	MD	Vermont	VT
Maine	ME	Washington	WA
Michigan	MI	Wisconsin	WI
Missouri	MO	West Virginia	WV
Mississippi	MS	Wyoming	WY
Montana	MT		

The subject line in the letter is one line that describes the purpose of the letter. This should be placed two lines down from the salutation and should be preceded with "RE:" This indicates the letter is "regarding" whatever follows. For example, "RE: Sally Luder." The subject line will be the name of a patient if the letter is being written with regard to a patient.

The body of the letter is the main part of the business letter. It should be placed two lines down from the subject line. Each paragraph should address only one issue.

The closing of the letter is typically placed two lines down from the body of the letter. The most common closing in a business letter is "Sincerely" though the medical office will

TABLE ■ 2-6 Guidelines for Using Courtesy Titles

- *Mr.* is the appropriate title to use for men.
- Professional titles, such as *MD* or *DO*, are used in place of the courtesy title. Example: John Aye, MD, rather than Mr. John Aye.
- *Ms.* is used when the marital status of the woman is unknown, or if the woman prefers that title.
- *Mrs.* is used for a married woman.
- *Miss* is used for an unmarried woman who prefers that title, or for young girls. When in doubt, use *Ms.* rather than *Miss.*
- Two persons at the same address should be listed separately. Example: Mr. Joseph Paterniti and Ms. Beth Dorio.

use whatever closing the physician prefers. Four or five lines should be left between the closing and the typed name of the physician the letter is from, in order to leave room for the signature (Figure ■ 2-6).

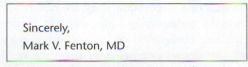

Sincerely,

Mark V. Fenton, MD

FIGURE ■ **2-6**   Example of a closing.

Reference initials are typically placed four to five lines down from the closing. The reference initials are of the physician who wrote the letter, followed by the medical professional who typed the letter. The physician's initials are in all caps, and the assistant's initials are in lowercase. The physician's and assistant's initials are separated by a diagonal (Figure ■ 2-7).

MVF/cmm

FIGURE ■ **2-7**   Example of reference initials.

Any information that may be enclosed with the letter should be indicated in the form of an enclosure notification. This should be placed two lines down from the reference initials and can be abbreviated as "ENC." or written out as "Enclosures." Following that, the number of items enclosed should follow in brackets. For example, if a letter has two enclosures, this may be indicated by "ENC. (2)" or "Enclosures (2)."

If the letter is to be copied to another party, this information may also be included on the letter. Typically, the notation "c:" is placed two lines down from the enclosure indication followed by the name of the person to whom the copy was sent. For example, if the letter is regarding Sally Luder, and the office is sending her a copy of the letter, the copy notation would state "c: Sally Luder."

On occasions, the business letter is more than one-page in length. When this happens, all subsequent pages must begin with the date of the letter, followed by the subject line. Pages after the first page do not require the letterhead, but should be printed on blank sheets that match the color and quality of the letterhead paper.

USE OF FONTS

Every word processing software program comes with a variety of fonts. These are the type styles of the lettering and are one way to set the letter off from others. Professional letters should be typed using a standard font, such as Times New Roman, Garamond, or Arial and should be typed in a 10- to 12-point font size. Use of a more informal font may be fun for certain patient letters or for making office informational sheets, but they are not considered appropriate for a professional business letter.

Sending Letters to Patients

Medical offices send written letters to patients for many reasons. Letters might be sent to all patients within a clinic to notify the patients of a change in an office policy or procedure. More personalized letters might be sent to patients to notify them of a need to schedule an appointment or to contact the patient regarding a missed appointment. Regardless of the reason, any letter sent to a patient should be professional, and attention to accuracy must be given to any correspondence that goes out of the office. A copy of any written correspondence sent to a patient should be filed in the patient's medical record.

Proofreading

Proofreading is the process of checking for spelling or content errors within the letter. As stated earlier in this chapter, most word processing software programs have the ability to check the spelling and grammar of a document. They are not, however, foolproof and are in no way a complete substitute for manually looking over the document to check for errors.

Today most documents are composed on a computer, which enables the medical professional to proofread the document prior to printing it. When proofreading, the medical professional should read slowly and check to be certain the letter flows and is not confusing to the reader. The letter should be read through a minimum of two times in order to catch all errors.

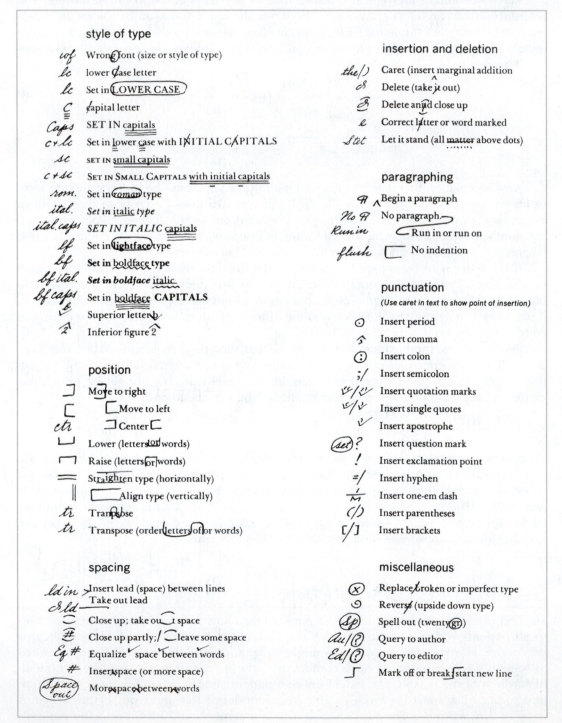

FIGURE ■ 2-8 Proofreader's marks.

Once the document has been through the proofreading process, it should be printed onto paper. At that time, it should be proofread one last time by the medical professional, who should determine if more or less space should be added between the lines in order to make the document more pleasant looking.

PROOFREADER'S MARKS

Proofreader's marks are used when one person is proofreading a document written by another person. These remarks are commonly used when proofreading printed documents. The proofreader uses a pen to make marks on the printed document to indicate the needed changes. See Figure ■ 2-8 for a list of proofreader's marks.

Accepted Abbreviations

When using abbreviations in the medical office, it is essential to use a list of accepted abbreviations. The Joint Commission publishes a list of standard accepted abbreviations that its members are required to use. Having a copy of this list in the medical office, and ensuring that all staff members are instructed to use *only* abbreviations from that list, will help to decrease any confusion or errors. If the medical professional is ever in doubt about an abbreviation, he or she should always err on the side of caution and spell the word out.

The Joint Commission has issued a list of medical abbreviations that its members should not use (Table ■ 2-7).

Memos within the Office

Memos are interoffice correspondence. They might be composed by the office manager as a way to relay a piece of information to the entire staff, or they might be composed by one staff member as a way to communicate something to another individual staff member.

Many medical offices have preprinted memo paper. Others may print memos from the computer. Memos are used to communicate with other members of the staff in a quick and efficient manner—they do not require postage, and the message is written so that the information it contains is communicated in a clear form.

TABLE ■ 2-7 Do-Not-Use List of Medical Abbreviations

Abbreviation	Potential Problem	Use Instead
U (unit)	Mistaken for "0" (zero), the number "4" (four) or "cc"	"unit"
IU (International Unit)	Mistaken for IV (intravenous) or the number 10 (ten)	"International Unit"
Q.D., QD, q.d., qd (daily) Q.O.D., QOD, q.o.d., qod (every other day)	Mistaken for each other. Period after the Q mistaken for "I" and the "O" is mistaken for "I" (q.i.d. is four times a day dosing)	"daily," "every other day"
Trailing zero (X.0 mg) Lack of leading zero (.X)	Decimal point is missed	X mg 0.X mg
MS	Can mean morphine sulfate or magnesium sulfate	"morphine sulfate" or "magnesium sulfate"
MSO4 and MgSO4	Confused for one another	

Source: The Joint Commission.

Most memos will begin with a "MEMO" or "MEMORANDUM" heading at the top of the page. Under the MEMO heading is a place for the date, a place to indicate to whom the memo is directed, and a place to indicate the author of the memo (Figure ■ 2-9).

MEMORANDUM:

Date:

To:

From:

FIGURE ■ 2-9   Sample interoffice memo.

Mailing Written Communications

Professional business letters should be mailed in business-size envelopes, also called size 10 envelopes. A standard size sheet of paper is 8 ½″ × 11″, and the standard size of a business envelope is 4 ⅛″ × 9 ½″. The size of a business envelope is designed to allow the business letter to easily fit inside when folded in thirds. The business letter should be folded from the bottom to approximately one-third of the letter length, and then folded again.

To properly address an envelope, the office address should appear in the upper left corner of the envelope. This is commonly preprinted on envelopes in the medical office, when supplies are purchased from a professional printer. The name and address of the recipient of the letter appears in the center of the envelope. The stamp or postage meter mark goes in the upper right corner of the envelope. If the piece of mail is of a personal nature, and the sender does not want anyone other than the recipient to open the mail, the sender should write "Personal" or "Confidential" on the envelope. This notation should be made to the left of the recipient's address.

USE OF WINDOW ENVELOPES

It is not uncommon for medical offices to use window envelopes for sending out certain types of mail. These are commonly used for mailing insurance billing forms or patient billing statements. When using window envelopes, it is important to check to be sure the address shows through the window prior to sealing the envelope.

POSTAGE METERS

Many medical clinics have postage meters, which are used to weigh the mail piece, determine the correct amount of postage required, and print the postage on the envelope or a label. These meters range in size and function from the most basic machine that will simply weigh the piece of mail and print the proper postage to meters that can accept a stack of mail, insert the pieces into envelopes, seal the envelopes, and affix the correct postage. Postage meters are extremely useful in the office. They cut down on wasted postage by taking the guesswork out of how much postage is needed, and they also eliminate the wasted time spent standing in line at a post office to purchase postage.

Resetting the Postage Meter

Most postage meters in the medical office are leased by the facility. The office will have a customer or user identification number assigned by the company that supplies the meter and the supplies (such as ink cartridges, ribbons, and labels). To refill the meter, the medical office can either place a credit card number on file with the postage meter company or send a check to the company prior to the need to refill. Either way, once the postage meter company has the funds in place to refill the meter, the medical professional calls the customer service number and keys in the user identification number, the clinic's password, the meter serial number from the postage meter, and the current access code from the meter. The postage meter will then be refilled automatically. Postage meters are generally designed to be very user friendly.

CLASSIFICATIONS OF MAIL, SIZE REQUIREMENTS, AND POSTAGE

The U.S. Postal Service (USPS) offers a variety of services for mailing letters and packages, depending on the urgency of the item and its value. Affixing a standard postage stamp ($0.44 as of 2012) to an envelope causes the letter to be sent via first-class mail. This service is available for items that weigh no more than 13 ounces. Mail weighing more than 13 ounces must be sent via Priority Mail.

Express Mail is the fastest service offered by the USPS. This service is guaranteed by the next day, 7 days per week.

Priority Mail is the second fastest service offered by the USPS, generally arriving 2 to 3 days after mailing to most destinations in the United States. The maximum weight for Priority Mail items is 70 pounds, and the maximum size of the package cannot exceed 108 inches when combining the length, width, and depth of the package. Priority Mail is available at a flat rate when using envelopes and packages provided by the USPS that clearly state "Flat Rate."

Media Mail, or Standard Mail, is the service offered by the USPS strictly for printed or bound materials, such as books or magazines, or for sound recordings, videotapes, CDs, and DVDs. This service is less expensive than the other services and it takes longer, usually 2 to 10 days, for the item to arrive at its destination. Media Mail cannot be used to send any type of advertising.

The USPS offers a variety of additional services for mailing a letter or package. Each option has an additional cost associated with it. Certified mail is a service that provides a mailing receipt and a record of the mailing at the local post office. This service is available only for First-Class and Priority Mail packages and letters. If the purchaser would like to receive a receipt once the package has been delivered, that service can be added.

Delivery confirmation is a service the USPS offers to allow the sender and receiver to track the piece of mail or package online by typing in the confirmation number. Registered mail offers the ability to purchase insurance up to $25,000 for the value of the item as well as track the item. It is only available for First-Class and Priority Mail packages and letters. A return receipt can also be added to this service. Insurance can be purchased for any item shipped via the USPS. The cost of the insurance is based on the declared value of the item.

BUYING POSTAGE ONLINE

The USPS allows consumers to purchase postage online. This can be done by any consumer who has a computer and a printer. This service is available for both domestic and international shipments and includes services such as insurance purchases (up to $500 value) and delivery confirmation.

RESTRICTED MATERIALS

The USPS prohibits the mailing of any item that is outwardly or of its own force dangerous or injurious to life, health, or property. In addition, most hazardous materials cannot be mailed. The USPS also places restrictions on other items—either prohibiting the items or allowing them to be mailed under certain circumstances. Such items include:

- Intoxicating liquors
- Firearms
- Knives or other sharp instruments

■ Odor-producing chemicals

■ Liquids and powders

■ Controlled substances.

If in doubt about the mailability of any item, the medical professional should call or stop by the post office to ask about the item in question.

OTHER DELIVERY OPTIONS

Packages and urgent letters may also be sent via Federal Express, United Parcel Service, or DHL. These services compete with the USPS in offering services such as tracking of packages, insurance, and proof of delivery.

Communicating with Patients via E-mail

Electronic mail, or e-mail, is an electronic way to communicate from one person to another via the use of a computer. Many offices use e-mail as a way to communicate with their patients. As a general rule, if a patient gives a medical office his or her e-mail address, then that person is considered to have given the office authorization to use it. However, it is very important to keep in mind that e-mail is far from a secure method of communication. E-mail addresses may be misspelled, causing the communication to be sent to an entirely different person. Also, employers have the right to view their employees' e-mail, causing e-mail sent to a patient at a work address to possibly be viewed by the employer. Because confidentiality is not guaranteed, it is a good policy to send only nonconfidential information to the patient via e-mail. This may include an appointment reminder or a happy birthday message.

Managing Incoming Mail and Correspondence

The receptionist is typically the person in charge of sorting and distributing the incoming mail in the medical office. Because many of the items received may be time sensitive, such as pathology reports or consultation letters, it is important to sort and distribute the incoming mail on a daily basis.

Each office should have a policy of how the mail is to be sorted and distributed, including a list of the items each staff member should receive. For example, the physician may receive all communications or reports regarding patients, any professional journals, and literature from professional organizations; the office manager may receive all bills to be paid by the office, advertisements for services or supplies, and samples from drug or supply companies; the billing office may receive all payments from insurance companies and patients and any correspondence from insurance companies; and the receptionist may receive the waiting room magazines.

In many offices, the person who sorts and distributes the mail is also asked to stamp the date received on each piece of mail. This allows the recipient to easily determine when the item was received within the office. Many medical offices have a policy requiring the person who sorts the mail to open each piece of mail. This allows the recipient to easily access the item inside the envelope without the need for a letter opener. Any items marked "Personal" or "Confidential," however, should not be opened.

Reading Body Language

Body language is nonverbal communication. It is the way people communicate with one another without using any words. When someone is bored, their body language may include yawning or slouching in the chair. When someone is scared, his facial expression will likely show widened eyes and raised eyebrows. When someone is in pain, her body language will show stiff or painful movements.

The medical office manager needs to maintain professional, respectful body language when interacting with others in the medical office. Remember that the actions of the medical office manager may be viewed by the patients, even when the conversation is between the manager and an employee. Whenever the medical office manager is in view of the patients in the facility, the manager must be poised and professional, with upright posture and attention to the way body language may be interpreted by others. Follow these tips on projecting a professional image during conversation:

body language
nonverbal communication, such as nodding the head, crossing the arms, and frowning

- Maintain eye contact. This conveys to the other party that the message is being heard.

- Do not cross the arms. Crossing the arms is interpreted as a closed position, rather than an open, relaxed image.

- Use a handshake when meeting someone. Whether the conversation is with a patient or a visitor to the medical office, beginning the conversation with a handshake is appropriate in a professional setting (Figure ■ 2-10).

- Smile as appropriate. In some conversations, smiling may not be appropriate, such as when hearing a complaint. It is also important to be sure the smile is genuine and does not appear manufactured or forced. Smiling should be seen as friendly and warm.

- Avoid frowning. Even if the speaker is relaying negative information, the medical office manager should not frown in response. Instead, she should have a look of concern on her face as she listens to the speaker.

- Maintain correct posture. When standing, stand up straight. When sitting, sit up straight. Slouching or leaning against a wall or desk portrays a less professional image.

- Maintain proper comfort zone distance. In the American culture, professional distance is about one arm's length from one person to the other (Figure ■ 2-11). Less distance than that may cause the speaker to be uncomfortable. Further distance than that sends the message that the medical office manager does not want to be too close.

- Be aware that how the manager dresses sends a nonverbal message to those around him. When the medical office manager dresses in professional office attire, and maintains proper grooming and hygiene, the message is sent that he cares about his appearance and does not wish to offend those around him.

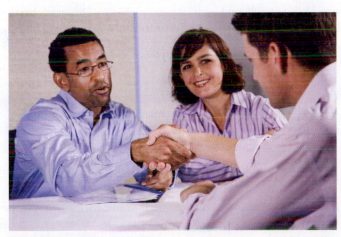

FIGURE ■ 2-10   Shaking hands is a common custom in the United States.
Source: © Goldenkb/Dreamstime.com.

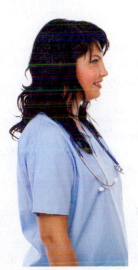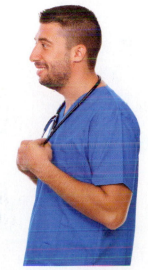

FIGURE ■ 2-11   In the medical setting, professional distance between two people is approximately one arm's length.
Source: © Justmeyo/Dreamstime.com.

Therapeutic Touch

therapeutic touch
use of touch to convey concern and compassion for another

The use of **therapeutic touch** is important when communicating with others in the medical office. Therapeutic touch is the use of touch to convey concern. An example would be a manager listening to a patient share frustration about his inability to pay a medical bill. If the patient becomes emotional, it is appropriate for the medical office manager to place her hand on the arm or shoulder of the patient. This touch conveys caring and concern (Figure ■ 2-12).

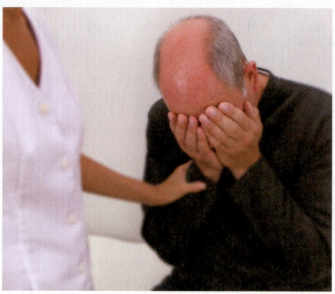

FIGURE ■ **2-12** When distressed, many patients appreciate a comforting touch on the hand or arm.
Source: © Nikki Zalewski.

In some cases, the use of therapeutic touch may not be appropriate. This may be the case with patients who have a history of abuse or who are extremely resistant to being touched by another.

THERAPEUTIC COMMUNICATION

Like therapeutic touch, therapeutic communication seeks to elicit some form of response from the patient, typically a calming or soothing approach. Many conversations that take place in the medical office are stressful to the patient or the employees. When these conversations occur, the medical office manager should employ therapeutic communication techniques. In practice, these techniques couple compassionate conversation and active listening skills with the use of words and a tone of voice that calm or soothe the patient or employee. Gestures and facial expressions are very important in a therapeutic conversation. The medical office manager must project compassion and concern, and those feelings must be perceived as sincere.

Therapeutic conversations also involve watching for body language and gestures from the patient or employee that may give additional information about how the person is feeling. As an example, a patient who has a furrowed brow is demonstrating irritation or concern. As the conversation proceeds, the medical office manager should watch those expressions to see when they lessen, indicating the patient has calmed.

Communicating with Physicians

The medical office manager will often be on a first-name basis with the physicians in the office. Even when this is the case, it is important to refer to the physician by her formal title when speaking in front of patients. As an example, if Sara, the medical office manager, is speaking with Dr. Rhonda Durant in the privacy of the physician's lounge, Sara may refer to the physician as "Rhonda." When the same two people are speaking within hearing range of patients, Sara should refer to the physician as "Dr. Durant." This conveys a message to the patient that the physician is a person of authority and the office manager is showing respect to the physician by using the formal title in this venue.

The relationship between the medical office manager and the physicians will differ slightly, depending on the type of practice. In some medical practices, the medical office manager reports to the physicians. In other settings, the manager may report directly to the organization and may have an equal footing with the physicians he works with. In either case, the medical office manager will need to have time set aside to speak with physicians in the practice.

Physicians are often very busy seeing patients when they are in the medical office. For this reason, medical office managers and physicians often set time aside to meet to discuss the needs of the practice. This may be done in a department meeting, with all physicians and the manager present to discuss any concerns. In some practices, it is common for one physician to be selected as a leader for the other physicians. In such a case, the manager may meet with all physicians once a month or so, and with the physician-leader more often.

The medical office manager and the office physician must maintain a professional relationship. Conversations between these parties must be professional, especially when within hearing range of patients or the staff.

Critical Thinking 2.5 ?

How might the patient view the physician differently if she overheard the office manager refer to the physician by his first name? Why might this be a problem?

Critical Thinking 2.6 ?

Imagine that a patient overhears a physician and the office manager in a heated discussion in the office. How might that affect the patient's view of the physician or the office? What would be a better venue for this physician and office manager to hold their conversation?

Communicating with Peers and Direct Reports

Peers to the medical office manager are other managers at the same management level, as well as physicians in some practices. The medical office manager may work in a facility where each department is managed by a different manager or within a facility where one manager oversees all departments.

direct reports
employee who reports directly to a particular manager

Direct reports are employees who report directly to the medical office manager. In a smaller practice, all employees may report directly to the medical office manager. In a larger facility, front-line staff may report to a supervisor, with the supervisors then reporting directly to the medical office manager.

To maintain proper flow of information in the medical office, the manager should have frequent conversations with those who work in the office. This can be done in a variety of ways. One common tool is the use of staff meetings (Figure ■ 2-13). These meetings may be held weekly, monthly, or even quarterly, depending on the needs of the practice. Staff meetings may be attended by just the employed staff in the medical office, or they may also include the physicians in the practice. In some practices, a department meeting is held with all staff and physicians and a separate meeting is held for just the physicians.

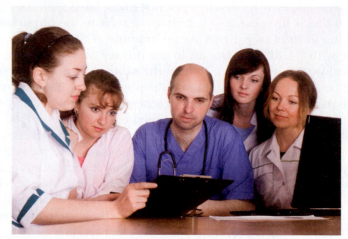

FIGURE ■ 2-13 A medical office staff meeting.
Source: © Aletia/Dreastime.com.

Another method of communicating with the staff is through one-on-one meetings between the manager and the staff member. One-on-one conversations may be used for formal performance evaluations (see Chapter 4 for information on employee evaluations) or in a more informal setting. When an employee is new, or undergoing a performance concern, the manager will want to meet with the employee more frequently (Figure ■ 2-14).

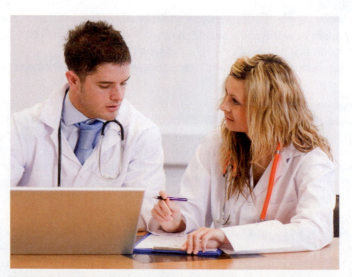

FIGURE ■ 2-14 Managers should meet in private with employees when the conversation may be personal.
Source: © Wavebreakmediamicro/Dreamstime.com.

When a conversation is about performance concerns, the medical office manager must have the conversation in a private location. This is done to maintain the privacy of the employee as well as to encourage open conversation. For example, the employee may not feel free to share the reason for his performance drop in front of his coworkers.

Many offices today hold daily meetings in the form of **huddles**. These are typically very short, ad hoc meetings, held in a central location, where information pertinent to the day's work will be shared. Huddles are an excellent way to communicate information quickly to everyone in the office. See Figure ■ 2-15 for an example agenda for a department huddle.

huddles
quick meetings in the medical office, most often done daily to share the important information for that day

---

Department Huddle Agenda

- Doctors who are seeing patients today and the medical assistant with whom they are working

- Exam rooms being used by doctors today

- Openings where patients may be seen if they call for an appointment today

- Any concerns about equipment that may be needed today

- Any concerns about interpreters needed for patients today

- Statistics for the practice, including number of prescriptions filled, patient satisfaction rating, staff satisfaction rating, telephone statistics for yesterday, number of patients seen, and number of no show patients

- Sharing of any patient compliments or complaints from yesterday

FIGURE ■ 2-15 Sample agenda for department huddle.

Huddles are commonly used in forward-thinking medical practices today as part of a **Lean process**. Lean processes were developed by the Toyota Manufacturing Corporation. Toyota has used Lean techniques to remove the unneeded steps from its manufacturing process, resulting in a more efficient, less costly system. Boeing has also adopted Lean thinking for its manufacturing processes. Healthcare leaders around the world have realized that the use of Lean thinking can benefit the way healthcare is managed and delivered. A large number of books are available on the use of Lean concepts in healthcare. See the end-of-chapter resources for a partial list.

Lean process
modeled after the Toyota Production System; a tool used to streamline and standardize processes

The Lean process also includes the use of a **Daily Management System (DMS)**, a communication tool used to relay important information about the practice to those who work there. Examples include statistics for the practice, including the number of prescriptions filled, patient satisfaction rating, staff satisfaction rating, telephone statistics for yesterday, the number of patients seen, or the number of no-show patients.

Daily Management System (DMS)
a Lean concept used to share information with staff on a daily basis

Any goals that management is working on with regard to patient satisfaction, productivity, or availability of appointments may be shared on the DMS board. Practices that use a DMS will often have a dedicated area within the practice where the information is easily seen and updated. This may be a bulletin board or a dry erase board and it may be located in the employee lounge or break room. In some practices, the DMS board is located where patients can view the information (Figure ■ 2-16). In these facilities, it is thought that by being transparent about what they are working toward, the staff will be more attentive to the stated goals.

When a medical office manager meets with her peers and direct reports, it is important to ensure that the lines of communication are open and flowing freely. The goal should be to manage the office in a more proactive, rather than reactive, form. By being aware of potential problems or concerns before they arise, the medical office manager is better poised to address the issues. Frequent communication with others in the medical office is the key to this goal.

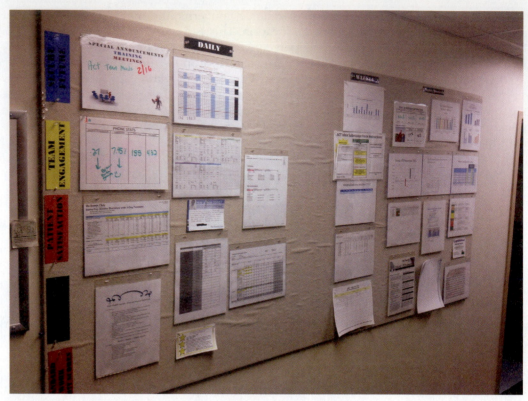

FIGURE ■ 2-16   A DMS board in a medical office.
Source: Christine Malone.

Critical Thinking 2.7 ?

How might the use of a DMS board help the medical office manager keep his staff on track toward office goals? How do you think tracking progression toward office goals affects employee engagement in the department?

Communicating with Patients

The medical office manager will commonly need to communicate with patients. Occasionally, this is done when the patient seeks out the manager to let them know of outstanding service or quality received. More commonly, it is a complaint about service or quality that causes the patient to contact the medical office manager (Figure ■ 2-17).

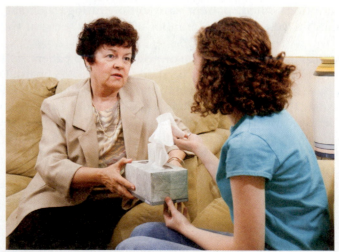

FIGURE ■ 2-17   The medical office manager will need to calm upset patients.
Source: © Lisa F. Young.

When meeting with the patient in person, the medical office manager should follow the guidelines presented in the Verbal Communication section earlier in this chapter. If the patient is upset, it is important to remove the patient to a private area. This is done not only for the privacy of the patient making the complaint, but also to avoid upsetting other patients and staff in the office. Most patients remain calm when they are faced with a calm, professional presence. The medical office manager must use open body language and affect an apologetic tone. Even though the medical office manager has not likely done anything personally to create the patient's distress, the manager is responsible for all that goes on within the facility. The manager must take that responsibility to heart and apologize when the patient is upset. An apology may be tendered without making it sound as if the manager was personally responsible. As an example, if patient states she is upset about a lengthy wait time for her appointment, the medical office manager could respond with, "Mrs. Jones, I am sorry you had to wait for your appointment. I can see that you are frustrated. My staff tells me that it will be another 15 minutes before Dr. Hagen is ready to see you. Can I get you something to make your wait more comfortable? Perhaps a cup of coffee?"

Remember that people who are upset do not want to hear excuses as to why a situation occurred. This merely tends to escalate the situation. As an example, if the medical office manager in the above situation responded to the patient by saying, "Mrs. Jones, I know you have had to wait, but you have to understand that we are short-staffed today with a medical assistant who called out sick. Dr. Hagen had a patient earlier this afternoon who had a very complicated case and he ran over his appointment time. We are sorry, but this is the way things happen in healthcare." In the second example, the patient is not likely to be sympathetic to the absence of a staff member, and the fact that another patient's appointment ran longer than expected simply tells the angry patient that her care is not as important as that of the other patient.

In keeping in line with HIPAA law, the medical office manager must ensure that conversations with patients are held in private locations, out of the hearing range of other patients and staff members. The following is a list of special situations regarding communication with patients in the medical office:

- Many patients who seek care in a healthcare facility are also employed in that facility. When the patient is also a coworker, the medical office manager must remain professional in the conversation with the patient. The manager must remember that when the person is in the office as a patient, he should be treated as any other patient. When that person is there as an employee, any mention of the conversation held while there as a patient is to be avoided.

- Many medical office managers work and live within the same community. When this is the case, sometimes the manager is faced with a patient who is also a neighbor. It is important for the manager to treat the patient as any other patient, and not to mention the conversation when she sees the neighbor in a social setting.

- Occasionally a family member or friend of the medical office manager may come into the facility for care. The American Medical Association discourages medical professionals from taking care of their own family members because it is thought to be difficult to remain unbiased in such a setting. The same may be true of the medical office manager. In some cases, the manager may need to defer the conversation to a peer or to a physician.

When dealing with patients who are upset about their care in the medical office, the medical office manager may need to perform some form of service recovery. This is done in the form of giving something to the patient to accommodate him for his inconvenience. In some cases, service recovery may take the form of financial considerations, when the office manager instructs the physician to treat the patient for no charge that day. In other cases, the medical office manager may give the patient a gift card for coffee or groceries to apologize for the inconvenience suffered.

Communicating with patients may mean using interpreters when the patient has a hearing impairment or speaks a language other than English (Figure ■ 2-18). When working with an interpreter, the manager must speak directly to the patient, even though the communication is going through the interpreter.

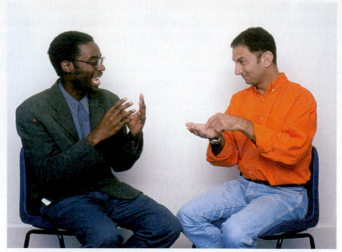

FIGURE ■ 2-18   Patients may need to communicate using an interpreter.
Source: Dylan Malone/Pearson Education.

Medical office managers will occasionally need to communicate with patients in written form. This may be the case when the need arises to send a letter to the patient on behalf of the clinic. See the guidelines in the Written Communication section earlier in this chapter for more on sending written correspondence to patients.

The telephone is often used for communicating with patients. Without visual representation, it is not possible to observe body language when speaking with someone over the telephone. See Chapter 5 for detailed information on speaking with patients via the telephone.

DEALING WITH DIFFICULT PATIENTS OR EMPLOYEES

Working with unhappy or disgruntled patients is a task that often falls to the medical office manager. Often, these patients have already spoken with another member of the healthcare team and, when their concerns are not addressed satisfactorily, the manager is called in.

The most important part of working with an unhappy patient is to remember that the patient is not irritated at the manager or employee. Rather than take the patient's irritation personally, the medical office manager must remain calm and stay focused on helping the patient to address the concern at hand. By allowing the patient to express his or her concerns, the manager demonstrates that he is compassionate and will hear out the complaint. Often, the patient simply wishes to have his concerns heard and no additional action is needed.

If the manager feels the situation needs further action, one way to find out what the patient wants is to ask. The manager may assume the patient wants something other than what it is the patient actually desires. By asking the patient, there is less room for confusion, and an amicable agreement or arrangement may be reached faster. Any conversation with an upset patient should be held in a private location, away from other patients or employees. In the event the manager feels the upset patient may pose a security risk, appropriate security should be called to intervene.

When an employee is upset and acting out in the medical office, the medical office manager will need to isolate that employee quickly. Allowing the employee to discuss his or her concerns in a private environment will often relieve the situation. If it does not, the employee may be sent home for the remainder of the day in order to get the tension out of the office. It is the medical office manager's responsibility to keep the office environment calm and free from patients or employees who are causing stress for others.

WORKING WITH DIFFERENT PERSONALITY STYLES

The medical office is as diverse an environment as any other workplace. People from various cultures and backgrounds will all work together to care for the patients seen. With many different personality styles, the medical office manager will need to keep the staff focused on a common goal or purpose. Proper training and clear expectations also assist the manager in assuring that different personality styles will work well together. In the event that differing personality styles cause conflicts in the work group, the medical office manager might put together a team-building event. These events may be driven by the company's human resource department, or they may be led by the office manager. A team-building event typically consists of a moderator encouraging everyone on the team to share their thoughts on how to work well together as a team. Questions include:

- How do the team members prefer to let each other know when they need assistance?
- How do the team members wish to be recognized for a job well done?
- How often do the team members want to receive communication about company initiatives?
- How do the team members want to receive communications?
- What are the team members' expectations for their manager?
- What are the manager's expectations for the team members?

Many personality style tests are available. As part of a team-building event, the medical office manager may wish to incorporate one of these tests so that all members of the team are aware of their personality style and how those styles interact with others.

Communicating Across Cultures

Medical office managers must realize that people from different cultures may have different styles of communicating. Gestures are a case in point. Although a gesture such as the "thumbs-up" signal may mean something is good in the United States, the same gesture in Iran and Iraq is considered obscene. When dealing with people from other cultures, the manager must understand how gestures may be interpreted differently and should strive to avoid them altogether. This is also important when it comes to using slang phrases. See Table ■ 2-8 for a list of slang phrases that may mean something different to people from outside the United States.

In the American culture, direct eye contact is seen as a sign of trustworthiness and honesty, and maintaining direct eye contact is preferred; however, in many Asian countries, direct eye contact is a sign of disrespect. Within some cultures, one member of the family may act as the speaker for others. As an example, in many Middle Eastern cultures, the man of the family speaks for his wife as well as his children. In some Asian countries, it is the eldest male member of the family who speaks for his younger relatives.

TABLE ■ 2-8 Slang Phrases and Their Meanings

Slang Phrase	American Meaning
Take the bull by the horns.	Take charge of the situation.
You can't get blood from squeezing a turnip.	You can't get money from someone who has none.
You need to get some shut-eye.	You need to get some sleep.
There is not enough meat on her bones.	She is too skinny.
We will farm out the medical transcription task.	We will hire someone outside the company to perform the medical transcription task.

Understanding how people from other cultures prefer to be addressed is important for all members of the healthcare team. Seniors often prefer to be called by their proper title (e.g., Mrs. Smith) rather than their first name (e.g., Sarah). This cultural preference is most common when being addressed by someone much younger. Because most cultures are very diverse today, the medical office will host patients, staff, and physicians from all over the world. For this reason, a good understanding of communication across cultures is important for all members of the healthcare team.

Case Study Questions

Refer to the case study presented at the beginning of this chapter to answer the following questions:

1. What methods of communication would work best for Sylvia to communicate with her team?
2. How can Sylvia make sure her communications are being understood by her group?

Chapter Review

Summary

- Verbal communication is the spoken form of communication. Verbal communication is used in the medical office by the medical office manager, other staff, physicians, and patients.

- Active listening involves noticing the body language of the speaker, as well as use of direct eye contact and avoiding distractions when listening.

- Written communication reflects on the entire office and must therefore be professional and free from errors. The use of spell checking and grammar checking software, as well as a manual proofread, is important before sending written documents out of the office.

- Medical offices often need to send letters to patients. These may include notices about laboratory findings or a simple letter to welcome the new patient to the practice.

- The practice of proofreading is done to be certain typographical, punctuation, and grammatical errors do not go unchecked. A list of symbols and notations is commonly used for the purpose of proofreading a document.

- Because some healthcare terms are lengthy, many are abbreviated to initials or shorter versions of the medical term. During the past several years, mistakes have been made due to misinterpretation of some of these abbreviations. To avoid these mistakes in the future, The Joint Commission has published a list of medical terms that should not be abbreviated.

- Memos are commonly used in the medical office to alert members of the staff to items of interest or importance.

- When mailing correspondence from the medical office, staff must be aware of what types of items are not legal to mail. Staff must also be aware of the costs associated with the various mailing methods available.

- Incoming mail should be managed by someone in the medical office. This task often falls to the receptionist. Managing the incoming mail includes sorting mail and giving the appropriate items to the appropriate people in the medical office.

- Body language is nonverbal communication in the form of gestures or facial expressions. Body language may be a more accurate portrayal of what a person is feeling and thinking.

- The use of therapeutic touch is appropriate on many occasions in the medical office. It can be used to comfort a distressed person. There are times, however, when touch may be considered inappropriate.

- The medical office manager's success in the office hinges on proper communications with those around her. This is important in dealing with physicians, coworkers, and patients alike. Professionalism in communication is key to success as a medical office manager.

- People from different cultures may require a different method or technique for communication. Gestures and phrases may be interpreted differently and, therefore, should be avoided if possible.

Multiple Choice

Choose the letter that best answers each question or completes each statement.

1. Which of the following is one of the five Cs of communication?
    a. Complicated
    b. Confusing
    c. Concise
    d. Cluttered

2. Which of the following is an example of the use of active listening?
    a. Watching the speaker's facial expressions as he talks
    b. Talking on the telephone while checking in patients
    c. Leading a departmental staff meeting
    d. Touching the patient in a comforting way

3. Which of the following is an example of body language?
    a. Frowning
    b. Smiling
    c. Walking as if in pain
    d. All of the above

4. When speaking to someone who talks slowly, what should you do?
    a. Ask them to speed up.
    b. Ask them to write their questions down.
    c. Slow down your own tempo.
    d. None of the above.

5. You are speaking with a patient and you see she has a furrowed brow. What does this tell you?
    a. She may not understand what you are saying.
    b. She is not actively listening to what you are saying.
    c. She is in acute pain.
    d. She has a hearing impairment.

6. Which of the following should be avoided when communicating with others?
    a. Chewing gum
    b. Pronouncing words correctly

    c. Matching your tempo to that of the other person
    d. Speaking directly to the other person

7. When speaking to a patient via an interpreter, which would be the most appropriate?
    a. Speak directly to the interpreter.
    b. Speak directly to the patient, but look at the interpreter while you are talking.
    c. Speak directly to the interpreter, but look at the patient while are talking.
    d. Speak directly to the patient while looking at the patient.

8. Which of the following is correct about interrupting someone when they are speaking?
    a. It conveys the message that what the person is saying is not important.
    b. Interrupting a person who is speaking is a good way to elicit feedback.
    c. It is appropriate to interrupt someone when you have heard enough to understand what the person needs from you.
    d. Interrupting another person is socially acceptable in American culture.

9. Why is it a good idea to ask for feedback during a conversation?
    a. Asking for feedback enables you to find out if your message was understood.
    b. Feedback helps you make sure you understood what the other person was saying.
    c. The use of feedback helps to avoid confusion in conversations.
    d. All of the above

10. Active listening involves:
    a. using proper grammar.
    b. use of feedback.
    c. listening.
    d. use of body language.

True/False

Determine if each of the following statements is true or false.

_____ 1. Active listening means avoiding distractions.

_____ 2. All written communication in the medical office is a reflection of the entire office.

_____ 3. The medical office manager rarely sends written correspondence.

_____ 4. The five Cs of communication are just as important in written communication as they are in verbal communication.

_____ 5. In a professional letter, a paragraph should be between one to three sentences in length.

_____ 6. The medical office manager needs to act in a professional manner at all times while in the view of patients.

_____ 7. The medical office manager must dress in a professional manner, including maintaining proper hygiene.

_____ 8. It is acceptable for the medical office manager to use a handshake when greeting patients in the medical office.

_____ 9. Crossing the arms when speaking to someone else is a sign of being open and warm.

_____ 10. The Joint Commission has issued a list of abbreviations that should not be used in the healthcare setting.

Matching

Match each of the following terms with its definition.

a. written communication   1. Listening as well as observing behaviors during conversation

b. feedback   2. A process modeled after the Toyota Production System

c. verbal communication   3. Use of touch to convey concern and compassion

d. huddles   4. Writing letters

e. Lean processes   5. Quick meetings in the medical office

f. direct reports   6. A Lean concept to share information in the office on a daily basis

g. active listening   7. Employees who report directly to a manager

h. body language   8. Frowning or smiling

i. therapeutic touch   9. Use of the spoken word

j. DMS   10. Asking for clarification when speaking to another

Chapter Resources

Black, J. (2008). _The Toyota way to healthcare excellence._ Chicago, IL: Health Administration Press.

Graban, M. (2008). _Lean hospitals: Improving quality, patient safety, and employee satisfaction._ New York, NY: Productivity Press.

Tapping, D. (2009). _Value stream management for lean healthcare._ Chelsea, MI: MCS Media.

PEARSON
myhealthprofessionskit™

Additional interactive resources for this chapter can be found at **www.myhealthprofessionskit.com.** Choose "Medical Assisting" from the discipline menu and then click on the book cover for _Medical Office Management._

CHAPTER 3

Legal and Ethical Issues in Managing the Medical Office

CHAPTER OUTLINE

- The Standard of Care for Different Healthcare Practitioners
- Checking the Credentials of Healthcare Professionals
- Maintaining Personnel Files for Physicians
- Medical Malpractice
- Reportable Conditions
- Maintaining the Physician–Patient Relationship
- Ethical Dilemmas
- Treating Minors in the Medical Office
- Receiving Subpoenas

LEARNING OBJECTIVES

Upon completion of this chapter, you should be able to:

- Spell and define the key terms in this chapter.
- Describe the *standard of care* concept as it applies to different members of the healthcare team.
- Understand the importance of checking the credentials of healthcare providers and describe the process of obtaining this information.
- Maintain personnel files for physicians.
- Understand how malpractice insurance protects the medical provider.
- List some of the common reportable medical conditions.
- Describe how the physician–patient relationship is designed.
- Define an ethical dilemma in the medical office.
- Understand the legalities involved in treating minors in the medical office.
- Describe the process of receiving and processing a subpoena for medical records.

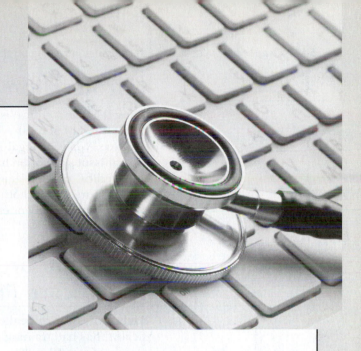

KEY TERMS

assumption of risk	duty	punitive award
claims-made policies	immunity	*res ipsa loquitur*
comparative negligence	informed consent	*res judicata*
compensatory award	malfeasance	*respondeat superior*
continuing education	malpractice	scope of practice
contributory negligence	malpractice insurance policy	settled
damages	misfeasance	standard of care
dereliction of duty	nominal award	statute of limitations
direct cause	nonfeasance	subpoena
discovery rule	occurrence policies	tort

Case Study

Take note of the following scenario and answer the case study questions that appear at the end of this chapter.

Bobbi Schessler works as the medical office manager of a large, multispecialty clinic in the inner city. One of Bobbi's physicians tells Bobbi that she does not see the need for hiring a registered nurse for an open position in the office; she wants Bobbi to save money and hire a medical assistant instead.

Introduction

Many legal and ethical issues can arise in the medical office. The medical office manager needs to stay abreast of current and pending legislation that may impact the medical practice. Whereas legal issues surround legislation, both on the state and federal level, ethical issues are often harder to define. To stay unbiased in the area of healthcare ethics, the medical office manager would be well-served to join and maintain membership in one or more medical office management professional groups. These groups keep abreast of and publish current ethical stands for their members.

The Standard of Care for Different Healthcare Practitioners

scope of practice
the skills practiced by a person who has received training in a particular profession

standard of care
the amount and type of care a reasonable and prudent person would provide, given the same training and circumstances

Each profession in healthcare, from medical assistants to nurses, from technicians to physicians, has had training for the tasks and duties they perform. This is referred to as their **scope of practice**. The scope of practice for any given profession includes the skills received in training for that profession, as long as those skills are permitted under the law. This is important to note because the scope of practice for a medical assistant, for example, may differ from one state to another. In other words, in one state, a medical assistant may be legally permitted to give certain vaccinations, whereas another state may disallow those same injections.

Each healthcare profession is held accountable for providing a certain **standard of care**. This standard may vary from one setting to another, depending on the equipment and staffing available. Per medical malpractice law, providers may be held liable for an injury to a patient if a determination is made that the standard of care was not met. The standard of care is the amount and type of care a reasonable and prudent person would provide, given the same training and circumstances. As an example of how this standard might differ from one location to another, imagine two physicians who each received the same medical training. One physician practices in a rural hospital, with limited staff and equipment available. The other physician practices in an urban hospital, with state-of-the-art equipment and an abundance of highly trained staff on hand. Two patients with the same complicated injury or illness presenting for care in each of these facilities may not receive the same standard of care because the rural setting may lack the equipment or staffing needed to provide the level of care necessary to treat the patient. The training of the healthcare professional is a large part of the standard of care determination—a nurse cannot be held to the same standard of care as a physician simply because the nurse does not have the same level of training.

Critical Thinking 3.1 ?

What does the medical office manager need to know about the scope of practice for a registered nurse as well as for a medical assistant?

Checking the Credentials of Healthcare Professionals

Many healthcare organizations check the credentials of nonprovider healthcare professionals only upon hire. This can be a risky policy because the licensure of those who work in healthcare may change over the years. When hiring nurses, technicians, phlebotomists, or medical assistants, many organizations require a copy of the current state licensure (if applicable) for that individual. An important follow-up process is to require all licensed employees to provide a copy of their license renewal each year for their employee personnel files. Organizations exist that will do this process for the medical facility on a yearly, quarterly, or even monthly basis. Although there is a cost involved in contracting for this verification process, it does take the task off the plate of the medical office manager.

When hiring or adding providers to the medical organization, it is important to go through a process of verifying credentials and work history. This process can be timely, especially for those providers who have an extensive work history. But because the healthcare facility may be liable for the actions of the providers it employs, this is a process that cannot be rushed or skipped. A copy of current licensure should be kept on file, as well as a copy of current medical malpractice insurance coverage (unless the medical facility is providing coverage). The medical facility will want to take the time to research any malpractice claims that may have been filed against a provider, and to check the status of licensure in other states in which the provider may have practiced.

Maintaining Personnel Files for Physicians

Along with keeping current with copies of providers' licenses and insurance coverage, the medical office manager needs to keep other important items in the providers' personnel files.

Nearly every state requires physicians, as well as midlevel providers (registered nurse practitioners and physician assistants), to maintain a certain level of **continuing education**. These continuing education opportunities are available to providers in many locations and range from seminars and professional association conferences to online courses. Although it is the physician's responsibility to track her own continuing education credits in order to maintain licensure in her state, many medical offices require a copy of these credits to be provided for the personnel file as well.

continuing education
educational courses or seminars taken by professionals to further knowledge or skills

malpractice
medical negligence that results in a patient being harmed in some way

---

Critical Thinking 3.2 ?

Do you think it would be important for a medical office manager to track the number of continuing education credits each employee, as well as the physician, accrues? Why or why not?

Medical Malpractice

Doctors are sued for varied reasons. Some are sued for making serious errors, such as giving the wrong medications, performing the wrong surgeries, or failing to properly diagnose or treat patients. Other doctors, though few in number, commit Medicare or insurance fraud or falsify patient records to conceal errors.

Malpractice falls into one of three types:

- **Malfeasance** occurs when an incorrect treatment is performed, such as operating on the wrong patient.
- **Misfeasance** occurs when a treatment is performed incorrectly, such as operating on a patient's arm and accidentally severing a nerve, leaving the patient without the use of the arm.
- **Nonfeasance** occurs when a treatment is delayed or not performed.

malfeasance
performing an incorrect treatment, such as operating on the wrong patient

misfeasance
performing a treatment incorrectly, such as operating on a patient's arm and accidentally severing a nerve, leaving the patient without the use of the arm

nonfeasance
delaying or failing to perform treatment

THE DOCTRINE OF *RESPONDEAT SUPERIOR*

Staff in the medical office can cause the office to be sued. If a medical assistant or nurse makes an error, for example, the lawsuit will usually be filed against the physician who

respondeat superior
the Latin phrase for "let the master answer"

malpractice insurance policy
liability insurance used to protect a physician in the event of a medical mistake or error

employs the medical assistant or nurse. This is called the doctrine of ***respondeat superior***, which is Latin for "let the master answer." Under this doctrine, physicians are responsible for the actions of their healthcare employees (Figure ■ 3-1). Note, however, that medical assistants, nurses, and other clinical staff can still be named in malpractice lawsuits, so each should seriously consider carrying a **malpractice insurance policy**. Because clinical staff have a low risk of injuring patients, insurance rates are generally low. Policies are available through local or state associations.

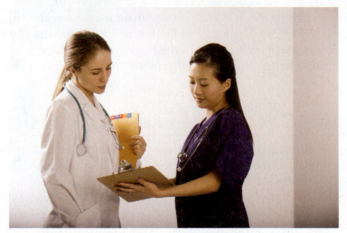

FIGURE ■ 3-1 Physicians work closely with their medical assistants and are responsible for their actions.
Source: © Iofoto/Dreamstime.com.

The doctrine of *respondeat superior* only covers employees performing within their scopes of practice at the time of injury. In other words, a healthcare worker performing a duty outside the scope of practice in the worker's state is not covered by the physician's malpractice insurance policy.

Borrowed Servant

The borrowed servant doctrine is a form of the *respondeat superior* application for malpractice cases. This doctrine may be used when an employee involved in a malpractice event is employed by a temporary agency, not the physician or facility where the event occurred. In these cases, the employee involved in the event is said to be a "borrowed servant" and therefore is covered by the physician or facility where the negligence occurred.

TYPES OF MALPRACTICE INSURANCE POLICIES

claims-made policies
policies that protect policyholders from malpractice claims only when the insurance company insuring the policyholders at the time of the alleged malpractice is the same company at the time the claim is filed in court

occurrence policies
policies that cover policyholders regardless of when claims are filed provided the policies were in effect at the time of the alleged malpractice events

Malpractice insurance policies are one of two types: **claims-made policies** or **occurrence policies**. Claims-made policies protect policyholders from malpractice claims only when the insurance company insuring the policyholders at the time of the alleged malpractice is the same company at the time the claim is filed in court. Assume, for example, that on June 1, 2013, Dr. Wisham is covered under a claims-made policy provided by Provost Insurance when she performs an alleged malpractice event. If Dr. Wisham is still covered by Provost Insurance when the claim is filed on December 10, 2013, she will be covered. If, however, she switches to a different insurance company before the filing date, Provost Insurance will not cover her. With her new plan, Dr. Wisham could purchase a "tail" to cover her for the alleged malpractice incidence. A *tail* is a rider on the new policy that states the new company will cover any events for a certain period before the policy's purchase.

Occurrence policies cover policyholders regardless of when claims are filed provided the policies were in effect at the time of the alleged malpractice events. If Dr. Wisham is covered by United Insurance under an occurrence-made policy on June 1, 2013, when an alleged malpractice event occurs, and then switches to a different company before the claim filing date of December 10, 2013, she would still be covered for the claim under her United Insurance policy.

Individual malpractice insurance policies are fairly inexpensive for nonphysicians. For clinical staff members working full time, rates are usually less than $100 per year for policies that cover up to $1 million per malpractice occurrence. For a quick online quote on malpractice insurance premiums, visit www.hpso.com.

Critical Thinking 3.3 ?

Look online for medical malpractice insurance policies for both registered nurses as well as medical assistants. Is there a difference in the cost of the coverage? If so, what is it?

PROVING MEDICAL MALPRACTICE

The vast majority of medical malpractice lawsuits fail to make it to court. They are either **settled**, meaning the two sides agree on a financial award to the injured patient, or they are dismissed due to lack of proof. To prove medical malpractice, the patient must prove the following "four Ds of negligence":

- **Duty**—Physicians have a duty to care for patients once they have taken those patients on. The patients must prove the physicians breached this duty.
- **Dereliction of duty**—Physicians must meet standard of care guidelines for a healthcare provider with the same training, in the same location, under the same circumstances. The patients must prove the physicians failed to perform to this standard.
- **Direct cause**—Patients must prove that the physicians' actions, or lack of actions, directly caused the patients' injuries.
- **Damages**—Patients must prove they sustained damages due to the negligence. Damages fall under a variety of categories, including:

    - Physical or mental disability
    - Loss of the enjoyment of life activities
    - Loss of financial earnings
    - Medical expenses
    - Pain and suffering
    - Loss of relationships.

TORTS

Malpractice law is found under civil law, rather than criminal law. Malpractice cases involve **torts**, which are defined as wrongful acts that lead to damages sustained by another. Most malpractice cases are negligent torts, which means the provider who caused the injury did not intentionally do so. Intentional torts are those that are proven to have been caused purposefully.

CATEGORIES OF MEDICAL MALPRACTICE AWARDS

Personal injury attorneys accept about 1 out of every 20 cases they review, but most cases are found in the physician's favor. Only 1 in 10 cases results in an award or a settlement for the patient. When injured patients win cases, judges or juries may make the three following types of awards:

- **Nominal award**—These are small awards or payments that are made when the negligence is proven, but the damages are minimal.

settled
a case is considered to be settled when the two sides in a lawsuit agree on a financial award to the injured patient

duty
Physicians have a duty to care for patients once they have taken those patients on

dereliction of duty
Physicians must meet standard of care guidelines for a healthcare provider with the same training, in the same location, under the same circumstances

direct cause
A patient must prove that the physician's actions, or lack of actions, directly caused the patient's injuries

damages
the actual costs associated with the injury sustained, such as medical care

tort
wrongful act that leads to damages sustained by another

nominal award
small award or payment that is made when negligence is proven, but the damages are minimal

compensatory award
money that is awarded to a patient or the patient's family to compensate for the cost of medical care, disability, mental suffering, any loss of income, and the loss of future income as a result of an injury

punitive award
award made when judges or juries feel that a healthcare provider should be punished for his or her actions

- **Compensatory award**—This is money that is awarded to a patient or the patient's family to compensate for the cost of medical care, disability, mental suffering, any loss of income, and the loss of future income as a result of an injury.

- **Punitive award**—Awards like these are made when judges or juries feel that a health-care provider should be punished for his or her actions. Courts may feel the provider was reckless or purposefully ignored signals that should have alerted the provider to the injuries. Several states, however, do not allow for punitive damages.

WRONGFUL-DEATH STATUTES

In medical malpractice cases where the patient dies as a result of the negligence of the provider, the surviving family may file a wrongful-death lawsuit. Typically, the monetary losses will be limited to the financial earnings the deceased patient would likely have earned throughout the rest of his working life. Payment may also be made for the cost of replacing the duties the deceased patient performed, such as child care, cooking, or cleaning services. Some states allow for the surviving family members to sue for pain and suffering in wrongful-death cases. Many states that allow for pain and suffering in these cases place a cap on the amount that may be awarded.

PREVENTING MEDICAL MALPRACTICE CLAIMS

Patients file malpractice lawsuits for many reasons, but lack of understanding is chief among them. Scientific advances in healthcare have allowed doctors to perform procedures that were considered too risky until recently. As procedures have become more complicated, patient risk has increased and increased the likelihood of both poor outcomes and malpractice lawsuits, especially when the physicians have failed to thoroughly explain the risks to patients. Physicians can help avoid lawsuits by completely explaining the risks of the procedures and obtaining the patients' **informed consent**. Informed consent should be documented in written detail and signed by both the patient and the healthcare provider (Figure ■ 3-2).

informed consent
physicians must give patients all information about a procedure, including risks and alternatives to the procedure

Another means of lawsuit reduction has been gaining popularity in recent years: If healthcare providers apologize to patients, those patients are less likely to file malpractice claims. Some believe that patients sue because they are angry and only pursue legal recourse because they failed to receive acknowledgment of the error and an apology. In research activities at the University of Michigan, healthcare providers were instructed to apologize to their patients when errors occurred. After 1 year, malpractice defense costs went from $3 million to $1 million. Today, 29 states have laws that allow healthcare providers to apologize to patients after injuries without those apologies being used as proof of malpractice in lawsuits.

DEFENDING AGAINST MEDICAL MALPRACTICE

Once a medical malpractice suit has been filed, the best defense is the medical record. Especially in the area of medical malpractice, an accurate and complete medical record is paramount. This record is the authoritative description of all care given to a patient. It includes all consent forms signed by the patient, as well as descriptions of the questions the patient asked and the answers the physician gave about needed care or treatment. For more on the medical record, see Chapter 7.

statute of limitations
the time within which an injured patient can file a malpractice lawsuit

discovery rule
the statute of limitations may begin from the date the injury was discovered or should have been discovered

THE STATUTE OF LIMITATIONS

Each state has a **statute of limitations** that sets the time within which an injured patient can file a malpractice lawsuit. Typically, this statute begins from the date of the injury. According to a legal term called the **discovery rule**, some states allow the statute to begin when the injury was discovered. This rule helps in cases in which the patient fails to discover the injury until several years after it occurred. Other states allow the statute to begin when a minor child turns age 18, allowing injured children to bring suits on their

MEMORIAL HEALTH

COMPLETE ORIGINAL IN INK FOR HOSPITAL CHART
PATIENT MUST BE AWAKE, ALERT AND ORIENTED WHEN SIGNING
DATE: _____ TIME: _____ ☐ AM ☐ PM

I AUTHORIZE THE PERFORMANCE UPON _____
OF THE FOLLOWING OPERATION (state nature and extent):_____
_____
_____

TO BE PERFORMED UNDER THE DIRECTION OF DR. _____

1. I HAVE BEEN ADVISED THAT THERE IS A FAVORABLE LIKELIHOOD OF SUCCESS, BUT I UNDERSTAND THAT A COMPLETELY SUCCESSFUL OUTCOME MAY NOT BE ACHIEVABLE, AND THERE ARE NO GUARANTEES REGARDING THE OUTCOME. I ALSO UNDERSTAND THAT CERTAIN ADVERSE EVENTS COULD OCCUR AS A RESULT OF THE PERFORMANCE OF THE PROCEDURE OR TREATMENT, INCLUDING PAIN, INFECTION, LACERATION OR PUNCTURE OF INTERNAL ORGANS, BLEEDING, NERVE DAMAGE OR EVEN IN RARE CASES, DEATH. I UNDERSTAND THAT HOSPITALIZATION OR OTHER INSTITUTIONAL CARE, HOME CARE OR CARE BY HEALTH PROFESSIONALS MAY BE NEEDED FOLLOWING THE PROCEDURE OR TREATMENT, RELATED TO FULL RECOVERY, RECUPERATION OR CONVALESCENCE. I UNDERSTAND THE ALTERNATIVES TO THIS PROCEDURE, INCLUDING MY RIGHT TO REFUSE TO CONSENT TO IT, AND I NEVERTHELESS HAVE DECIDED TO CONSENT TO PERFORMANCE OF THE PROCEDURE OR TREATMENT.

2. I CONSENT TO THE PERFORMANCE OF OPERATIONS AND PROCEDURES IN ADDITION TO OR DIFFERENT FROM THOSE NOW CONTEMPLATED, WHETHER OR NOT ARISING FROM PRESENTLY UNFORESEEN CONDITIONS WHICH THE ABOVE NAMED DOCTOR OR HIS/HER ASSOCIATES OR ASSISTANTS MAY CONSIDER NECESSARY OR ADVISABLE IN THE COURSE OF THE OPERATION.

3. I CONSENT TO THE DISPOSAL BY HOSPITAL AUTHORITIES OF ANY TISSUES OR PARTS WHICH MAY BE REMOVED.

4. THE NATURE AND PURPOSE OF THE OPERATION/PROCEDURE, POSSIBLE ALTERNATIVE METHODS OF TREATMENT, THE RISK AND BENEFITS INVOLVED, AND THE COURSE OF RECUPERATION HAVE BEEN FULLY EXPLAINED TO ME. NO GUARANTEE OR ASSURANCE HAS BEEN GIVEN BY ANYONE AS TO THE RESULTS THAT MAY BE OBTAINED.

5. I UNDERSTAND AND AGREE WITH THE ABOVE INFORMATION. I HAVE NO QUESTIONS WHICH HAVE NOT BEEN ANSWERED TO MY FULL SATISFACTION. I UNDERSTAND THAT I HAVE THE RIGHT TO ASK FOR FURTHER INFORMATION BEFORE SIGNING THIS CONSENT.

I have crossed out any paragraph above which does not apply or to which I do not give consent.

PATIENT SIGNATURE: _____ WITNESS SIGNATURE: _____
(OR PARENT OR GUARDIAN IF PATIENT IS UNDER 18 YEARS OF AGE) (OF PATIENT, PARENT OR GUARDIAN SIGNATURE)
PATIENT DATE OF BIRTH: _____ WITNESS SIGNATURE: _____
RELATIONSHIP: _____ ☐ **TELEPHONE CONSENT** (2ND WITNESS NEEDED FOR TELEPHONE CONSENT)

FIGURE ■ 3-2 Sample informed consent form.

own behalf once they reach adulthood. Table ■ 3-1 outlines the statute of limitations for each state.

ASSUMPTION OF RISK

Assumption of risk is a defense to medical malpractice that physicians can use to prove they made the patients aware of the risks of their procedures. Under this defense, patients cannot sue the physicians when one of those risks occurs. This defense relies, however, on a detailed consent form having been signed by the patient.

Every member of the healthcare team is responsible for patient safety. Any team member who witnesses something that seems wrong is compelled to speak with the physician about it out of the patient's hearing range. Team members who remain silent may be considered partly responsible for patients' injuries.

CONTRIBUTORY AND COMPARATIVE NEGLIGENCE

The **contributory negligence** defense is one in which physicians may have been at fault for patients' injuries but can prove that the patients aggravated their injuries or in some way worsened them. For example, assume a physician sends a patient home with a sling

assumption of risk
a defense to medical malpractice that physicians can use to prove they made the patients aware of the risks of their procedures

contributory negligence
a malpractice defense in which a physician may have been at fault for a patient's injury but can prove that the patient aggravated the injury or in some way worsened it

TABLE ■ 3-1 Statute of Limitations in Each State

State	Statute of Limitations for Medical Malpractice
Alabama	2 years from the date of injury or 6 months from the date the injury was discovered to a maximum of 4 years from the date of injury.
Alaska	2 years from the date of injury.
Arizona	2 years from the date of injury.
Arkansas	2 years from the date of injury.
California	3 years from the date of injury or 1 year from the date the injury was discovered or should have been discovered. In the event a foreign object is found inside the plaintiff, the statute begins at the date the object was discovered or should have been discovered.
Colorado	2 years from the date of injury or date the injury was discovered or should have been discovered to a maximum of 3 years from the date of injury.
Connecticut	2 years from the date of injury or date the injury was discovered or should have been discovered to a maximum of 3 years from the date of injury.
Delaware	2 years from the date of injury or within 3 years if the injury was unknown and could not reasonably have been discovered.
Florida	2 years from the date of injury or date the injury was discovered or should have been discovered to a maximum of 4 years from the date of injury.
Georgia	2 years from the date of injury.
Hawaii	2 years from the date of injury or reasonable date of discovery. In the event an object is left inside a patient, a claim may be filed up to 1 year from the date of discovery. All claims must be filed within 6 years of the injury.
Idaho	2 years from the date of injury.
Illinois	2 years from the date of injury or up to 4 years if the injury could not reasonably have been discovered within 2 years.
Indiana	2 years from the date of injury.
Iowa	2 years from the date of injury or discovery of the injury. All claims must be filed within 6 years of the injury.
Kansas	2 years from the date of injury or up to 4 years if the injury could not reasonably have been discovered within 2 years.
Kentucky	1 year from the date of injury or up to 5 years if the injury could not reasonably have been discovered within 1 year.
Louisiana	3 years from the date of injury.
Maine	3 years from the date of injury.
Maryland	5 years from the date of injury or 3 years from the date the injury was discovered, whichever is greater.
Massachusetts	3 years from the date of injury or 3 years from the date of discovery. All claims must be filed within 7 years of the date of injury.
Michigan	2 years from the date of injury or 6 months from the date of discovery. All claims must be filed within 6 years of the date of injury.
Minnesota	4 years from the date of injury.
Mississippi	2 years from the date of injury or 2 years from the date of discovery. All claims must be filed within 7 years of the date of injury.
Missouri	2 years from the date of injury or date of discovery up to 10 years from the date of injury.
Montana	3 years from the date of injury or discovery up to 5 years from the date of injury.
Nebraska	2 years from the date of the injury or 1 year from the date the injury was discovered. All claims must be filed within 10 years of the date of injury.
Nevada	4 years from the date of injury.
New Hampshire	2 years from the date of the injury. In the event a foreign object is left inside a patient, the claim must be filed within 2 years of the discovery.
New Jersey	2 years from the date of the injury or 2 years from the date the injury was discovered or should have been discovered.
New Mexico	3 years from the date of injury.
New York	30 months from the date of injury. In the event a foreign object is left inside a patient, the claim must be filed within 1 year of the discovery.

State	Statute of Limitations for Medical Malpractice
North Carolina	3 years from the date of injury or the date the injury was discovered or should have been discovered. All claims must be filed within 10 years of the injury.
North Dakota	2 years from the date of injury or the date the injury was discovered or should have been discovered. All claims must be filed within 6 years of the injury.
Ohio	1 year from the date of injury. In the event a foreign object is left inside a patient, the claim must be filed within 1 year of the discovery.
Oklahoma	2 years from the date of injury.
Oregon	2 years from the date of injury or the date the injury was discovered or should have been discovered. All claims must be filed within 5 years of the injury.
Pennsylvania	2 years from the date of injury.
Rhode Island	3 years from the date of injury.
South Carolina	3 years from the date of injury or the date the injury was discovered or should have been discovered. In the event a foreign object is left inside a patient, the claim must be filed within 2 years of the discovery. All claims must be filed within 6 years of the date of injury.
South Dakota	2 years from the date of injury.
Tennessee	1 year from the date of injury.
Texas	2 years from the date of injury.
Utah	2 years from the date of injury or the date the injury was discovered or should have been discovered. In the event a foreign object is left inside a patient, the claim must be filed within 1 year of the discovery. All claims must be filed within 4 years of the date of injury.
Vermont	3 years from the date of injury or 2 years from the date the injury was discovered or should have been discovered. All claims must be filed within 7 years of the injury.
Virginia	2 years from the date of injury or the date the injury was discovered or should have been discovered. In the event a foreign object is left inside a patient, the claim must be filed within 1 year of the discovery. All claims must be filed within 10 years of the date of injury.
Washington, D.C.	3 years from the date of injury.
Washington State	3 years from the date of injury or 1 year from the date injury was discovered or should have been discovered. All claims must be filed within 8 years of the injury.
West Virginia	2 years from the date of injury or the date the injury was discovered or should have been discovered.
Wisconsin	3 years from the date of injury or 1 year from the date the injury was discovered or should have been discovered. All claims must be filed within 5 years of the injury.
Wyoming	2 years from the date of injury or the date the injury was discovered or should have been discovered.

Source: Expert Law.

instead of a cast and tells the patient to limit the motion of the arm to avoid aggravating the injury. If the patient then lifts groceries, worsening the fracture, that patient could be proven to have contributed to negligence.

Because the law assumes a reasonable person would not have done the act that contributed to their injury, most states do not give patients awards in contributory negligence cases. When awards are allowed, the court will typically assign a percentage of the award based on how responsible the patient was for the injury. For example, if the court finds the physician is 50 percent responsible for an injury and the patient is also 50 percent responsible, the physician will be ordered to pay 50 percent of the damages. These types of cases are normally called **comparative negligence**.

IMMUNITY FROM NEGLIGENCE SUITS

The Federal Tort Claim Act of 1946 prohibits lawsuits against any U.S. governmental facility, such as veterans' hospitals or military bases. This provides **immunity** for ordinary negligence, not intentional injury.

comparative negligence
when both the physician and the patient are found to be responsible for an injury

immunity
protection from being held responsible monetarily in a lawsuit

RES JUDICATA AND *RES IPSA LOQUITUR*

Res judicata is Latin for the phrase "the thing has been decided." If patients lose their malpractice lawsuits, they cannot bring other suits against the physician for the same injuries. Once a case has been decided in a physician's favor, the case must be dropped. Conversely, when the court awards a patient damages, the physician can appeal the decision in the hope that the patient will settle for less than the awarded amount or the case will be found in the physician's favor.

Another malpractice doctrine is ***res ipsa loquitur***, Latin for "the thing speaks for itself." Cases of *res ipsa loquitur* are ones in which the malpractice is obvious. For example, a wrong limb may have been amputated or an instrument left inside a patient. In such cases, physicians must prove that what they did was correct, as opposed to other types of malpractice cases, where the patient must prove the physician's negligence.

FRAUD

Fraud is a deliberate act to conceal facts in order to receive illegal or unfair gain. In the healthcare setting, fraud may take a number of different forms. Billing for services that were not rendered or intentionally charging for more extensive services than those actually performed are types of fraud. Physicians or medical facilities who take payments for sending referrals to other physicians or facilities are guilty of receiving kickbacks, another form of fraud. Because fraud can and does result in criminal charges against those involved, it is vital that the medical office manager be aware of what constitutes fraud and watch for the appearance or presence of such activities. Many medical insurance carriers do not differentiate between intentional fraud and nonintentional fraud—that is, providers as well as staff members involved may be charged with a crime even if a billing error was made by mistake. Healthcare providers who intentionally falsify medical records, or who attempt to cover up errors in the medical record, may be guilty of fraud.

Reportable Conditions

Physicians have certain responsibilities surrounding the reporting of certain events. Physicians who deliver babies must report birth certificates, for example. Physicians who are the last to care for patients who have died are normally responsible for completing death certificates. All states list reporting requirements in the event of certain infectious or communicable diseases. Such lists can be obtained from state or local health departments and should be updated yearly.

REPORTING VACCINE INJURIES

According to the 1986 National Childhood Vaccine Injury Act, vaccine injuries must be reported by physicians' offices to alert other physicians to possibly contaminated batches of vaccine. To report a vaccine injury, the medical office manager should obtain the patient's name and age, as well as the name and lot number of the vaccine. The call must be documented in the patient's file.

REVOKING MEDICAL LICENSES

Each state has its own medical practice acts. These acts list the duties and responsibilities of the physician and outline the actions that may be cause for disciplinary action, including suspension or revocation of the physician's license. In general, the more serious the action, the more serious the disciplinary action. For example, physicians who are convicted of felonies or who have been proven to have abused patients may face license revocation.

Maintaining the Physician–Patient Relationship

Both physicians and patients have responsibilities in their relationships. Patients are free to choose their physicians within the guidelines of their managed care plans. They can also choose whether they want to begin care or limit their care. Patients have the right to understand their treatments' components, as well as any side effects or benefits. All of this information must be detailed for the patient before the procedure. In cases where an invasive procedure is needed, patients must be given complete information about the procedure and should sign an informed consent form indicating they understand all risks.

Physicians have the right to refuse treatment to new patients, or even existing ones, unless those patients have life-threatening, emergent conditions. With proper notification, physicians can change their policies or their availabilities. When physicians are away from their practice for a period of time, for instance, if they go on vacation, they must arrange for other physicians to cover their practices in the event of an emergency. To simply close an office, with no emergency referral, may be seen as abandonment of the patient.

TERMINATING THE PHYSICIAN–PATIENT RELATIONSHIP

Physicians are allowed to terminate a physician–patient relationship for any legal reason. Many physicians choose to terminate a relationship with a patient due to noncompliance with healthcare orders. The relationship may also be terminated for nonpayment of medical bills, for drug-seeking behavior, or for not showing up for scheduled appointments.

Regardless of the legal reason chosen by the physician to terminate the relationship, the patient must be given sufficient notice of termination. This may be done by sending the patient a letter (often by certified mail) alerting the patient to the termination of the relationship. The letter should also offer to refer the patient to another physician, and to transfer the patient's medical records to the new physician (Figure ■ 3-3).

Critical Thinking 3.4 ?

How might the employees in the medical office help to maintain the physician–patient relationship? What sort of activities would enhance this relationship? What activities would harm the relationship?

USE OF PATIENT SATISFACTION DATA

Healthcare today is a competitive environment, and most patients have the freedom to choose where they will seek medical care. To attract and retain patients, healthcare organizations look to provide a high level of customer service to the patients they serve. One method for determining what constitutes good customer service is to conduct a patient satisfaction survey. These surveys are sent randomly to patients through the mail, or they may be handed to patients at the time of their healthcare visit. The surveys ask the patient to rate her satisfaction with various aspects of her visit, from the pleasantness of the staff, to the cleanliness of the facility, to the amount of time spent waiting for the physician, to the explanation the physician gave regarding the patient's condition. Healthcare organizations use the data collected from these surveys to make changes to the facility or to counsel staff and physicians regarding improvements.

Critical Thinking 3.5 ?

Most patient satisfaction surveys inquire about the patients' satisfaction with the care provided by the healthcare staff as well as the physician. How might a medical office manager work to help her staff to provide outstanding service to the patients they care for?

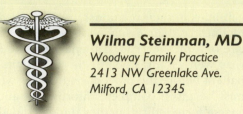

Wilma Steinman, MD
Woodway Family Practice
2413 NW Greenlake Ave.
Milford, CA 12345

August 25, 2013

Gloria Sanchez
891 NW Wallingford Ave.
Milford, CA 12345

Dear Ms. Sanchez:

Because you have missed your last four follow-up appointments to monitor your condition, I will no longer be able to provide you medical services. I believe your condition requires attention and strongly encourage you to seek care with a physician. When you have chosen a new physician, please advise this office by requesting, in writing, the transfer of your medical records.

If you wish, I would be happy to give you a referral. I will be available to treat you for no longer than 30 days from the receipt of this letter.

Sincerely,

Wilma Steinman, M.D.

Wilma Steinman, M.D.

FIGURE ■ 3-3 Sample termination-of-care letter.

Ethical Dilemmas

Medical ethics govern the behavior of healthcare professionals. Each professional association has its own code of ethics that details the actions that are considered ethical by that profession. These ethical codes may be found on the websites of each professional organization.

All healthcare professionals can expect to face legal and ethical situations that may require them to act to protect a patient, yet remain within the bounds of law and the scope of practice. Sometimes, physicians may ask medical staff to perform duties outside their scope of practice. Because this is illegal, the medical staff member should be comfortable about not accepting the task. To do so could cause patient injury and a lawsuit against both the medical staff member and the physician. When a physician makes a request like that, it is often a result of the physician not understanding the medical staff member's scope of practice. The medical staff member should alert the office manager so the manager is able to have a conversation with the physician about the scope of practice of the various medical team members.

An unethical physician may ask a staff member to break the law. Although this is very rare, members of the medical team must respond by staying within their scope of practice and the law according to the medical practice laws of that state. Medical professionals are legally bound by law and scope of practice to treat patients lawfully and ethically and to document correctly in patients' charts.

Critical Thinking 3.6 ?

Imagine that a physician convinces his medical office manager to hire a medical assistant instead of a registered nurse. What should the medical assistant do if the physician encourages her to perform duties that are outside the medical assistant's scope of practice?

If medical professionals wonder whether their actions cross ethical or legal boundaries, they should consider the following questions based on the Blanchard and Peale ethical model:

1. Is the action legal?
2. Is the action ethical?
3. How will the action make me feel?
4. How would I feel if the action, and my involvement, was published in the local newspaper? If I had to explain my actions to my child/spouse/parent?

If the medical professional is uncomfortable with any of the answers to these four questions, the action likely crosses an ethical or legal boundary and the medical professional should decline to participate.

The American Medical Association (AMA) has outlined several areas surrounding ethics in the management of patient care. These include:

- With regard to organ transplantation, physicians must not consider age in the decision of who gets the organ. Priority must be given to the patient who has the strongest chance of obtaining long-term benefit; a person's individual worth to society must not be considered.

- With regard to clinical research, physicians must fully inform any patient involved in research and must give those patients the highest level of respect and care. The goal of any research program must be to obtain some type of scientific data.

- With regard to obstetrics, physicians must perform abortions within the boundaries of state and federal laws. If physicians do not wish to perform abortions, they must refer patients to physicians who will perform the procedure. If a patient undergoes genetic testing, the physician must give the results to both parents.

Other ethical viewpoints by the AMA involve the area of finances in the healthcare setting:

- Patient care should not be dictated by the patient's ability to pay. In other words, a physician should not order expensive tests for a patient who can pay and skip tests for those who cannot.

- Physicians can charge for missed appointments only when they notify the patients ahead of time.

- Patients must be able to receive copies of their medical record, regardless of any amounts owed the office. The physician cannot hold the medical record hostage for payment of a bill.

- Physicians can charge interest on medical bills in accordance with state law if they notify patients ahead of time.

- Fees for service must be reasonable and fair and must be based on Current Procedural Terminology (CPT) code guidelines regarding the nature of the care involved.

Treating Minors in the Medical Office

In most states, children under age 18 may receive certain types of medical treatment without their parents' consent. Such treatments are limited to those for family planning (i.e., birth control or abortion), sexually transmitted infections (STIs), mental health, HIV/AIDS, or alcohol or drug rehabilitation. Because laws for releasing minors' information vary from state to state, medical office managers must be very clear about the laws in the states where they work.

Minors may receive copies of only those documents their parents cannot see. For example, minors could request and receive copies of their STI treatments, but they could not receive copies of the vaccines they received. Parents, in contrast, could receive only copies of their children's vaccinations, not their STI treatments.

Receiving and Processing Subpoenas

subpoena
a legal document that requires a medical office to release medical records or provide court testimony

Occasionally, medical offices may receive **subpoenas** for patients' medical records. Subpoenas may arise from lawsuits due to injury, such as from a car accident. A judge must sign a subpoena, which authorizes the physician to release the information without the patient's signature. Medical facilities are not required to notify the patient of the subpoena or release the information, but many will as a courtesy. HIPAA requires medical facilities to keep records of all patient-record disclosures, however, and to make those records available to patients upon request.

Case Study Questions

Refer to the case study presented at the beginning of this chapter to answer the following questions:

1. How might Bobbi respond to the physician about hiring a medical assistant instead of a registered nurse?
2. How would you suggest Bobbi find out what the scope of practice is for a medical assistant, as well as a registered nurse, in the state where the practice resides?
3. What information should Bobbi collect before she discusses this with the physician?

Chapter Review

Summary

- The standard of care is the care determined by the type of training a provider has obtained, in addition to where the provider practices, and the equipment and facilities that are available.

- The credentials of healthcare professionals should be checked prior to an offer of employment. To ensure that credentials are maintained, a copy of updated licenses should be kept in employee personnel files.

- Physicians are required to obtain continuing education credits in order to maintain their licensure. The medical office manager will need to keep copies of these education credits, as well as insurance information, in physician personnel files.

- Physicians must maintain malpractice insurance to protect them in the event of a claim of medical malpractice. There are two types of insurance policies covering medical malpractice claims, and several defenses to these claims.

- Each state requires healthcare professionals to report certain medical conditions. In addition to medical conditions, other conditions, such as vaccine injuries and cases of abuse, are reported as well.

- The patient–physician relationship must be maintained in order to achieve optimum patient care. This relationship includes accurate record keeping, as well as good communication on behalf of both the physician and the patient.

- Various ethical dilemmas may present in the medical office. Although some of these dilemmas may be easy to address, others may be more unclear. Most associations, such as the American Medical Association, maintain codes of ethics that guide members in times of ethical uncertainty.

- Minors are those people under the age of 18 years. In the event a minor is seeking treatment for certain conditions, such as pregnancy or HIV testing, the minor may obtain these services without the need for consent from the parent.

- Subpoenas are documents signed by a judge in a court of law. These documents are typically used to demand copies of medical charts to be used in a court case. When subpoenas are received, the medical office manager will want to consult with the physician regarding the case and the documents to be copied.

Multiple Choice

Choose the letter that best answers each question or completes each statement.

1. Nearly every state requires which of the professions below to obtain continuing education credits in order to renew their license?
   a. Physicians
   b. Medical office managers
   c. Medical assistants
   d. All of the above

2. Which of the following has the authority to revoke a physician's medical license?
   a. The hospital where the physician is employed
   b. The physician's local medical society
   c. The state where the physician is licensed
   d. The physician's malpractice insurer

3. Which of the following is true about the *standard of care* concept?
    a. It is the care that a provider has seen provided while in training.
    b. It is the care that the provider has been trained to do and is part of that provider's scope of practice.
    c. It is the care the provider wishes she knew how to perform.
    d. It is the care the patient demands.

4. George Savanna signed a consent form prior to having surgery on his hand. The physician discussed with George all portions of the consent form prior to surgery, including the possibility of prolonged numbness in his fingers after the surgery. If George experiences this numbness after the surgery, what defense would the physician have in a malpractice suit?
    a. Assumption of risk
    b. Denial
    c. Contributory negligence
    d. Comparative negligence

5. Where might a physician obtain continuing education credits?
    a. At a medical seminar
    b. Online via medical conferences
    c. Through their local professional association
    d. All of the above

6. Which of the following is the best defense against medical malpractice?
    a. An accurate and well-kept medical record
    b. Pleasant interactions between the physician and his patient

    c. Admission by the physician that she has done something wrong
    d. Hiring an attorney as soon as a claim is filed

7. A minor is a person under what age?
    a. 25
    b. 20
    c. 18
    d. 16

8. Which of the following type of malpractice award is given to pay for actual medical costs?
    a. Nominal
    b. Compensatory
    c. Contributory
    d. Punitive

9. Which of the following is NOT an area for which the AMA has issued an ethical guideline?
    a. Financial
    b. Clinical research
    c. Organ transplants
    d. Location of medical practice

10. Which of the following parts of a medical record can be released to a 16-year-old without parental permission?
    a. Vaccination record
    b. Results of HIV test
    c. Copy of operative report for surgical repair of the arm
    d. Lab results from routine physical exam

True/False

Determine if each of the following statements is true or false.

_____ 1. The doctrine of respondeat superior only covers employees performing within their scopes of practice at the time of injury.

_____ 2. Because clinical staff have a high risk of injuring patients, medical malpractice insurance rates are generally high.

_____ 3. According to a legal term called the discovery rule, some states allow the statute of limitations in malpractice cases to begin when the injury was discovered.

_____ 4. *Res judicata* is Latin for the phrase "the thing speaks for itself."

_____ 5. Punitive damages are awarded to punish the defendant.

_____ 6. HIPAA requires medical facilities to keep records of all patient-record disclosures.

_____ 7. Veterans' hospitals have immunity from ordinary negligence suits.

_____ 8. Medical ethics are what govern the behavior of healthcare professionals.

_____ 9. When a medical malpractice case is settled, it means the two sides agreed on a financial award to the injured patient, or the case was dismissed due to lack of proof.

_____ 10. *Respondeat superior* is Latin for "the thing has been decided."

Matching

Match each of the following terms with its definition.

a. assumption of risk

b. claims-made policies

c. compensatory damages

d. continuing education

e. contributory negligence

f. discovery rule

g. immunity

h. informed consent

i. misfeasance

j. direct cause

1. A defense to medical malpractice that physicians can use to prove they made the patients aware of the risks of their procedures

2. Money that is awarded to a patient or the patient's family to compensate for the cost of medical care, disability, mental suffering, any loss of income, and the loss of future income as a result of an injury

3. A patient must prove that the physician's actions, or lack of actions, directly caused the patient's injuries

4. Educational courses or seminars taken by professionals to further knowledge or skills

5. The statute of limitations may begin from the date the injury was discovered or should have been discovered

6. A malpractice defense in which physicians may have been at fault for a patient's injury, but can prove that the patient aggravated the injuries or in some way worsened it

7. Protection from being held responsible monetarily in a lawsuit

8. Protect policyholders from malpractice claims only when the insurance company insuring the policyholders at the time of the alleged malpractice is the same company at the time the claim is filed in court

9. Physicians must give patients all information about a procedure, including risks and alternatives to the procedure

10. Performing a treatment incorrectly, such as operating on a patient's arm and accidentally severing a nerve, leaving the patient without the use of the arm

Chapter Resources

American Medical Group Management Association – an organization that supplies medical offices and physicians with tools for better managing their practices: www.amga.org

Provider Trust – an organization that will perform monthly licensure checks for healthcare employers: www.providertrust.com

PEARSON
myhealthprofessionskit™

Additional interactive resources for this chapter can be found at **www.myhealthprofessionskit. com.** Choose "Medical Assisting" from the discipline menu and then click on the book cover for *Medical Office Management.*

CHAPTER 4

Personnel Management

LEARNING OBJECTIVES

Upon completion of this chapter, you should be able to:

- Spell and define the key terms in this chapter.
- Determine appropriate staffing needs in the medical office.
- Write a job description for positions in the medical office.
- Compose an advertisement for job positions in the medical office and describe the various venues for placing advertisements.
- Screen résumés from job applicants.
- Describe techniques for interviewing job applicants.
- Understand the task of calling for references for job applicants.
- Outline the reasons for performing background checks on job applicants.
- List the steps for calling to offer employment.
- Describe orientation of the new employee.
- Develop training programs for new employees.
- Define *employment at will*.
- Understand the various supervisory styles to use with different personalities.
- Compose an evaluation of an employee.

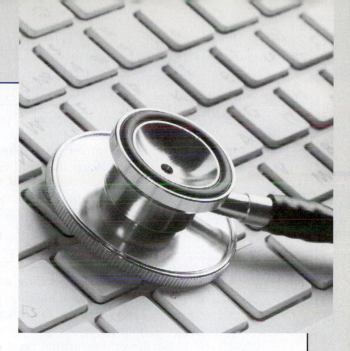

- Describe steps for performing disciplinary action with employees.
- Understand employee assistance programs.
- Outline the processes for terminating employment of an employee.
- Understand how the employer must deal with sexual harassment in the workplace.
- Understand the process for both calling for and giving employee references.
- Maintain the employee personnel file.

Case Study

Take note of the following scenario and answer the case study questions that appear at the end of this chapter.

Svetlana Pilat is the medical office manager in a busy family practice clinic. Her clinic is adding two new physicians and Svetlana needs to determine the appropriate support staff needed for the physicians. She is not sure if she will need to hire nurses or medical assistants and whether each physician will need his or her own staff or if the physicians can share. She also needs to determine if her current reception staff will be sufficient to cover the workload of two new physicians.

Introduction

The management of personnel in the medical office typically falls to the medical office manager. Whereas some medical clinics may be large in size and have a human resources department, other clinics are smaller in size and all human resource tasks fall to the manager. Regardless of the size of the clinic, or the presence or absence of a separate human resources department, the medical office manager must be aware of the concepts of managing employees, including state and federal laws that may apply.

Determining Staffing Needs

The goal in staffing the medical office is to have enough staff members to perform all tasks, yet not have too many staff members. Having too few staff members to support the physicians in the practice limits the physician in the number of patients she can see. A situation of too few staff members will also create a stressful environment for the staff working in that facility. Having too many staff members costs the practice financially; typically personnel costs are the highest category of expenses in the medical office.

The type and number of medical office staff members depend on several factors, from the specialty of the physician to the type of services offered. Physicians who perform in-office surgical procedures will need support staff to set up the equipment needed, assist during the procedure, and clean up after the procedure. This process can be time consuming, and the physician may be ready to move on to the next patient before the medical assistant is ready to assist with the second patient.

An example of a physician who commonly needs two medical assistants is a dermatologist. These physicians may have one medical assistant take a patient to an examining room and assist during a minor skin procedure (Figure ■ 4-1). While that assistant is cleaning the equipment and the room used for that patient, a second assistant may be doing the same tasks for the next patient so the physician can continue. Another example of a physician who may work with two medical assistants is a pediatrician. While one medical assistant is administering immunizations to a child, the second medical assistant may be getting the physician's next patient ready for the physician. By having multiple support staff, physicians are able to leave the work medical assistants and nurses are trained to do to those staff members, while the physicians tend to those things only a physician is trained and licensed to do.

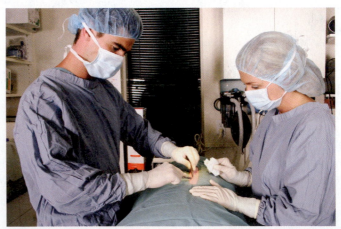

FIGURE ■ 4-1 Physicians are often assisted by medical assistants during minor in-office procedures.
Source: © Trish23/Dreamstime.com.

Medical practices where the physicians work with each patient for an extended period of time may not require as much support staff. An example is a neurology practice. Neurologists typically spend 30 to 40 minutes with each patient. During that time, their medical assistant is able to set up for the next patient and also take care of other tasks. Having two medical assistants may not be practical for this type of physician.

Critical Thinking 4.1 ?

What are some of the drawbacks of having too many staff members in the medical office? What are the drawbacks of having too few?

DETERMINING THE TYPE OF STAFF NEEDED

Most medical offices will have staff working as receptionists, medical assistants, and nurses. In larger facilities, staff will also work in the medical records department, laboratory, and billing office. In smaller offices, the office manager, medical assistants, and nurses may perform these tasks. Typically, the registered nurse earns a higher wage than the medical assistant, who earns a higher wage than the receptionist.

The medical office manager will need to be aware of the laws in the state where he is working in order to determine the skills each clinical staff member is trained and/or licensed to perform. As an example, in many states medical assistants are not permitted to **triage** and offer medical advice to patients. In these states, this task must be performed by a registered nurse. If a physician needs a clinical staff person to triage and offer medical advice in such a state, that physician will need to employ a nurse for this task. Running a medical office is similar to any other business in that it is important to spend money on staffing wisely. If a receptionist can do a task, it would not make good business sense to have a higher paid nurse performing that task (Figure ■ 4-2).

triage
the process of determining the medical nature and urgency of a patient's condition

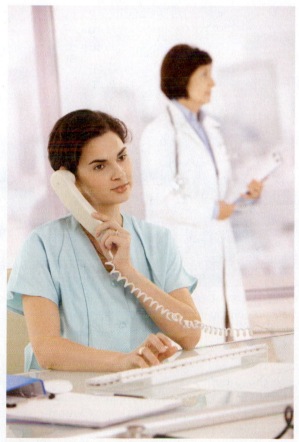

FIGURE ■ 4-2 Nurses commonly perform telephone triage with patients.
Source: © Nyul/Fotolia.com.

Critical Thinking 4.2 ?

What might happen if a medical office had nonmedically trained staff offering triage services and information to patients?

The first step in determining the type and number of staff to employ is to compose a list of the services the physicians offer. For each service offered, the office manager will need to determine the type and number of staff needed to support the physician. Next, the office manager will need to determine the number of patients seen on an average day. In a busier practice, patients may be scheduled to come in at appointment times close to one another, with the physician moving from one patient to the next, leaving the support staff to start and end the visit with the patient. With several employees trained to do the same job, the physician is able to see more patients in less time. The goal is to have the physician busy seeing patients and not slowed down waiting for his clinical support staff to finish their tasks and move to the next patient.

In determining the number of administrative support staff to employ, the medical office manager will again need to determine the number of patients being seen and the **administrative duties** that need to be performed. Administrative support staff are those who perform tasks such as billing and coding for medical services, scheduling appointments, answering telephones, and greeting patients. In a small medical office, one person may perform all of those tasks. In a larger facility, such as one with multiple physicians, it may be necessary to employ several receptionists for the telephone and front-desk tasks, as well as additional staff to perform the billing and coding tasks (Figure ■ 4-3). In some facilities, the office manager may perform some of these tasks, in addition to managing the office.

administrative duties
clerical duties, such as answering the telephone and scheduling appointments

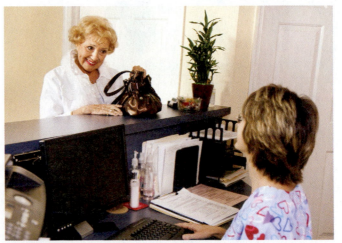

FIGURE ■ 4-3   Receptionists manage incoming calls as well as patients coming in for their appointments.
Source: © Lisa F. Young/Fotolia.com.

clinical duties
back-office duties, including hands-on patient care

Clinical duties are those duties performed in the medical office by medical assistants, phlebotomists, technicians, or nurses. These tasks include taking a patient's medical history and the recording of the patient's vital signs. Clinical tasks include education of the patient regarding treatments, preparing the patient for examinations and studies, and assisting the provider during examinations and procedures. Clinical duties also include performing certain laboratory tests in the medical office, sterilizing medical equipment, and administering medications at the direction of the healthcare provider.

Writing a Job Description

When writing a comprehensive job description, the office manager must include the physical requirements of the position, as well as the skills and skills requirements needed to perform the job. The best job descriptions are those that are more inclusive, rather than vague, when it comes to describing the actual work required of the position. See Figure ■ 4-4 for an example of a comprehensive job description for a receptionist. By describing all physical requirements of the job, applicants are able to determine if they are capable of these requirements. For example, if an applicant is unable to lift more than 10 pounds due to a physical condition, and the job description lists a lifting requirement of 20 pounds, the applicant knows right away that he is not physically able to perform the tasks required of the position.

Medical office receptionist job summary: Serves visitors to the medical office by greeting them both in person and on the telephone.

Duties:

- Answers the telephone and helps callers with their needs
- Welcomes patients and visitors to the medical office
- Schedules appointments for patients
- Checks patients in as they arrive for appointments and alerts the clinical staff to the patient's arrival
- Collects payments from patients as needed
- Alerts patients to any delays in the office
- Records any updates to patient demographics in the electronic medical record
- Follows all policies and procedures as outlined for this position

Qualifications:

- Must be able to sit for up to four hours at a time
- Must be able to lift up to 25 pounds
- Must be fluent in English
- Must be able to multi-task, have attention to detail, and be organized
- Must be flexible in taking on new tasks
- Must have outstanding customer service skills
- Must be comfortable using a computer and multi-line telephone system

---

FIGURE ■ 4-4 Medical office receptionist job description.

THE JOB DESCRIPTION USED IN DISCIPLINARY ACTION

Having the majority of the tasks required of the position listed in the job description is helpful to the office manager in the event disciplinary action is required. For example, if the employee is consistently unable to perform a task listed on the job description, the office manager is able to use the job description to aid with the disciplinary process. In such an event, the office manager would counsel the employee on the work needed, and reference the job description where those tasks are listed.

USING THE JOB DESCRIPTION DURING THE INTERVIEW PROCESS

When conducting **interviews** with potential employees, the office manager should provide the applicant with a copy of the job description. Reviewing the job description with the applicant provides the opportunity for discussion of the required duties of the position, including any physical work required. Of course, the **Americans with Disabilities Act** (ADA) prohibits exclusion of an applicant based solely on a disability. However, if the job requires the applicant to perform physical tasks that are outside the ability of an applicant with a disability, the employer is legally able to turn the applicant away.

interview
the process of asking and answering questions of an applicant to determine suitability for hire

Americans with Disabilities Act
a federal law that outlines the legal rights of persons with disabilities

Advertising for Employees

employment firm
agency that specializes in matching job applicants with employers

Medical office staff members are recruited in a variety of ways. Prior to the Internet, most employers sought staff in one of two ways: placing an advertisement in the local newspaper or using an **employment firm**. Both of these ways continue to be used for recruitment of medical office staff; however, the Internet now allows medical offices to place advertisements for employees at little or no cost in some cases. Many medical offices have their own websites on the Internet and place employment advertisements online (Figure ■ 4-5).

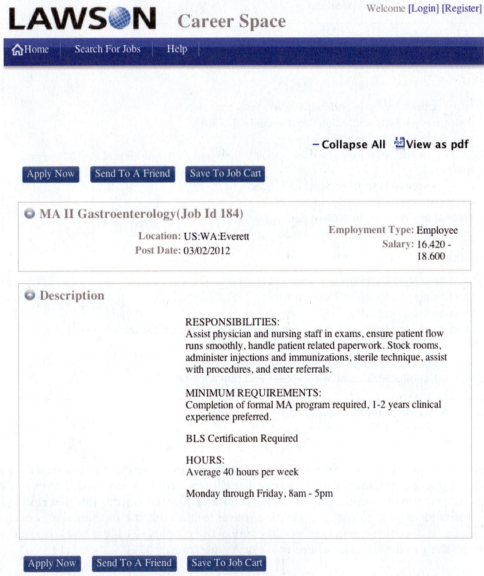

FIGURE ■ 4-5 An online advertisement for a medical assistant. Reprinted with permission of Career Space.

Most newspapers today have an online presence and employment advertisements placed with that paper may be placed online as well. Having an employment advertisement online enables the medical office to reach a wider audience, including applicants who live out of the area and are seeking employment prior to an upcoming move.

Employment firms are still commonly used when seeking medical office staff. These firms recruit applicants and perform a variety of tasks, such as calling past employment references, testing of the applicants' skills, and coaching the applicant on interview techniques. The employment firm will contact medical facilities in the area regarding the possibility of sending an applicant for an interview. These firms are paid for their services in one of two ways: payment is either made by the applicant, or it is made by the employer once an applicant is offered a position. Using an employment firm alleviates the burdens of testing for required skills and calling for references and may result in a faster time to hire.

Critical Thinking 4.3 ?

A busy medical office manager advertised for a billing office specialist. She received nearly 75 résumés in response to the advertisement. Some of the applicants are skilled and some are not. How might this manager have saved time by using an employment firm in her pursuit of hiring for this position?

Many medical facilities today advertise for positions with local colleges. In the event the medical office is located near a school where nurses or medical assistants are trained, this may be a great resource for potential employees. In these situations, the employer will need to be aware that applicants will not typically possess any prior experience in the medical office job. With some community colleges offering certificate programs in areas such as billing and coding or front-desk reception, the medical office manager may find success in placing advertisements for such positions with the college.

Most clinical positions, such as those of medical assistants and nurses, have local associations to which they belong. These associations will often have their own websites, as well as an e-mail list of members. Medical office managers may submit an advertisement for an open position with these associations in order to reach a larger audience.

Screening Résumés

After advertising an open position in the medical office, the manager will need to begin to screen the **résumés** received. This process may be lengthy, depending on the number of applicants for the position. In some cases, applicants may not meet the minimum qualifications for the position. For example, if the manager is seeking to employ a registered nurse with a minimum of 5 years of nursing experience, the résumés of applicants who do not meet that requirement may be discarded. Résumés for qualified candidates will then need to be reviewed to determine which candidates to call for interviews.

With the prevalence of word processing software today, any job applicant has the opportunity to assemble a professional résumé. Typically, résumés that are unprofessional, such as those that contain typographical errors or handwritten corrections, will be discarded even if the applicant is qualified for the position.

Items that may be of concern to look for when screening résumés include:

- Short stays of employment in the past. Does the applicant have several past employers, all of which were for less than 1 year? In this case, the applicant may not be a good fit if the manager is looking for a long-term employee.

- Gaps in employment listed. While gaps may indicate an applicant has taken time off for family or to return to school, gaps may also signify missing information. In the event an applicant has been fired from a position, a gap in employment on the résumé may exist. Although this may not be cause for exclusion from an interview, the office manager should inquire about the gap when meeting with the applicant.

Items that may cause candidates to stand out when screening résumés include:

- **Volunteer** work. Employees who spend time doing volunteer work indicate a desire to help out in their community. These people often make very good healthcare employees.

résumé
a job applicant's list of educational and work experience, including skills and talents

volunteer
to offer time to or perform services for an agency or organization without payment

- High grade point average (GPA) for recent graduates. Applicants who are new to their field may have recently graduated from their training program. Those who earned high grades may list that on their résumé. Good students often make for good employees.

- Long terms of employment with prior employers. Staying with the same employer for years before moving to a different job indicates stability and loyalty to the employer. Employees who stay with the same employer long term are those who typically can get along well with others.

Critical Thinking 4.4 ?

A medical office manager receives two résumés for an open position. One résumé contains spelling and grammatical errors and the other does not. If the position is for a registered nurse, how might the first applicant pose a problem for this practice?

TELEPHONE SCREENING INTERVIEWS

Some medical office managers perform a telephone interview with potential employees prior to an in-person interview. This may be particularly appropriate in situations where the applicant lives out of the area. Telephone interviews may also be performed in clinics where a large number of people have applied for the same position. By performing short telephone interviews, the manager is able to screen out those applicants who do not sound like a good fit for the practice. Because telephone screening interviews do not take place face to face, the manager is unable to gather certain visual details about the candidate. These details include how professional the candidate appears, her ability to maintain eye contact, and how the candidate performs under the stress of an interview. Many of these visual details are important to the job; therefore, most managers will arrange for in-person interviews for those candidates who pass the telephone screening interview.

Critical Thinking 4.5 ?

What are the downfalls of the telephone interview? What sort of information is the office manager unable to collect in this type of interview?

USING THE HUMAN RESOURCES DEPARTMENT TO SCREEN APPLICANTS

In larger healthcare facilities, the screening of job applicants may be done by the human resources (HR) department. In this type of facility, the applicants will apply for a position and interview with an HR representative prior to meeting the department or clinic manager. Sometimes, the HR representative will call for references and verify education of the applicants prior to sending the applicant to the department or clinic manager. For large clinics that may receive a large number of applicants, using the HR department to screen applicants is a time-saver for the department or clinic manager.

SCHEDULING THE INTERVIEWS

Once the medical office manager has reviewed the résumés, she will need to call candidates to set up an interview. Applicant interviews may be performed by the manager only, or they may be performed by including other members of the medical office team. For example, many medical offices perform group interviews with applicants, involving the manager, a physician, and some of the other medical office staff. This type of interview allows the manager to obtain input about other group members' perceptions of the candidate. Group interviews also give the manager the opportunity to view the candidate in a high-pressure situation—group interviews tend to make applicants more nervous than one-on-one interviews. Some managers may decide to interview applicants individually, and then bring back the best applicants for group interviews.

After deciding on the type of interview to be performed (individual or group), the office manager will need to set aside time in her schedule to perform the interviews. Applicant interviews should be performed in a quiet location, and the manager's schedule should be arranged so that the interviews can be conducted without interruption.

The office manager or another member of the staff may call applicants to set up interviews. If the applicant is reached, an interview is scheduled. In the event the applicant is not available, a message should be left with a direct call-back telephone number for the applicant to call to schedule an interview. If there is any information the applicant may need to know about the interview, such as where to park, or the address of the office where the interview will occur, that information should be shared at the time of the telephone call.

Interviewing Applicants

When interviewing applicants, the medical office manager should note the mannerisms of the applicant. This will include the type of dress the applicant wears—is he in professional attire or is he wearing jeans and a sweatshirt (Figure ■ 4-6)? The manager will want to note any mannerisms, such as extreme nervousness, or evidence that the applicant is not telling the truth.

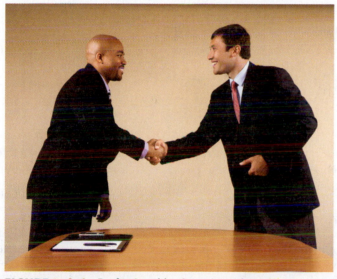

FIGURE ■ 4-6 Professional business interview attire.
Source: © iofoto/Fotolia.com.

The best way to interview potential employees is to use a preprinted sheet of questions (Figure ■ 4-7). Using the same questions for all applicants allows the manager to judge the applicants using the same information for all. Preprinted questions also allow the manager to remember important questions and to maintain the scheduled interview timeline.

While interviewing applicants, the office manager will want to look for the applicant's energy level and mood. Does the applicant seem at ease and friendly? Does he make eye contact during the interview? At the end of the interview, the medical office manager should ask the applicant if he has any questions. At this point, the manager may

1. What interests you about working in this clinic?
2. What do you enjoy about working in healthcare?
3. Tell me about the biggest challenge you have ever faced in a job.
4. Tell me about a situation where you have had conflict in the work place. How did you resolve this?
5. How would your current (or former) co-workers describe you? How would your current (or former) supervisor describe you?

FIGURE ■ 4-7 List of job applicant questions.

be wary of applicants who ask questions about pay, benefits, or time off. Asking these types of questions may be reason to believe the applicant is looking for a job simply for the paycheck, rather than because he enjoys working with patients.

Once all questions have been answered, the medical office manager should take the applicant on a tour of the clinic or department and introduce the applicant to other members of the team. During this time, the manager will want to watch for signs that the applicant is stressed—does he flinch when a child is crying in an exam room? If the manager feels the applicant may be a good fit, it may be appropriate to ask the applicant if he would like to stay and **shadow** another person in the department for an hour or so. This gives the applicant, as well as members of the office staff, the opportunity to get a feel for the fit of the applicant.

> **shadow**
> to watch another person perform his or her job in order to learn how to do that job

ILLEGAL INTERVIEW QUESTIONS

Medical office managers need to ensure that they do not ask applicants any questions that are illegal. Illegal questions are those relating to protected classes under the Civil Rights Act of 1964:

- Race, color, ethnicity, or country of origin
- Religion
- Marital status
- Birthplace
- Age
- Disability.

Employers who ask questions related to these protected areas may be sued for discrimination by an applicant who is not hired for the position. An applicant may contend that the lack of offer of employment was based on the applicant's answer to the illegal question.

Critical Thinking 4.6 ?

What are some of the benefits to the applicant in shadowing another person in the department? What are some of the benefits to the office staff?

Calling for References

Once a candidate has been screened and the medical office manager wishes to pursue employing the individual, the medical office manager must check the candidate's previous employment references. This important step is skipped all too often, and managers may find that the information on the résumé and gathered at the interview was untrue. If the applicant has not provided names and numbers for former employers on the application or résumé, the office manager should ask for this information at the conclusion of the interview.

When calling for references, the medical office manager should speak to the person to whom the applicant reported. This person is in the best position to provide information about how the employee performed, her dependability, and her ability to work in a stressful healthcare environment. Note that some employers do not give out much information when called for a reference; they may be willing to supply only the dates of employment.

More than one reference should be called on any applicant. For applicants who have worked in healthcare previously, all employers for the past 5 years should be called, at a minimum. For applicants who have recently graduated from healthcare programs, former instructors may be called for a reference. The way a student behaves and performs in the classroom is often indicative of how that student will behave and perform as an employee as well.

Background Checks

Applicants being considered for a job in a healthcare facility should be run through a **background check**. Background checks verify that the applicant has no criminal record. If the healthcare facility does not perform a background check, and hires an employee with a criminal record, that facility may be liable should the employee cause harm to a patient while working in that facility in the future.

In the event the background check comes back indicating a criminal record, the employer may still choose to discuss employment with the individual. If, for example, the applicant has a single, minor item on his record from an event many years in the past, the employer may make the decision to offer employment regardless of the infraction. If, however, the applicant has numerous items on the background check, or if the items are serious in nature or very recent, the employer will want to think strongly of turning that applicant away. With medications, financial records, and personal patient information being available to medical office staff, hiring an applicant with a known criminal record is risky to the medical facility. In many states, it is not possible to license or certify an individual who has a criminal record. This may preclude the individual from performing all aspects of the job, including giving injections or administering medications.

Background checks may be done at the state and/or federal level. These checks may include criminal offender record information (CORI) and sexual offender recorder information (SORI) reviews.

background check
verification of any arrests or criminal convictions in an applicant's history

VERIFYING EDUCATION

In the event the applicant will hold the position of nurse, medical assistant, or other licensed or certified position, the medical office manager should verify the individual's education, license, or certification prior to offering employment. For positions that require a certain level of education, such as a master's degree, the manager will want to verify that level of education as well.

> **Critical Thinking 4.7 ?**
>
> Why is it important to verify the education of a potential employee? If a medical facility wishes to hire a manager with a master's degree, how might the lack of such a degree affect the clinic?

Calling to Offer Employment

Once the applicant has been approved by the interviewer or interviewing committee, has had his references called and verified, and has been through a background check, an offer of employment may be made. If **salary** has not yet been discussed with the applicant, it should be discussed at the time of an offer of employment is made.

salary
wages for the job performed

Once the applicant has accepted the offer of employment, a start date should be confirmed. At this time, any other applicants who have come in for an interview should be called to let them know another candidate was selected. The medical office manager will want to keep the résumés of any other good applicants in the event the hired applicant does not work out or another position opens within the clinic or department.

Orientation of the New Employee

orientation
a period of time for training new employees

mentor
an established employee who is assigned to train a new employee

When the new employee is hired, he should spend his first days (or even weeks) in **orientation**. During this period, the employee will be trained on the computer systems in the office and given information on safety, HIPAA compliance, and customer service. Each new employee should be given a **mentor** to work with while in training (Figure ■ 4-8). The mentor should be a person who performs the same job the new employee will be performing. The new employee will shadow his mentor until comfortable with the new position. At that time, the new employee should be in proximity to the mentor so that the mentor can step in to answer questions or give guidance when needed.

A clear and concise orientation plan should be written for every new employee, with a copy provided to the employee and his or her mentor. These plans should include any training that is scheduled, including the dates of the training and where it will occur. At the time of hire, the new employee should go over the policy and procedure manual with the medical office manager to be certain the new employee understands the policies of the medical office and is given the opportunity to ask any questions he or she may have.

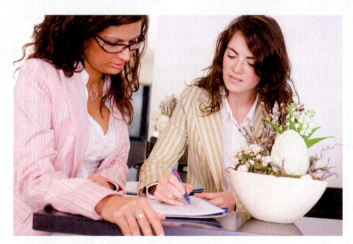

FIGURE ■ 4-8 New employees will typically be trained by existing employees in the same job role.
Source: © Nyul/Dreamstime.com.

All new employees should be given a copy of the employee handbook or information as to the location of this information if it exists in electronic format only. New employees must be made aware of the various processes in the department. These include:

- How to use the time clock
- How to request time off
- How to call in ill
- What to do in the event of an emergency
- How to exit the building in the event of a fire.

PROBATIONARY STATUS

Most employers have a set period of time after hire of a new employee called a *probationary period*. During this time, the employee is considered to be in training, learning the skills of the new job. Probationary status is typically 90 days in length and is the period of time during which either the employer or the employee may come to the conclusion that the employee is not a good fit for the company or the position. When this occurs, the employee is dismissed from employment at the end of the probationary period. With most employers, employees undergo a 90-day evaluation at the end of the probationary period. Any need for performance improvement is reviewed at that time and documented in the employee's file.

Developing Training Programs for the New Employee

All new employees should be made aware of the various tasks for which they need training. Although the mentor may do most of the training, this may not always be the case. In larger healthcare facilities, the staff in a training department may take on the task of training all new employees. The employee and the trainers should be clear on the goals of the training. This is best achieved by following a clear and concise written orientation plan.

No matter who takes on the task of training new employees, a mechanism for tracking the training that has been performed should exist. In some facilities, this takes the form of a training checklist, with both the new employee and the mentor or trainer checking off tasks as the training is done. Any time an employee is trained in using equipment, some formal tracking system, including the date and signatures of the employee and trainer, should be used.

Critical Thinking 4.8 ?

Describe how you would use a training checklist in evaluating the need for further training of a new employee.

Employment at Will

State law dictates whether the state is an employment-at-will state. In these states, employers may terminate the employment of any employee, at any time, for any legal reason. This means the employer does not have to have an actual reason to fire the employee, but can terminate employment at will. In these states, no contract needs to be signed by employees. Employers are not able to terminate employment of an employee for any legally protected reason, such as ethnicity, marital status, or age.

Different Supervisory Techniques for Different Personalities

Just as there are different learning styles, there are also varying styles of managing or supervising employees. Most managers have a dominant management style. See Chapter 1 for a list of three management styles.

Rarely does a medical office manager use just one management style. Instead, the manager will use the style that is most appropriate for the situation, or the employee, at hand. It is important for medical office managers to adopt different leadership styles. Constant use of the autocratic leadership style, for example, may inspire staff to resign or resist making decisions on their own. The laissez-faire style, in contrast, may lead to a disorganized office if used all the time. The ability to balance all of these styles is critical to addressing issues on a case-by-case basis.

The medical office manager should also adopt his management style to the employee, depending on the personality of the employee. For example, with an employee who is very serious and who takes her job very seriously, the manager may keep conversations about performance serious, addressing facts and data, rather than feelings. With an employee who is very emotional, or prone to having her feelings hurt, the manager may use a more gentle approach in discussing an issue and discuss how the situation makes that employee feel.

Critical Thinking 4.9 ?

Describe a situation where each of the three management styles previously discussed would be used best.

Employee Evaluations

Generally, all new employees should be evaluated after 90 days of employment. This evaluation will typically consist of going over the details of the job and updating the employee of any areas of deficit. Prior to the 90-day evaluation, the medical office manager should gather feedback and details from the mentor and from other coworkers if appropriate. If any performance concerns need to be addressed, the manager will need to come up with an improvement plan for the employee. This may entail additional training. Performance improvement plans must list a date by which the employee is to have shown the necessary improvements.

Any evaluation of the employee should include written documentation, and the signatures of both the employee and the manager, along with the date of the evaluation, should be included. A copy of the evaluation should be provided to the employee and a copy kept by the manager. In organizations with HR departments, a copy of the evaluation may be sent to that department as well.

Some employers choose to perform a second performance evaluation with new employees at 6 months post-hire. This evaluation, similar to the 90-day evaluation, will include feedback from the mentor or coworkers. If the employee had any performance improvement items left from the 90-day review, they will be addressed again during the 6-month evaluation.

With some employers, the 6-month evaluation is performed as a midyear review with all employees. Using this tool, employers are able to give feedback to employees twice per year, rather than only once. Many employees today prefer frequent feedback on performance, and employers will find that giving frequent feedback is the best tool for altering and guiding performance in their employees (Figure ■ 4-9).

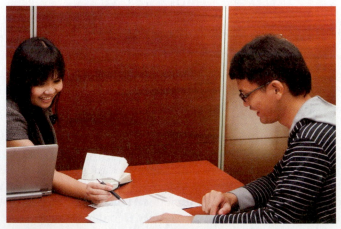

FIGURE ■ 4-9 Performance appraisals should take place in a private location.
Source: © Ampyang/Dreamstime.com.

All employees should be given a yearly performance evaluation. It is not possible to know what is expected in the workplace without a performance evaluation to guide the employee. A performance evaluation is a review of a certain time period (90 days, 6 months, or 1 year) and should never contain information that is new to the employee. The evaluation is a review, and any performance concerns listed should have been gone over with the employee prior to the meeting. During the evaluation, feedback is given regarding performance, and goals are set for the next evaluation period.

For yearly performance evaluations, many healthcare facilities use a 360-degree evaluation. With this type of evaluation the manager solicits feedback on performance about the employee from various members of the healthcare team. Those solicited should be both coworkers, as well as persons who may report to the staff member being evaluated. Performance appraisals should also consist of the gathering of feedback about performance from the employee herself.

> **Critical Thinking 4.10 ?**
>
> How might providing frequent feedback benefit the employer? How might this practice benefit the employee? Do you think giving frequent feedback is worth the effort?

Employee Discipline

Employees may be disciplined for performance issues or because certain behaviors need to be altered. The medical office manager who provides clear expectations to his staff members will typically need fewer disciplinary meetings than the manager who does not provide clear expectations. Every employer must have policies and procedures that guide employees' actions. Employees must know what is expected of them regarding performance, and how they are to behave in the workplace. These expectations include:

- Shift time. Employees need to know what time they are to arrive for their shift, how long to take for breaks and lunch, and what time they are to leave at the end of the shift.
- Dress code. Employees need to know what attire is to be worn in the workplace. This expectation must be clear, and should include examples of acceptable and unacceptable attire, including shoes and jewelry.
- Use of equipment. Employees need to be fully trained on the use of any equipment, including the maintenance and ordering of supplies or repair requests.

Expectations begin with a robust job description and continue with proper training of employees. Any time an employee deviates from the expectations, communication between the medical office manager and the employee should occur as soon as possible (Figure ■ 4-10). In some cases, the employee may not have completely understood the expectation. In this event, the goals of the meeting with the office manager are to counsel the employee on the expectations and to make sure the employee understands what is expected going forward.

VERBAL WARNINGS

If an employee has been counseled about the expectations required and fails to perform as expected the second time, a **verbal warning** may be appropriate. A verbal warning must be documented, and a signed copy of receipt of the warning placed in the employee's file (Figure ■ 4-11).

The warning should consist of the employee's name and the date. A description of the infraction is listed, along with the ramifications of this action on the employee's coworkers or patients. The employee's response to the warning is documented, including the action plan for improvement. A follow-up date should be set for the office manager and employee to meet to discuss progress toward improvement.

verbal warning
the process of giving notice of disciplinary action to an employee verbally

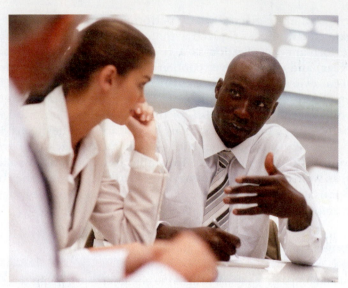

FIGURE ■ 4-10   The medical office manager must counsel employees on performance issues as they arise.
Source: © Yuri Arcurs.

March 15, 2012

Employee: Donna Depner

Subject: Verbal Warning

Issue/Concern:

On March 10, 2012, Donna was asked to assist her co-worker and room a patient. Donna became visibly upset at the request and began to throw things at her desk. Though Donna did eventually room the patient as requested, her attitude and inflexible nature made it obvious both to her co-workers and to her patient that she was not pleased at being asked to do this task.

How does this affect others?

By being inflexible and having a negative response when asked for assistance, Donna is not being a team player in the office. When Donna displayed this negative response, her co-workers get the message that she is inflexible and should not be asked for assistance. When patients see this response in the office, they do not get a sense of good customer service and are less satisfied with their visit.

Action needed:
In the future, when Donna is asked for assistance, she will either decline if she is unable to assist or she will assist. Either way, Donna will maintain the high level of professionalism, team work, and customer service that is expected of all employees in this facility.

By signing below, I acknowledge receipt of this verbal warning. I realize this will become part of my permanent employee file. I realize that discussing this warning with my co-workers may be considered retaliation and, should that occur, I may be subject to further disciplinary action, including possible termination from my position with this organization.

_____   _____

Employee signature   Date

FIGURE ■ 4-11   Acknowledgment of verbal warning.

written warning
the process of giving notice of disciplinary action to an employee in written form; typically more severe than a verbal warning

WRITTEN WARNINGS

In the event the employee commits another breach of policy or procedure, it may be appropriate to issue the employee a **written warning**. This warning, much like the verbal warning, consists of a meeting between the employee and office manager. If the medical facility employs HR representatives, this person may be present as well. A written warning is more severe than a verbal warning. The employee must be made aware of the expectations for performance improvement, and the consequences that will result if the employee fails to improve must be listed. The employee signs the warning and is given a copy. As with any performance improvement plan, a follow-up date should be set for the employee and manager to meet to discuss improvement.

Employee Assistance Programs

During discussions with an employee about performance, the employee may admit to the office manager some form of personal issue that is contributing to the performance concern. This issue may be due to divorce, a death in the family, or even substance abuse. Most mid- to large-sized employers have some form of employee assistance program available for employees. These programs may range from offering professional counseling to the employee at no cost, to setting up drug or alcohol rehabilitation programs, to offering to arrange for a leave of absence. The goal in offering assistance to the employee is to help the person take care of what may be a temporary stressor in her life. If, after availing herself of the assistance offered by the employer, the employee still fails to perform as expected, disciplinary action will proceed.

Critical Thinking 4.11 ?

How might utilizing an employee assistance program benefit the employer?

Employee Termination

When employees have been given warnings and sufficient time to show improvement in performance, yet still have not reached the desired level of performance, it may be time to terminate employment. Termination of employment should be done in a respectful manner, with care taken to provide the employee the opportunity to leave without undue embarrassment. In many cases, the employee will know the termination is about to happen. This is especially true if the manager has been clear about expectations and the timeline for improvement.

Certain actions by the employee may result in immediate termination of employment. These include:

- The use of drugs or alcohol while working or arriving at work under the influence of drugs or alcohol.
- Abuse or assault of a patient or coworker.
- Stealing office supplies.
- Intentionally misusing or damaging equipment.
- Breach of patient privacy (HIPAA violation).

When one of these events occurs, the employee will be told his employment has been terminated. The employee should then be escorted from the building. In the event the employee becomes combative, security or the local police may need to be called.

Once any employee has been terminated from employment, any identification cards and keys must be collected before the employee leaves the premises. The employee's access to the computer systems must also be removed so that no patient content may be viewed by the employee. The employee should be given the opportunity to collect any personal items from his workstation. This collection of items should be done with the manager, HR representative, or security person present to ensure the employee collects only what belongs to him.

Sexual Harassment and the Workplace

Federal law contains protections against sexual harassment in any workplace. The medical office manager will need to be sure all employees are educated about what conduct is defined as sexual harassment.

Sexual harassment is defined as any unwelcome sexual advances, requests for sexual favors, or verbal or physical harassment of a sexual nature. Sexual harassment can also include offensive remarks about a person's gender, and the person guilty of sexual harassment can be either male or female.

When an employee feels he or she is being sexually harassed in the workplace, it is that employee's responsibility to report the behavior or situation to the manager. Once the report has been made, the manager must investigate the allegation. If harassment occurs in the workplace, the manager must be quick to act to protect employees, or the medical practice is at risk of being sued. It is important to note that sexual harassment may include an employee who is offended by another employee's display of a sexually explicit item, such as a wall calendar. If an employee finds the material offensive, that employee may make a claim of sexual harassment.

Providing Employee References

litigation
the act of filing a lawsuit against someone

slander
the act of harming another person's reputation by stating something untruthful

Employees will leave employment for a number of reasons, from moving out of the area to the acceptance of a job with another facility. When employees look for new employment, their former employers may be asked to provide a reference. As mentioned earlier in this chapter, employers may choose to give reference information or they may not. For those who choose to give out limited information, the reference may simply consist of the dates the employee worked for the organization. Employers may choose to give out limited information due to fear of **litigation** from the former employee. If the employer gives out information that is untrue or information that is subjective in nature or consists of unproven allegations, that employer may be sued for **slander** by the former employee.

Any information given in an employee reference must be factual. If the former employer says anything that may be construed as negative about the former employee, it must be something that was proven and documented in the employee's review or file. For example, if an employee was terminated due to theft of drugs, and that theft was proven and documented, the former employer may legally give that information to the caller. If, however, the employee was suspected of drug use, but the allegation was never proven, the former employer may be sued for giving that information to the caller. Anytime a former employer is providing reference information about a former employee, that employee's file should be reviewed to be sure the information being given is factual.

WRITING LETTERS OF RECOMMENDATION

Occasionally employees will leave their jobs due to a move out of the area or to go back to school. Many of these employees will request a letter of recommendation from their employer, which they will use in seeking employment in the future (Figure ■ 4-12). These letters should contain only factual information and should not be written for any employee who was terminated due to performance concerns. Potential employers may view these letters of recommendation as endorsements of the employee and if it is later discovered that the employee was fired due to serious performance concerns (such as theft of drugs), the new employer may seek legal action against the person who wrote the letter of recommendation.

January 18, 2012

RE: Kay Cee Reeves

To Whom It May Concern:

I had the pleasure of working with Kay Cee Reeves here at Woodinville Pediatrics.

Kay Cee demonstrated a tremendous drive to do whatever needed to be done to take care of her patients throughout the day. Her ability to work both alone and within groups was unsurpassed, and her attention to detail, especially in the area of patient confidentiality will serve her future employer well.

I would recommend Kay Cee Reeves for any position she is applying for. She will make a valued asset to the medical office that recognizes her talents and abilities, and the patients she cares for will be fortunate to have her as their advocate.

Sincerely,

Christine Malone

Christine Malone, MHA
Medical Office Manager, Woodinville Pediatrics
(425) 555-9872

FIGURE ■ 4-12 Sample reference letter for an employee.

Maintaining the Employee Personnel File

To comply with federal and local laws, the employer must keep certain items in the employee's personnel file. These items include:

- A copy of the employee's Social Security card, passport, or other proof of citizenship
- The employee's application and/or résumé
- All performance evaluations
- Any disciplinary actions and performance improvement plans
- Copies of certifications or licenses
- Information about the employee's continuing education credits (if applicable)
- Information about Family Medical Leave Act (FMLA) leaves.

Employee personnel files are confidential and should not be accessed by anyone other than the manager. These files should be kept in a locked file cabinet, or in a secure area within the facility. When the employee is no longer employed at the facility, the personnel file should be moved to another location, but should not be destroyed. In the event the employee makes a legal allegation against the employer, or another employer calls for a reference, the personnel file must be accessed.

Case Study Questions

Refer to the case study presented at the beginning of this chapter to answer the following questions:

1. Once Svetlana has decided she needs to hire one medical assistant and a part-time receptionist, how should she go about finding those employees?
2. Would Svetlana use a different venue to advertise for the medical assistant than she would for the receptionist?
3. Who should Svetlana involve from her office in the interviewing process?

Chapter Review

Summary

- Determining staffing needs in a medical office is an exercise in knowing the scope of practice of employees and the abilities each employee will bring to the clinic.

- When writing a job description, the medical office manager should include both physical as well as mental tasks.

- Advertising for employees for the medical office may be done in newspapers, online, or by contacting local schools.

- The medical office manager will want to screen résumés of applicants to determine the best candidates to bring in for an interview.

- The medical office manager may choose to interview applicants individually or may choose to convene an interviewing committee for this task.

- Once candidates have been approved through the interviewing process, past employment or school references should be called.

- Background checks should be performed on all medical office staff members to ensure the safety of the patients.

- After determining the best candidate for a job, the office manager will need to call the candidate to make an offer of employment.

- Proper orientation of new employees helps prevent misunderstandings and errors in the future.

- When developing a training program for new employees, the medical office manager may choose to have the training done by one person or the training may be shared by multiple staff members.

- The medical office manager should use different supervisory techniques with different employees, depending on the needs of the employee and the situation. Sticking with only one management style may not work in all situations.

- Providing employee performance evaluations is key to giving appropriate feedback and direction to employees. These evaluations may be done once per year, or more frequently with newer employees.

- Disciplining employees for performance concerns must be done in a fair and respectful way. The goal is to improve performance, not to drive the employee away from the clinic.

- Employee assistance programs exist to provide employees help in times of crises. The programs may offer mental health counseling, financial counseling, or other forms of assistance at no cost to the employee.

- Immediate termination of an employee may be done for egregious things, such as abuse or theft. Other performance concerns should be first addressed with a disciplinary action, with termination considered only as a last resort.

- Responding to claims of sexual harassment is something the medical office manager will need to do in a timely manner. If these claims go unmanaged, the medical office is in danger of being sued by the person making the allegation.

- When giving references for former employees, the medical office manager must remain objective and provide only factual information.

- Employee personnel files are confidential and must be maintained even when the employee leaves the medical clinic's employment.

Multiple Choice

Choose the letter that best answers each question or completes each statement.

1. Which of the following items should be found in the employee's personnel file?
   a. A photograph of the employee
   b. A copy of the employee's application or résumé
   c. A copy of the employee's bank statement
   d. All of the above

2. When determining the staffing needs of the office, which of the following should the office manager consider?
   a. The length of time the physician spends with his patients
   b. The number of parking spaces available for staff
   c. The amount of time each employee has been working for the clinic
   d. The age at which each employee will retire

3. Which of the following items on a background check may be cause to reject an applicant for a job in a medical office?
   a. Two speeding violations in the past year
   b. An arrest for drunk drinking in the past year
   c. A conviction for drug possession two years ago
   d. An arrest for jay walking in the past 6 months

4. When interviewing applicants for a nursing position, which of the following behaviors might the office manager be concerned about?
   a. An applicant who arrives with her small child due to lack of daycare
   b. An applicant who arrives for the interview wearing sweatpants and a t-shirt
   c. An applicant who does not make eye contact during the interview process
   d. All of the above

5. Which of the following is a reason for giving an employee performance evaluation at 90 days of employment?
   a. To develop an improvement plan for any skills that have not been perfected yet
   b. To determine the appropriateness of a raise for the employee
   c. To give the mentor feedback about the employee's performance
   d. None of the above

6. The medical office manager is called for an employment reference for Bernard King. This employee was suspected of stealing drugs from the medical office and was subsequently fired for poor performance. Which of the following comments is **not** appropriate for the office manager to tell the caller?
   a. "Mr. King worked for this clinic from January 2009 to December 2010."
   b. "I'm sorry, we do not give out employee references."
   c. "We suspected Mr. King of stealing drugs in the clinic."
   d. "Mr. King was let go due to performance concerns."

7. When disciplining an employee for a performance concern, which of the following tasks should be completed?
   a. Meet with the employee in a private area.
   b. Have the employee participate in coming up with a performance improvement plan.
   c. Have the employee sign the warning and give him or her a copy.
   d. All of the above

8. Employee assistance programs may be used for which of the following employees?
   a. An employee who admits she has a drinking problem and would like help
   b. An employee who is stressed about her husband's unemployment
   c. An employee who has recently adopted a child from Brazil
   d. All of the above

9. When screening résumés, which of the following applicants should the office manager consider calling for an interview?
   a. An applicant who has held three jobs in the past 3 years
   b. An applicant who has made corrections on her résumé with ink
   c. An applicant who has misspelled a few words on the résumé
   d. An applicant who has had a 5-year gap between two jobs listed on the résumé

10. When terminating an employee's employment, which of the following should the office manager do?
   a. Let the employee know at the beginning of the day that he will need to work his shift and that this will be his last day.
   b. Accompany the employee to his work area to collect his things before escorting him from the building.
   c. Announce the employee's termination at the daily office meeting.
   d. Ask the employee to explain the reason for his termination to his coworkers.

True/False

Determine if each of the following statements is true or false.

_____ 1. All employers are required by federal law to give references on former employees.

_____ 2. Employees should be allowed to keep their own personnel files at their desks.

_____ 3. The same management style should be used with all employees in order to remain consistent.

_____ 4. The same interview questions should be asked of all applicants for the same position.

_____ 5. It is only necessary to call for references on employees who will be working with medications or money.

_____ 6. Only clinical staff members should be involved in group panel interviews.

_____ 7. A job description should contain information about the physical requirements of the position.

_____ 8. Training of new employees should be recorded.

_____ 9. Employee assistance programs are required of all employers.

_____ 10. Background checks are only required of physicians.

Matching

Match each of the following definitions with the appropriate statement or term.

a. a reason for an employee to be terminated immediately

b. a 90-day performance evaluation

c. a place to advertise for medical assistants

d. listed on the job application

e. the purpose for calling references

f. a way to determine staffing needs in the medical office

g. a job interview

h. a reason for a verbal or written warning

i. something kept in the employee personnel file

j. a reason for setting up a training program for new employees

1. Local medical assisting program

2. Consuming alcohol while working

3. Excessive tardiness

4. A copy of the employee's Social Security card

5. To make certain employee's understand the expectations for certain tasks

6. A venue to set up a performance improvement plan

7. Listing the amount of time a physician needs for each type of patient

8. To determine an applicant's prior work performance

9. The physical requirements of the job

10. Sitting down with and asking questions of a job applicant

Chapter Resources

Americans with Disabilities Act (ADA): www.ada.gov

Equal Employment Opportunity Commission (EEOC): www.eeoc.gov

Occupational Safety and Health Administration (OSHA): www.osha.gov

U.S. Department of Labor (DOL): www.dol.gov

PEARSON
myhealthprofessionskit™

Additional interactive resources for this chapter can be found at **www.myhealthprofessionskit. com.** Choose "Medical Assisting" from the discipline menu and then click on the book cover for *Medical Office Management.*

CHAPTER 5

Managing the Front Office

CHAPTER OUTLINE

- Telephone System Features
- Telephone Etiquette in the Medical Office
- Types of Incoming Calls to the Medical Office
- Telephone Triage
- Prioritizing Telephone Calls
- Emergency Telephone Calls
- Handling Difficult Callers
- Calls from Emotionally Upset Patients
- Documenting Calls from Patients
- Using an Answering Service
- Personal Phone Calls

- Calling Patients
- Using a Telephone Directory
- Making Long Distance or Toll Free Calls
- Calling in Prescriptions and Prescription Refill Requests
- Arranging for Translation Services
- Telecommunication Relay Systems
- Maintaining the Reception Area
- Greeting Patients in the Medical Office
- Visitors to the Medical Office

LEARNING OBJECTIVES

Upon completion of this chapter, you should be able to:

- Spell and define the key terms in this chapter.
- Describe the various features of telephone systems.
- Describe proper telephone etiquette in the medical office.
- Understand the types of incoming calls to the medical office.
- Outline how telephone triage is utilized in the medical office.
- Prioritize telephone calls according to urgency.
- Understand how to manage emergency telephone calls in the medical office.
- Describe various techniques for dealing with difficult callers in the medical office.
- List various ways for dealing with calls from emotionally upset patients.
- Document telephone calls from patients.
- Describe the purpose and function of using an answering service in the medical office.
- Understand the importance of incorporating a policy on employee use of the telephone for personal calls in the medical office.

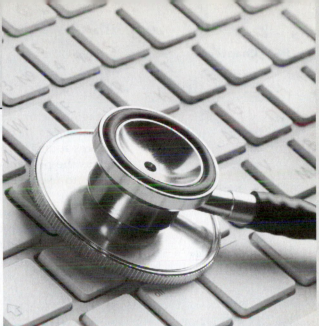

- Discuss protocol for caling patients, leaving messages, and calling other healthcare facilities.
- Describe the use of various telephone directories.
- Discuss office policy regarding long distance calls.
- Call in prescriptions via the telephone.
- Arrange for translation services in the medical office.
- Describe the functions of a telecommunication relay system.
- Understand the front office function of maintaining the reception area in the medical office.
- Describe how to greet patients in the medical office in a way that provides good customer service.
- Describe how to handle visitors who arrive in the medical office.

KEY TERMS

automated system	direct telephone line	new patient
automatic dialer	established patient	speaker telephone
automatic routing unit	hands-free headset	teletypewriter (TTY) system
call forwarding	hold feature	voice messaging system
conference call	last number redial	

Case Study

Take note of the following scenario and answer the case study question that appears at the end of this chapter.

Roxanne Martin is the office manager in a busy pediatric office. She has had several issues of patients complaining about the comfort of the waiting area. The complaints involve the issues of trash being left on the tables and the lack of magazines to read. In addition, patients have complained that they are not being kept aware of delays in their appointment times.

Introduction

Managing the front office of a medical facility includes thinking about both those patients who are seen in person and those who call on the telephone. The types of telephone features found in the medical office vary according to the size and type of practice, as well as the preferences of the physicians and management. Many telephone systems are simple to use and include features that are similar to those people have on their home telephones. In a larger healthcare facility, the telephone features tend to be more elaborate. Although these systems are more costly, they are often helpful in the management of calls, which improves patient satisfaction.

Another important part of managing the front desk in the medical office is the facility itself. Attention must be paid to the number and size of chairs for patient use, the type of reading material provided, and other details that may affect patients' experiences.

Telephone System Features

The telephone system features found in medical offices today are advanced, sophisticated units that require training before use. The telephone is often a patient's first point of contact with the medical office, so the person who answers the telephone must have a professional voice. The office should have a policy in place indicating when to answer the telephone—on the first ring, second ring, etc. In many medical offices, the telephone is set to ring no more than four times before the call is automatically transferred to a **voice messaging system**. This feature keeps the patient from waiting on the line indefinitely while the telephone rings. Because the person assigned to answer the telephones in the medical office may be occupied with other tasks, having a feature that allows the caller to go to a voice messaging system is one way to manage the workflow in the office.

In large medical offices, callers will be greeted by an **automated system**. This system typically plays a recorded message for the caller while the caller waits for the receptionist to pick up the line. Some systems offer the helpful feature of estimating for the patient how long the wait may be before his call is answered. Some medical offices may play recorded advertisements for services offered, such as smoking cessation classes, or the availability of evening and weekend appointments.

voice messaging system
an automated system that allows callers to leave a voice message for the intended recipient

automated system
a telephone answering system that automatically picks up a telephone call electronically

---

Critical Thinking 5.1 ?

What do you think the advantages are of having a receptionist answer the phone, as opposed to using an automated system?

---

hands-free headset
a telephone answering system that allows the user to have his or her hands free while talking on the phone

For the person who answers calls frequently in a medical office, a **hands-free headset** is an appropriate piece of equipment. With this device, the user is able to answer calls without having to pick up a handset. This device also allows for less stress on the body because the user is not required to hold a telephone handset between the ear and the shoulder—a common cause of neck and shoulder pain (Figure ■ 5-1).

Hands-free headsets may be wired directly to the telephone, or they may be wireless. With the wireless type, the user is able to get up and move around the office while using the telephone, rather than be tethered by the telephone cord. Wireless devices are especially helpful in a facility where the user may need to move from one location to another while using the telephone, such as a medical assistant, nurse, or office manager (Figure ■ 5-2).

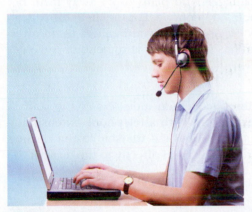

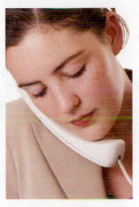

FIGURE ■ 5-1b
Holding the telephone
between the face and
shoulder may cause
neck and shoulder pain.
Source: © Nspimages/
Dreamstime.com.

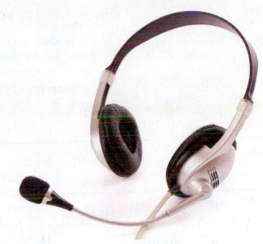

FIGURE ■ 5-2 A wireless telephone headset allows
users to move away from their desk while on the
telephone.
Source: © Jiri Hera/Fotolia.com.

FIGURE ■ 5-1a   Using a hands-free
headset.
Source: © Valuavitaly/Dreamstime.com.

LAST NUMBER REDIAL

The **last number redial** telephone feature offers the user the ability to press one button
when choosing to redial the last number called. With some telephone systems, this feature enables the user to continue to dial the last number until the call is answered. In very
sophisticated systems, the user may have the telephone system continue to dial the number and then alert the user when the call is eventually answered. This allows the user to
move on to other tasks, rather than wait for the call to be answered.

> **last number redial**
> a telephone feature
> that allows the user to
> redial the last number
> by pressing one button,
> rather than redialing the
> entire telephone number

CONFERENCE CALL

The **conference call** feature allows two or more parties to speak on the telephone at the
same time. This function is helpful in cases where the parties are unable to be in the same
location at once, yet verbal communication is required to avoid miscommunication. An
example would be a physician who wishes to give test results to a patient, and the patient
wishes to have a third party on the call to hear the results. When using this feature, especially if there are more than three parties on the call, each party should identify herself
before speaking in order to avoid confusion.

> **conference call**
> a telephone feature
> that allows numerous
> people to be on the same
> telephone call

SPEAKER TELEPHONE

Using the **speaker telephone** feature, two or more parties may be in the same room
while conversing with another party on the telephone. The physician may use this feature
to consult with another healthcare professional, while the patient is in the room listening.
When using the speaker telephone feature, it is common courtesy to alert the person on
the other end of the call to the presence of others in the room. HIPAA laws must be
observed while using this feature. If personal patient information is to be shared, all
persons involved must be authorized to hear the information, either by the patient or a
court order.

> **speaker telephone**
> a type of telephone that
> allows multiple people in
> a room to participate in
> the phone conversation

Critical Thinking 5.2 ❓

When using the speaker telephone feature, why do you suppose it is common courtesy to alert
the person on the other end of the call to the presence of others in the room (other than for
HIPAA reasons)?

CALL FORWARDING

call forwarding
a telephone feature that allows users to automatically forward calls to a different telephone number

The **call forwarding** feature is used to automatically route incoming calls to another telephone number. As an example, the office manager who plans to be away from her desk in meetings may forward her calls to her mobile telephone. For the main office telephone number, the call forwarding feature may be used to forward callers to an after-hours answering service once the reception team has gone home at the end of the day.

DIRECT TELEPHONE LINES

direct telephone line
a feature that allows callers to dial directly to the desk of a person in the office

Most medical offices assign **direct telephone lines** to certain members of the staff. A direct telephone line differs from a telephone extension. With a telephone extension, a caller calls the main office telephone number, then requests a transfer to the desired extension. With a direct telephone line, the caller is able to dial directly to the desk of the person he is trying to reach.

Critical Thinking 5.3 ?

What reasons can you think of for the medical office manager to give his direct telephone line number to a patient?

HOLD FEATURE

hold feature
a telephone feature that allows the receptionist to place the caller in a queue in order to take another call

The **hold feature** of telephone systems allows staff to place a caller on hold. This may be done prior to transferring the call to a particular extension, or it may be done when staff is occupied with other patients or callers and needs to place the newest caller on hold until free to take the call. Because callers cannot see what is going on in the medical office when they call, it is important to check back with callers when they are on hold, especially if the wait time will be longer than a minute.

Prior to placing any caller on hold, staff must make sure the call is not an emergency, and they must ask permission of the caller to be placed on hold.

MUSIC ON HOLD

Many telephone systems offer the ability to play music to callers while they are on hold. Some medical offices play recorded messages, such as advertisements for services offered in the facility. In the event the medical office chooses to play music to callers on hold, the music should be generic so as to avoid offending callers in any way. Religious music, for example, may be considered offensive by some callers and therefore should be avoided. If the medical office chooses to use a radio station for music while callers are on hold, staff should ensure that the station is dialed in clearly, so there is no static on the line to annoy callers while they hold.

SPECIAL FEATURES

automatic dialer
a telephone feature that allows users to automatically redial a number until someone answers the line

automatic routing unit
a telephone system that electronically answers and routes telephone calls after receiving a prompt from the caller

An **automatic dialer**, or speed dialer, is a telephone system feature that allows users to dial up to 100 programmed numbers with the push of one or two buttons, rather than dialing the entire number (Figure ■ 5-3). This is especially time-saving for those users who dial many of the same numbers frequently.

Automatic routing units are used in many medical facilities to allow callers to reach their desired party using only the automated system. These systems allow callers to choose an extension from a menu within an electronic system once their call is answered. With no receptionist answering the call, this type of system may seem less personal than others. Automatic routing units are efficient, however, and numerous callers may be assisted at the same time, without waiting for a receptionist to answer the call.

Larger healthcare facilities will often have telephone systems that allow managers to track the number of calls an individual is receiving and making during the day. This feature also allows the manager to see how long each call is in duration, and to compare employees to determine who is performing at the expected level and who may need additional training on the telephone system.

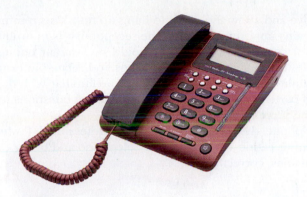

FIGURE ■ 5-3 Many office telephones feature an automatic dialer.
Source: © Johnkasawa/Dreamstime.com.

Voicemail

In many medical offices, voicemail is used for collecting telephone messages after hours or when the office staff is occupied with other patients. If the medical office manager chooses to use a voicemail feature, the message callers hear should start with a disclaimer asking them to hang up and dial 9-1-1 if the call is regarding a medical emergency. The following example is a typical recording for an office using voicemail: "You have reached Cedarwoods Family Practice. If this is a medical emergency, please hang up and dial 9-1-1. Our office hours are Monday through Friday from 9 a.m. to 5 p.m. Please leave your name, number, and reason for the call after the tone. Your call will be answered as soon as possible. Thank you and have a good day."

A staff member should be assigned to retrieve any voicemail messages as soon as the workload allows, and return calls in a timely manner.

Telephone Etiquette in the Medical Office

Because the telephone is often the caller's first contact with the medical office, serious attention must be paid to being professional when speaking with callers. Good telephone etiquette in the medical office includes answering the telephone by the fourth ring. This gives callers the impression that their call is important. When callers experience lengthy wait times on the telephone, they may become irritated and may even hang up.

The person answering the telephone in the medical office should answer the telephone with a smile. Because callers can determine the mood of a person answering the phone simply by the sound of the voice, the person answering the call must remain calm and professional at all times while on the telephone.

Proper telephone etiquette includes the use of good manners. Addressing the caller as "Mr. Jones" instead of by the caller's first name shows the caller that he is due a level of respect. The person answering the telephone in the medical office must use proper grammar and speak in a moderate tone at a moderate speed. Even if the caller is upset, the medical office staff must remain calm and professional and help seek solutions to assist the caller.

Answering calls professionally is an art form that all members of the medical office staff should master. Before answering any calls, the receptionist should obtain a pen and paper for taking notes, and answer the telephone with a cheerful, yet professional greeting. The receptionist should speak clearly and identify the office and herself. Some offices use physician names, whereas others use the names of their offices. Some offices even use original greetings, such as "It's a great day at Mountain View Clinic. This is Sara."

As soon as callers give their names, the receptionist should write those names down. Throughout patient calls, receptionists should refer to the callers by name, reinforcing that the callers are important. When a call has been completed, the receptionist should always say good-bye and allow the caller to hang up first. This reinforces the impression that the caller remains important and that the receptionist is in no hurry to move on.

In terms of call content, receptionists should be familiar enough with their office locations to be able to give most callers directions and related information such as parking fees and availability. Receptionists should also be familiar with the insurance plans in which their offices participate so they can answer patient questions in that arena. Printed lists near the phone serve as a good reference.

Even over the phone, the receptionist must be professional. Professionalism includes never chewing gum or eating while using the telephone and being careful to pronounce words, including names, correctly.

Types of Incoming Calls to the Medical Office

Although most of the calls received in a medical office are from patients or potential patients, other callers may include outside physicians or medical facilities. Vendors and suppliers are occasional callers to the medical office as well. Though the practice of receiving personal telephone calls should be discouraged, staff may receive these calls throughout the day. Understanding how to route these calls, and the urgency with which they may need to be routed, is something the medical office manager will need to properly train staff about.

SCREENING TELEPHONE CALLS

As part of their telephone duties, receptionists are charged with screening calls, which involves determining a call's purpose and whether that purpose is an emergency. To give receptionists solid guidelines, every medical office should have a written policy for screening calls.

DIRECTING PATIENT CALLS TO PHYSICIANS

Occasionally, the calls receptionists take are from parties who ask to speak with physicians directly. As a result, physicians should outline criteria for when they will accept patient calls. In addition to meeting physicians' needs and desires, such policies give receptionists guidelines for telephone use. Many physicians accept no telephone calls, even when not with patients. When a patient asks a physician to return a call, the receptionist should place the message with the patient's chart on the physician's desk.

In offices with several physicians, typically only one physician will be "on call" after hours, a role the physicians serve on a rotating basis. Any physician who is on call after hours must have some way of being reached. Due to the nature of the occupation, physicians must be available at all times, whether by telephone or pager. In addition to being readily available to the receptionist or other member of the medical staff, such numbers must be readily available to the office's answering service. When physicians do accept calls, the receptionist should gather a caller's name and reason for calling before transferring the call to the physician.

Telephone Triage

The ability to triage patient telephone calls, or place them into priority order, is something everyone who answers the telephone in the medical office must be trained to perform. To triage calls properly, those who answer calls must know the types of complaints that may be life threatening and, therefore, know when to transfer the call to a medical staff person, such as a nurse, or to call 9-1-1 for emergency services. Some life-threatening emergencies include:

- Chest pain
- Heavy bleeding after an injury
- Bleeding in a pregnant woman

- High fever in an infant or very young child
- Severe asthma attack
- Severe shortness of breath
- Possible poisoning or allergic reaction
- Obvious broken bone
- Sudden confusion, loss of consciousness, or change in mental status
- Mention of suicide or harm to themselves or others.

When answering telephone calls, staff should have a triage notebook available to them (Figure ■ 5-4). This notebook may be in printed form, such as in a three-ring binder, or it may be electronic and located on the office computer systems. Regardless of its form, the triage notebook is an algorithm for use in determining the severity of the call, which allows staff to properly route the caller. Included in the telephone triage notebook is a triage form (Figure ■ 5-5) that should be followed to ensure all appropriate questions are asked of the caller.

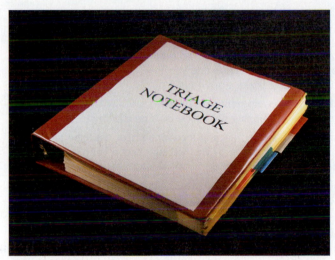

FIGURE ■ 5-4   A triage notebook.
Source: Dylan Malone/Pearson Education.

(Receptionist fills out this part) Message intake by:			
Date	Time	Patient Name	
Caller's Name (if not patient)		Reason for the call	
Relationship to patient		Other Medical Problems	
Phone #		Patient's Age	Weight
Work Phone #		Pregnant?	Primary Care Physician
Cell Phone #		From_____am/pm To_____am/pm	
Patient can be reached ☐ at home ☐ on cell ☐ at work			
(Nurse or Medical Assistant fills out this part) Problem/Assessment			
Medication refill (circle)		Medication	
Pharmacy Name		Phone #	
Follow up: ☐ ER referral ☐ Appointment made for _____ at _____. ☐ Physician to call. Physician called on _____ at _____. ☐ Pharmacy called. Refill ready at _____. ☐ Home health referral ☐ Specialist referral ☐ File			
Call returned by		Date/Time	Provider consulted

FIGURE ■ 5-5   Telephone triage form.

Prioritizing Telephone Calls

established patient
a patient who has established care in the medical office

new patient
any patient who has never been seen or has not been seen within the past 3 years by a provider in the facility

When taking more than one call at once, staff must be trained on how to prioritize calls. As a general rule, it is more efficient to take care of short telephone calls before longer ones. Shorter calls may be those from **established patients** calling to schedule an appointment or calls that merely need to be routed to another staff person. Longer calls may include those from **new patients** to the clinic or angry callers who may take up staff time in answering questions. A new patient is any patient who has never been seen or has not been seen within the past 3 years by a provider in the facility. Calls from angry patients should typically be addressed prior to other nonurgent callers. This is due to the nature of the call—remaining on hold, even for short periods of time, may cause an angry caller to become more agitated. Figure ■ 5-6 describes four calls to the medical office and the rationale for prioritizing them.

- ❏ **Line 1:** A mother is calling to schedule her 4-month-old child for a well-child checkup and vaccines. The office has not seen this child as a patient previously.
- ❏ **Line 2:** An equipment salesperson wants to speak with someone about equipping the office with new billing software.
- ❏ **Line 3:** An extremely angry patient states that she has been placed on hold twice by the "billing person" and has been disconnected both times.
- ❏ **Line 4:** A patient is calling to confirm the preoperative instructions he was given last week. His surgery appointment is for tomorrow morning.
- ❏ **Line 5:** A patient is calling for the results of her laboratory work done yesterday.

The receptionist should address Line 3 first, because the patient is very angry. To minimize the damage, the receptionist should apologize for the patient's inconvenience, secure the patient's return number, and advise the patient to expect a return call within an hour. The receptionist should contact the billing department immediately upon handling all other calls and make the request for a return call.

After the angry caller, the callers on Lines 4 and 5 take priority. The receptionist should route both to a clinical medical assistant or the nurse on staff. Line 2 is the next call in priority order. The receptionist should route this call to the office manager, and then turn to the caller on Line 1. The Line 1 caller comes last in this situation, because a new-patient call takes the longest to resolve.

FIGURE ■ 5-6   Prioritization of telephone calls.

Emergency Telephone Calls

When patients call their medical office while experiencing a true medical emergency, the reception staff must be trained in how to handle these emergent calls. Using the triage notebook, the receptionist will determine if the caller needs emergency assistance, rather than transfer to a clinical staff member. If a determination is made that the caller needs emergency help, the receptionist must stay on the line with the patient, while alerting a coworker to the need for assistance. While the receptionist gathers information from the patient, the coworker calls emergency services to request transport for the caller to the hospital. The receptionist should remain on the line with the caller until emergency transport services arrive. At that time, the receptionist should document the call in the patient's medical chart and alert the physician about the call.

Handling Difficult Callers

No matter how a caller behaves on the telephone, the staff member who answers the telephone must remain professional. On occasion patients will call their medical office while very upset. The most important thing the staff member who takes the call must do is remain calm. By speaking politely and remaining calm, the staff member should be able to disarm the angry caller. An apology should be made to the angry caller. This can be done without accepting blame for the actions that have caused the caller to be angry. For example, a staff member might say, "Mr. Jones, I am sorry you are upset about your bill. Let me see what I can do to help you." This language does not indicate that the person answering the call is at fault for the bill Mr. Jones has received. Apologizing to the caller is the easiest way to keep the patient's anger from escalating, and the apology often causes the caller to calm down and state her case without anger.

No one in the medical office is required to take abuse from patients—either in person or on the telephone. Therefore, if a caller continues to remain hostile on the telephone, or if he is calling the staff member names or swearing, the call may be ended. The language to use would be "Mr. Jones, I need you to stop yelling and calmly let me know what I can do to help you. If you do not stop yelling at me, I am going to have to end this call." If the abuse continues, the staff member should hang up the telephone, document the call in the patient's chart, and alert the physician or office manager about the call. In some cases, the office manager or physician may choose to call the patient back to see if the issue can be resolved.

Calls from Emotionally Upset Patients

Emotionally upset patients include those who are grieving or who have been in an accident. These patients may present a communication challenge when they call the medical office. In some cases, additional time is required to determine the purpose of the call and possibly even the identity of the caller. The staff member who receives such a call must first determine if the caller is experiencing a current medical emergency. If so, the call should be handled as outlined in the previous section.

HARD-TO-UNDERSTAND CALLERS

Part of acting like a professional includes listening to patients speak without interruption. When patients have speech impediments or their English is unclear, receptionists may have to ask those patients to repeat themselves. When confusion persists, receptionists should try repeating what they heard to see if the patients' messages were understood correctly.

Documenting Calls from Patients

Audio recording of telephone calls may only be done if the caller has been told of the recording. If a caller opts out of having her voice recorded, the medical office staff must respect that wish and cannot record the telephone call. Any time a patient calls the medical office and the call pertains to the patient's medical treatment, that call should be documented in the patient's medical record. Examples include:

- A patient calls to state he has been unable to take his medication due to side effects.
- A patient calls to say she has not filled her prescription due to financial restrictions.
- A patient calls to cancel upcoming appointments because he is feeling better.
- A patient's spouse calls to say the patient is in the hospital.
- A patient's daughter calls to say the patient is recently deceased.

In addition to documenting the call, the staff member should ensure that the physician sees the documentation. The physician may choose to contact the patient or the patient's family in these situations.

TAKING TELEPHONE MESSAGES

In medical offices where each staff member has his or her own extension, the receptionist need only transfer the call for a caller to leave a message. In clinics where direct extensions do not exist for all staff members, the receptionist will need to take a telephone message if a caller is asking for a particular individual on the staff. When taking a telephone message, all staff should be trained to take down the date and time of the call, the name of the caller (verifying spelling), the name of the person the caller wishes to reach, and the number where the call should be returned. As an added customer service touch, the staff member taking the call should alert the caller to any possible delays in the return call. For example, if the person the caller wishes to reach is out of the office on vacation for the next 2 weeks, the caller should be told that the call will not be returned until the person is back in the office.

Critical Thinking 5.4 ?

What problems can occur if a telephone message is missing important information?

Using an Answering Service

The telephone is an extremely important portal to the medical office. It is the mechanism by which patients and other customers and suppliers reach the office. Just as it is important to hire and train professional receptionists to answer the telephone, it is equally important to choose a professional answering service when the medical office chooses to use one. Many answering services specialize in medical office telephone services. The answering service must have current information on how to contact the physicians, including any information on the physician who is on call during off-hours. Many answering services will take messages from patients after hours, whereas others will simply offer information on the office hours or page the physician if the call is urgent.

Personal Phone Calls

Studies on businesses across the United States have found that the average employee spends 65 hours each year on personal telephone calls during work hours. This is very expensive for employers and, therefore, this practice is frowned on. Many employers feel that employee use of the telephone for personal calls during paid work hours is theft, and the activity may result in disciplinary action. The key to avoiding this practice is for the office manager to compose a policy on personal use of the telephone during paid office work hours. With such a policy on file, employees may be disciplined if their use of the telephone for personal calls exceeds what is allowed. From a customer service perspective, patients do not wish to see or hear a medical staff member on the telephone with a personal call while they wait to be assisted (Figure ■ 5-7).

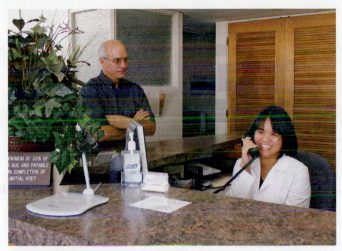

FIGURE ■ 5-7   Receptionists should not make personal calls while patients wait.
Source: Dylan Malone/Pearson Education.

Critical Thinking 5.5 ?

Why do you think patients may frown on medical office staff using the telephone for personal use?

Calling Patients

Before calling patients, medical staff should have all materials and information at hand, including the patients' medical charts. Staff who are calling patients to schedule appointments should be well versed in the times procedures take, as well as any special patient instructions, such as not eating for 12 hours before a particular visit. Any patient calls that are medically relevant must be charted in the patients' charts.

LEAVING MESSAGES

To be HIPAA compliant, medical staff must maintain confidentiality at all times, including while on the telephone. When leaving messages, for example, staff must remember that the people taking those messages, such as the patients' spouses or parents of minors seeking treatment for pregnancy, sexually transmitted infections, mental illnesses, or drug and alcohol counseling may lack the patients' permission to know the nature of the calls.

When medical staff must leave messages for patients, those staff members should leave their names, the physicians' names, and the appropriate telephone numbers. When an office's name self-identifies, such as "Marysville Oncology Specialists" or "Monroe Women's Care and Family Planning Clinic," the medical staff should not leave the office name as part of the message, because doing so discloses some of the patient's confidential information. Instead, medical staff should leave the names of physicians only, as in "This is John calling from Dr. Waddelow's office. I'm leaving a message for Jose. Please call me at 555-123-4567."

CALLING OTHER HEALTHCARE FACILITIES

Medical office staff often need to call other healthcare facilities involved in the care of mutual patients, whether to schedule appointments with specialists or obtain information from patients' primary care providers. Whatever the reason for the call, the medical staff must maintain patient confidentiality at all times. This means disclosing only absolutely necessary information to the other office staff when placing the call. If the medical staff member is scheduling a patient with a specialist, for example, that staff member will need to provide the patient's contact and insurance information. Other private patient information, like lifestyle habits and payment history, should not be disclosed.

Using a Telephone Directory

In the past, a "telephone directory" usually meant a "telephone book," but today several different companies produce telephone books. The medical office may have one book for white pages and one for yellow pages, for example. When a medical office is in a large metropolitan area, it may have several books to cover its surrounding areas. Listings in the white pages are alphabetical by a person's last name. In the yellow book they are alphabetical by business type. Most telephone books create sublistings for business types, as well. For example, under the directory for physicians there may be an alphabetical listing of physicians by type, such as pediatricians or oncologists.

Most telephone directories are color coded for ease of use. Many precede their white pages with business sections in different colors. Directories typically have listings for local ZIP codes at their beginnings and a government section that includes listings for federal, state, and local agencies. These pages are typically colored differently; very often they are blue.

USING AN ONLINE DIRECTORY

Many medical offices today use the Internet to look up telephone numbers. Many websites, for example, www.Yahoo.com, can search local and national telephone directories for both personal and business information.

USING A ROLODEX™ SYSTEM

Every medical office should keep a directory of commonly called telephone numbers on the computer or in a Rolodex card file (Figure ■ 5-8). Such tools make it easier to locate the number for the cardiac specialist the physician refers patients to, for example.

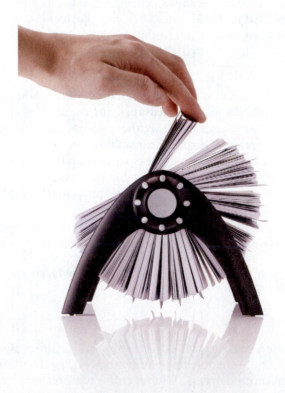

FIGURE ■ **5-8**   Rolodex™ systems may be used to store commonly used numbers.
Source: © Mingusen/Dreamstime.com.

Making Long-Distance or Toll-Free Calls

The medical staff may frequently make long-distance telephone calls on behalf of the medical office. Some offices require staff to log the purpose of any long-distance telephone calls, as well as the names and numbers of the parties being called. To comply with such requests, medical staff should familiarize themselves with their offices' policies.

Most suppliers and businesses the medical office buys from will have toll-free telephone numbers, which means they typically begin with 1-800, 1-888, or 1-866 and impose no charges on callers.

Calling in Prescriptions and Prescription Refill Requests

Many medical offices today require patients to call their pharmacy for medication refills, rather than call the office directly. The purpose for this practice is to eliminate the possibility for any confusion regarding the medication the patient needs refilled. When the patient calls the pharmacy directly for a refill, the pharmacy either calls or faxes the medical office with a prescription refill request. When this happens, the medical assistants or receptionists can forward the refill request to the physician for approval or denial.

In the event the patient calls the office directly for a prescription change or refill request, the staff member who takes the call must write down all important information. This would include:

■ Name and telephone number of the patient

■ Birth date of the patient

■ Name of the medication

■ Name and telephone number of the pharmacy.

This information should be given to the physician so she can make a decision about whether the prescription should be filled.

Arranging for Translation Services

Some patients coming in for medical care do not speak English. This is more common in areas where the population includes large groups of immigrants. Typically, it is the medical office's responsibility to arrange for translation services for the patient. When scheduling such a patient, the receptionist must determine the language the patient speaks in order to arrange for an interpreter. Contact information for local interpretation services should be kept near every receptionist desk station. The receptionist is the one who typically calls to arrange for this service.

In communities where there is a large population of immigrants from a certain area, the office manager may consider hiring staff who speak both English and the language of the immigrant group. This enables the medical office to use the staff member for translation in the event the official translator does not arrive on time or at all.

Ethical and legal problems can arise when patients use a family member or friend as a translator during a medical visit. The friend or family member has no legal or ethical obligation to translate exactly what the patient and the provider say and, therefore, may choose to edit certain items out of the conversation. This can pose a problem if the patient is not given the exact information she needs for proper care. Because of this possible conflict, most medical offices do not allow friends or family members of the patient to perform translation services during a medical visit.

Telecommunication Relay Systems

Patients who have hearing or speech impairments may use a telecommunication relay system to contact the medical office. The Americans with Disabilities Act requires that telephone companies have telecommunication relay systems available 24 hours per day, 365 days per year. A telecommunication relay system works in the following way:

1. The caller types a message into a special telephone.

2. The message transmits to the relay service.

3. An operator calls the medical office.

4. When the receptionist answers, the operator self-identifies and identifies the caller.

5. The operator then mediates between the receptionist and the caller, reading messages to the receptionist and typing responses to the caller.

6. When the call is complete, the receptionist says goodbye to the patient, then hangs up.

teletypewriter (TTY) system
a telephone system that allows for communication with a person who has a hearing impairment

Any medical office with a large number of patients with hearing impairments (e.g., an audiology practice) may have a **teletypewriter (TTY) system** (Figure ■ 5-9). TTY systems connect to the telephone, allowing both parties to the call to type their responses and thereby eliminate the need for a telecommunication relay service.

When using services such as these, note that conversations are aimed at the caller, not the operator. The operator will type every word exactly as spoken. In other words, the receptionist should not say, "Tell Monique that her appointment will be Thursday, the second, at noon." Instead, the receptionist should say, "Monique, your appointment will be Thursday, the second, at noon."

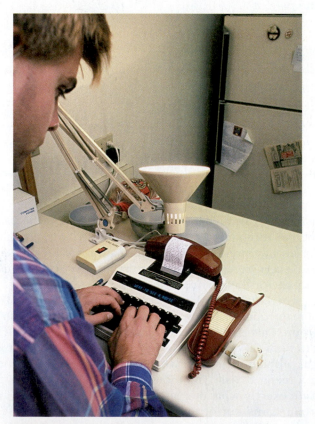

FIGURE ■ 5-9   Callers who have hearing impairments may use a TTY system for telephone calls.
Source: Michael Newman/PhotoEdit, Inc.

Maintaining the Reception Area

The reception room should be quiet and peaceful. Patients who are waiting for appointments should be able to sit calmly, undisturbed by loud noises and other distractions. In addition to being quiet, the reception area must be kept clean and free of hazards. To attain this goal, receptionists should be trained to check the reception area to be sure it is clean, free from odors, and clutter-free throughout the day, and to retrieve any lost or forgotten items. The receptionists may need to ask children to be quiet or instruct patients to take food outside.

Most medical offices play some form of relaxing music in their reception areas. In many medical offices, sick patients may be segregated from those who are not sick. This is done to reduce the spread of infectious viruses. In medical offices where children are seen, a separate waiting area, or portion of the main waiting area, may exist for children. These areas will often be populated with toys and books for children or a television that plays children's movies. Care must be taken to ensure that any toys kept in the reception room are safe for children of all ages. Toys must be large enough so that small parts cannot be swallowed by very young children, which could create a choking hazard. Toys must be easy to clean and must not contain any sharp edges. Many states have passed legislation regarding mandatory cleaning of toys. In Washington State, for example, toys must be cleaned with a 10% bleach solution after every use. Laws such as these are designed to limit the spread of germs from one child to another.

READING MATERIAL IN THE RECEPTION AREA

The material available for patients to read while they wait for their appointment should reflect the demographic of the patients seen. In a pediatric office, reading material might consist of magazines catering to parents or working women. In a geriatric practice, magazines might be those catering to retired persons, such as travel and cooking magazines. Many medical offices keep educational material in the reception area for patients to read. This material will be geared toward the medical conditions most commonly seen in a particular practice. For example, an orthopedic practice may display educational material about sports injuries or how to care for a cast or arm splint.

SEATING IN THE MEDICAL OFFICE RECEPTION AREA

To ensure patient comfort, the reception room should have an adequate amount of comfortable, easy-to-clean furniture. Experts in medical office space planning believe medical offices should have enough seating to accommodate at least 1 hour's worth of patients per physician, as well as the friends or relatives who accompany those patients. The furniture should be at a level from which most patients can rise easily and without assistance. Many offices have coat racks for patients' coats or umbrellas.

Practice type dictates the reception room's décor. For example, a pediatrician's practice would have a very different reception room than a practice that caters to the elderly. A pediatric practice should have videos and toys, whereas a practice that caters to geriatric patients might have a fish tank or other soothing decorations.

Critical Thinking 5.6 ?

Why might a medical office choose to have a separate waiting area for patients who are accompanied by children?

Greeting Patients in the Medical Office

When patients arrive in the reception area of the medical office, the receptionist should greet them right away. If the receptionist is busy with other tasks when the patient arrives, the receptionist should look up and smile at the patient and hold up an index finger to indicate a slight delay in service (Figure ■ 5-10).

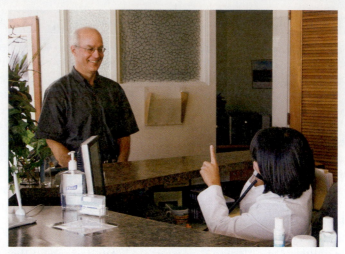

FIGURE ■ 5-10   The receptionist indicates she will be with the patient momentarily.
Source: Dylan Malone/Pearson Education.

To maintain patient privacy in the reception area, the reception desk should be slightly away from the seated patients. This way, the patient can converse with the receptionist without being overheard by other patients.

When greeting a new patient to the practice, the receptionist should orient the patient to the office by offering information on the location of the restroom and coat rack, and where to find reading materials. When greeting established patients, the receptionist should confirm that all information on file remains the same as the last visit. When patients' insurance information has changed, the receptionist may photocopy the new insurance card for routing to the billing office staff.

Critical Thinking 5.7 ?

Why do you suppose the receptionist should greet the patient right away? How might the patient feel if the receptionist does not look up when the patient approaches the desk?

ADMINISTERING PAPERWORK AT THE FRONT DESK

When patients arrive in the medical office, the receptionist gives them any necessary paperwork to complete, noting the location for any signatures. New patients will typically be given a history form (Figure ■ 5-11) to complete. This form provides the medical office with the patients' medical, personal, and family health history. When giving patients any paperwork to complete, the receptionist should also supply the patient with a clipboard and a pen.

Critical Thinking 5.8 ?

How might the receptionist handle a patient who arrives without his glasses and, therefore, cannot fill out the needed paperwork?

COLLECTING PAYMENTS AT THE FRONT DESK

The best time to collect payment from the patient is while the patient is in the office. (See Chapter 13 for more information on collections in the medical office.) If the patient has a known copayment of a certain amount, the receptionist should be trained in collecting that copayment at the time of the patient's visit. A script such as "Mrs. Velazquez, your

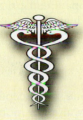

Victory Medical Center
4100 SW Highway 6
Victorville, WA 12345
(509) 555-9832

Patient Name: _____
    Last Name   First Name   Middle Initial

Address: _____
    Street   City   State   Zip

Home Phone: _____ Work Phone: _____

Mobile Phone: _____ Birthdate: _____

Social Security Number: _____ Age: _____

Sex: _____ Marital Status: S M D W Children: _____

How do you prefer to be addressed? _____

Spouse's Name: _____

Primary Care Physician: _____ Phone No.: _____

Name of Person Responsible for Bill: _____

Relationship to Patient: _____ Phone No.: _____

Address of Person Responsible for Bill: _____

Patient's Employer: _____ Phone No.: _____

Occupation: _____

Spouse's Employer: _____ Phone No.: _____

Occupation: _____

INSURANCE INFORMATION

Primary Insurance: _____ Policy No.: _____

Name of Policyholder: _____ Birthdate: _____

SS#: _____ Relationship to Insured: _____

Secondary Insurance: _____ Policy No.: _____

Name of Policyholder: _____ Birthdate: _____

If Injured: Date: _____ Place: _____

Claim Number: _____ Nature or Cause of Injury: _____

Employer at Time of Injury: _____ Phone No.: _____

EMERGENCY INFORMATION

In case of emergency, local friend or relative to be notified (not living at same address)

Name: _____ Relationship to Patient: _____

Address: _____ Phone No.: _____

I hereby authorize the healthcare professionals in this clinic to diagnose and treat my condition. I clearly understand and agree that all services rendered me are charged directly to me and that I am personally responsible for payment. I agree that I am responsible for all bills incurred at this clinic. I hereby authorize assignment of my insurance rights and benefits directly to the provider for services rendered. I also authorize the healthcare professionals to discuss my care with other healthcare providers who I am currently treating with.

_____   _____
Patient's Signature   Date   Parent or Guardian Signature   Date

FIGURE ■ 5-11 Patient history form.

insurance copayment today will be $30. Would you like to take care of that via cash, check, or credit card?" Most medical offices ask patients to pay their copayment prior to being seen by the physician. This prevents the possibility of the patient leaving the office after the visit without having paid the amount due.

NOTIFYING PATIENTS OF DELAYS

When a delay occurs and the patient will not be seen at her appointed time, the receptionist should alert the patient to that delay. Some medical facilities use a wait-time monitor (Figure ■ 5-12) to indicate any delays on behalf of the physician. Even if this system is used, the receptionist should be proactive and verbally alert patients if the provider is running behind. This practice lets the patients know that their time is important, and it offers patients the opportunity to get a cup of coffee or go to the car to get a book if they want to. If the physician is running far behind schedule, patients who have not yet arrived should be called and given the opportunity to reschedule or come at a later time. This is done as a courtesy to the patient and an acknowledgment that the patient's time is considered valuable.

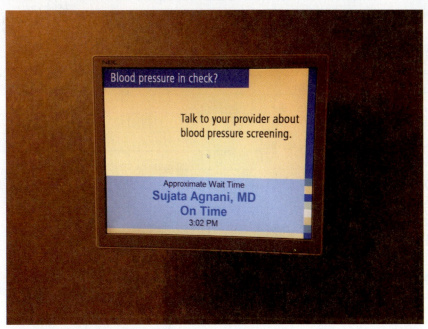

FIGURE ■ 5-12 A wait-time monitor.
Source: Christine Malone.

Visitors to the Medical Office

Staff entertaining visitors in the medical office should be kept to a minimum. HIPAA legislation dictates that any personal patient information shared in the medical office is kept confidential. Having visitors in the patient care areas could be considered a HIPAA violation. If staff needs to entertain a visitor while they are working, the staff member should go to the waiting area or outside the building to have the needed conversation. Visitors should be not allowed in patient care areas if they are not there as patients themselves.

Case Study Question

Refer to the case study presented at the beginning of this chapter to answer the following question:

In what ways might Roxanne address the patients' issues about garbage in the waiting area and the lack of reading materials?

Chapter Review

Summary

- The telephones in the medical office offer a host of features, including last number redial, conference calls, speaker telephone, and call forwarding.

- Proper telephone etiquette is important for anyone on the medical office team who uses the telephone.

- Although most calls coming into the medical office are from patients or potential patients, other types of calls are also received. The receptionist should be aware of how to handle each type of call in order to process the calls properly.

- Telephone triage is the practice of determining the urgency of a caller's needs.

- Telephone calls should be prioritized according to the needs of the caller, as well as the time it will take to accomplish the call.

- Emergency telephone calls must be handled with the patient's safety at the forefront of thought.

- Difficult callers may present a challenge to the medical office team. By remaining calm, these callers may be disarmed.

- Calls from emotionally upset patients may require more of the receptionist's time to determine the purpose of the call.

- Any calls from patients that pertain to the patient's medical care should be documented in the patient's medical chart.

- Choosing an answering service should include research into the type of clients the service works with. Answering services that work with other medical providers are typically good choices to work with in that they will better understand patients' needs.

- A policy should be written for employee use of the office telephone for personal use. Allowing employees to use the telephone during patient hours may offend patients who are waiting to be helped.

- Medical staff members must pay great attention to patient privacy when calling patients. No medical information must be shared with anyone other than the patient.

- Medical office staff should be trained in the use of telephone directories in order to efficiently and accurately find the desired information.

- Patients are typically required to call their pharmacy to ask for prescription refills, rather calling the medical office directly.

- Arranging for translation services is a task required of the medical office. For ethical and legal reasons, the patients' family or friend should not perform this task.

- Telecommunication relay systems are used to enable patients with hearing impairments to communicate with the medical office.

- The reception area must be maintained as a professional environment. This includes picking up garbage and ensuring that appropriate and adequate reading material is available.

- A professional receptionist should greet patients in the medical office. Patients must know that they are important to the office and be treated in a respectful manner.

- Visitors to the medical office must not be allowed into clinical areas in order to maintain patient privacy.

Multiple Choice

Choose the letter that best answers each question or completes each statement.

1. The best time to collect a patient copayment is:
   a. when the patient arrives at the front desk.
   b. when the physician enters the exam room.
   c. when the patient is leaving the office.
   d. via the mail.

2. Which of the following patients may be asked to sit in the sick patient area of the reception room?
   a. A pregnant patient
   b. A mother bringing in her 4-month-old baby for vaccinations
   c. A patient coming in to have a cast removed
   d. A patient with symptoms of influenza

3. A non–English-speaking patient comes into the office for care. Which of the following persons is appropriate to use for translating during the visit?
   a. The interpreter who was scheduled by the office receptionist prior to the visit
   b. The patient's spouse
   c. The patient's parent
   d. All of the above

4. An emotionally upset patient calls into the medical office. What is the first thing the receptionist must do?
   a. Ask the caller to calm down.
   b. Place the caller on hold and transfer the call to the office manager.
   c. Alert a coworker to call for emergency services on another telephone line.
   d. None of the above.

5. A patient calls the medical office requesting a refill of his prescription. He does not remember the name of the medication. How might the receptionist handle this call?
   a. Ask the patient to call his pharmacy to begin the refill process.
   b. Let the patient know the receptionist cannot help him unless he provides the name of the medication.
   c. Tell the patient the policy is to have 48 hours notice for any prescription refill.
   d. Call the patient's pharmacy to ask what medications the patient is taking.

6. The physician is running 1 hour behind schedule. What is the best way for patients to be told of the delay?
   a. The receptionist should alert the patients to the delay as the patients arrive at the front desk.
   b. The receptionist should update the wait-time monitor in the reception room so patients will see there is a delay when they enter the office.
   c. The receptionist should call patients who have not yet arrived to alert them to the delay and give them the opportunity to reschedule or arrive later.
   d. The medical assistant should go out to the reception room every few minutes to make an announcement about the delay.

7. A caller to the medical office is abusive and begins cursing at the receptionist. What should the receptionist do?
   a. Hang up on the caller without saying anything.
   b. Place the caller on hold and check back every few minutes to see if the caller has calmed down.
   c. Let the caller know he cannot be helped if he does not calm down.
   d. Curse back at the caller.

8. The average worker spends how many hours a year on personal telephone calls during work hours?
   a. 45   b. 55
   c. 65   d. 75

9. Which of the following types of music is most appropriate for playing while callers are on hold?
   a. Religious music
   b. Rap music
   c. News talk radio
   d. Easy listening music

10. Which of the following patient telephone calls to the medical office should be charted in the patient's medical record?
    a. A patient who calls to make arrangements to pay her bill in monthly installments
    b. A patient who calls to reschedule her appointment from this Friday to next week
    c. A patient who calls to say she cannot afford to fill her prescription and therefore will not be able to take her medication
    d. A patient who calls to complain that there are not enough handicapped parking spaces in the clinic parking lot

True/False

Determine if each of the following statements is true or false.

_____ 1. An established patient is one who has never been seen in the medical office previously.

_____ 2. Typically, it is the medical office's responsibility to arrange for translation services for the patient.

_____ 3. A call from an emotionally upset patient may take longer to process than a call from a calm caller.

_____ 4. Whenever using the speaker telephone feature, it is common courtesy to alert the person on the other end of the call to the presence of others in the room.

_____ 5. Hand-free headsets may be wired directly to the telephone or they may be wireless.

_____ 6. No matter how the caller behaves on the telephone, the staff member who answers the telephone must remain professional.

_____ 7. Chewing gum while answering the telephone in the medical office is considered unprofessional.

_____ 8. Audio recording of telephone calls may only be done if the caller has been told of the recording.

_____ 9. Prior to placing any caller on hold, staff must make sure the call is not emergent and they must ask permission of the caller to be placed on hold.

_____ 10. When answering telephone calls, staff should have a triage notebook available to them.

Matching

Match each of the following terms with its definition.

a. automated system

b. automatic dialer

c. speaker telephone

d. triage

e. last number redial

f. conference call

g. automatic routing units

h. hands-free headset

i. direct telephone lines

j. hold feature

1. A telephone feature that allows users to automatically redial a number until someone answers the line

2. A telephone answering system that automatically picks up a telephone call electronically

3. A telephone feature that allows numerous people to be on the same telephone call

4. A system of allowing callers to dial directly to the desk of the person in the office

5. A telephone system that electronically answers and routes the telephone call after receiving a prompt from the caller

6. An automated system that places callers in a queue until the receptionist is free to pick up the call

7. A telephone answering system that allows the user to have his or her hands free

8. A system that allows the user to redial the last number by pressing one button, rather than redialing the entire telephone number

9. A system of determining if the patient's needs are life threatening

10. A telephone system feature that allows multiple people in a room to participate in a phone conversation

Chapter Resources

Documenting patient telephone calls: www.rmf.harvard.edu

Medical center telephone systems: www.hcwt.com/

PEARSON
myhealthprofessionskit™

Additional interactive resources for this chapter can be found at **www.myhealthprofessionskit. com.** Choose "Medical Assisting" from the discipline menu and then click on the book cover for _Medical Office Management._

CHAPTER 6

Appointment Scheduling

CHAPTER OUTLINE

- Scheduling New Patient Appointments
- New Patient versus Established Patient Appointments
- Allowing the Appropriate Amount of Time for Appointments
- Convenient Scheduling
- Computer Scheduling versus Paper Appointment Books
- Types of Appointment Scheduling
- The Appointment Schedule as a Legal Document
- Allowing for Unforeseen Appointments

- Triage and Appointment Scheduling
- Appointment Reminder Systems
- Making Corrections to the Appointment Schedule
- No-Show Appointments
- Achieving the Most Efficient Scheduling System
- Managing the Physician's Professional and Travel Schedule
- Scheduling Hospital Services and Admissions
- Arranging Transportation for Patients

LEARNING OBJECTIVES

Upon completion of this chapter, you should be able to:

- Spell and define the key terms in this chapter.
- Describe the process of scheduling new patient appointments.
- Define a new patient and an established patient.
- Understand the purpose of allowing the appropriate amount of time for patient appointments.
- Describe techniques for scheduling patients at times that are best for the medical office.
- Outline the pros and cons of paper versus computer appointment scheduling.
- Define the various types of appointment scheduling in the medical office.
- Understand the concept of the appointment schedule as a legal document.
- Allow for unforeseen appointments when scheduling.
- Describe how triage works in scheduling appointments.
- Describe how appointment reminder systems are utilized.

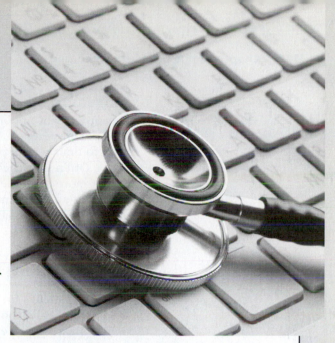

- Discuss the procedure for correcting the appointment schedule.
- Define a no-show appointment, and outline the steps for following up on no-show appointments in the medical office.
- Understand how to achieve an efficient scheduling system.
- Manage the physician's professional and travel schedule.
- Schedule hospital services and admissions.
- Arrange transportation for patients.

KEY TERMS

appointment reminder cards	fixed appointment scheduling	slack time
buffer time	matrix	wave scheduling
cluster scheduling	modified wave scheduling	
double booking	open hours scheduling	

Case Study

Take note of the following scenario and answer the case study questions that appear at the end of this chapter.

Tully West is a medical office manager working with a group of pediatric physicians. Each physician has a different schedule for clinic hours, and each physician has different requirements for how long they would like to see a particular type of patient.

Introduction

The process of appointment scheduling will vary with the type of practice, as well as provider preference. Whereas some providers prefer longer appointment types or may want to limit certain patient or visit types, other providers may have very different preferences. Often the scheduling of appointments in the medical office requires the coordination of more than one schedule. For example, a patient may need to see the provider and also have an x-ray and blood work done. These three portions of the patient's one visit may require coordination of three schedules.

Scheduling New Patient Appointments

The new patient's first encounter with the medical office is typically over the telephone. When these calls come in, they should be answered in a timely manner and the receptionist must be professional as well as friendly. Each medical office will have a list of items that must be collected from a new patient at the time an appointment is scheduled. Most commonly, these items are:

- The patient's legal, full name—with spelling verified
- The patient's birth date
- The patient's home, work, and mobile telephone numbers
- The reason for the patient's visit to the office
- The length of time the patient has had the condition
- The name of the patient's referring physician, if applicable
- The patient's insurance type
- The patient's need for directions to the medical office.

While on the telephone, the receptionist should alert the new patient to any policies that apply in that medical office. These policies may include:

- The need for the patient to provide photo identification at the time of the visit
- The need for payment from the patient at the time services are rendered
- The need for a copy of the patient's insurance identification card at the time of the visit
- The need for copies of laboratory reports or x-rays, if applicable
- The expected arrival time for the patient for the appointment.

The receptionist should let the new patient know of any specifics regarding parking for the facility, including the costs, as well as the location of the office in the event the clinic is not located in its own freestanding building. Most of this information can be gathered in a few minutes on the telephone, and it is important for the patient to not feel as if their type of insurance or ability to pay is the most important item of information collected.

Critical Thinking 6.1 ?

Why is it important for the patient to not feel as if his or her type of insurance or ability to pay is the most important item of information collected?

After collecting the needed information from the patient, the receptionist should verify the date and time of the appointment once again before ending the call. Once the call is complete, the receptionist may begin building the patient information in the paper or electronic medical record. This will typically include verification of the patient's insurance information so that an accurate copayment amount can be collected from the patient at the time of the visit.

Many medical offices choose to mail information to the new patient prior to his visit. This may include any necessary paperwork that the new patient will be required to complete for the physician. If the medical office has a brochure, it should be included when mailing information to the new patient (Figure 6-1). When offices send information to the patient prior to the first visit, the receptionist should alert the patient to this at the time of the telephone call. Patients should be told to complete the paperwork and to bring it with them to their scheduled visit.

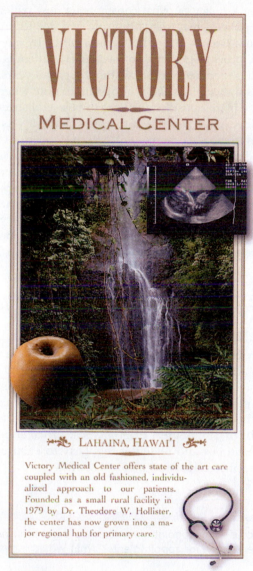

FIGURE ■ 6-1 Sample medical office brochure.
Source: Christine Malone.

Today, many medical offices have their own website on the Internet. These websites are a convenient place to host any paperwork that patients will need to fill out. Callers with access to a computer and printer may then be directed to the website and asked to download any necessary forms for completion prior to the first visit. It is also possible for patients to fill out information online and submit forms electronically in some medical facilities, thereby eliminating the need for paper to be printed or mailed.

New Patient Versus Established Patient Appointments

Most medical offices have a policy on what constitutes a new patient versus an established patient. However, those policies may vary from one practice to another. Generally, a new patient is one who has not been seen in the medical office by any of the providers in the same specialty within the previous 3 years. An established patient is one who has been seen by one of the providers in the same specialty within the past 3 years. This rule applies when billing patients' health insurance plans and is important to note when assigning billing codes to patient visits. Insurance plans consider a patient to be established, even if the patient was seen by a different provider in the practice, if the previous visit was within the past 3 years.

An exception to this applies to the patient who has been involved in an accident or injury, such as a car accident or on-the-job injury. Those patients will need to undergo a full examination as if they are new to the practice, in order to fully determine the extent of their injuries. Many medical offices that use paper medical charts keep patients' accidental injury files separate from those patients' general medical files. Then, when insurance companies request copies of patients' medical records due to accidental injury, the copying task is far easier. With electronic medical records, this separation can still be accomplished by electronically indicating which information belongs with the injury portion of the patients' files.

Allowing the Appropriate Amount of Time for Appointments

The amount of time needed for patient appointments depends on the type of practice and the preference of the healthcare providers. Table 6-1 lists general appointment types and the times allowed for each type of appointment. In typical offices, new patients are normally seen for longer periods than established patients. For example, a new patient appointment may be scheduled for 45 minutes, whereas an established patient appointment may be for only 10 or 15 minutes. Each medical office should document its policy for allotting appointment times and review it regularly to ensure that it continues to be appropriate for patients, physicians, and medical staff.

TABLE ■ 6-1   Time Allotted for Patient Appointments

Appointment Type	Allotted Time (in minutes)
New patient	30
Physical exam	60
Routine checkup	15
Well-child checkup	15
Blood pressure check	5

Many physicians prefer to limit certain types of appointments on any given day. For example, a pediatrician may only want to see one or two sports physicals in a day. An OB/GYN physician may only want to see one or two new maternity patients in a day. Again, documented policies are beneficial because they can clarify physicians' preferences and help the receptionist schedule appointments properly. If, for example, the pediatrician will only allow two sports physicals a day, the office may schedule those appointments for 10 a.m. and 3 p.m. Once those appointments are filled, the receptionist can easily see that the schedule will support no more sports physicals that day.

Critical Thinking 6.4 ?

Why do you think some physicians would want to limit certain appointment types seen on a particular day?

CREATING AN APPOINTMENT MATRIX

The process of scheduling medical office appointments begins with an appointment **matrix**. An appointment matrix, which can be used with both paper and computerized appointment schedules, depicts the appointment times available in the medical office. Receptionists block out the times on the matrix when physicians are unavailable due to hospital rounds, vacations, or holidays. When appointment matrices are paired with appointment systems, receptionists can also block times for certain pieces of equipment so equipment conflicts do not arise.

matrix
a system for mapping out the appointment times available in the medical office

Depending on the type of practice or the specialties of the physicians, receptionists use certain abbreviations in their matrix notations. Within an office, however, these abbreviations must be standard so that all members of the healthcare team can interpret the abbreviations accurately.

Critical Thinking 6.5 ?

Why do you think it is important for the medical office staff to use the same abbreviations throughout the office? What could happen if different abbreviations were used by various staff members?

Every office has a few patients who need extended appointment times due to disability or complex health issues. Staff should note these unique requirements on the patients' paper or electronic records so that the staff member who is scheduling appointments can allot appropriate amounts of time.

Convenient Scheduling

When receptionists schedule appointments, they must pay attention to patients' needs. For example, receptionists should schedule patients who need fasting blood draws at the beginning of the day. Just as receptionists should heed patient needs, they should factor in what is appropriate for the office. For example, if the office has only one electrocardiogram (ECG) machine, it would be inappropriate for the receptionist to schedule two patients who need the machine at once. When only one staff member performs a certain procedure or test, the receptionist must keep that person's availability in mind when scheduling appointments.

Computer Scheduling Versus Paper Appointment Books

Today, most large medical offices use computer software to manage their patient appointments (Figure 6-2). Electronic appointment scheduling offers many advantages. With computerized systems, several staff members can access the appointment schedule at once and from different locations in the office. Some computerized systems allow staff and/or physicians to access the appointment schedule from outside the office.

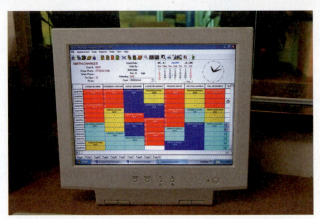

FIGURE ■ 6-2 Computerized appointment book screenshot.
Source: Michal Heron/Pearson Education.

Another advantage of using an electronic appointment book is the ability to easily read the information. With paper appointment books, handwriting may sometimes be difficult to discern.

Critical Thinking 6.6 ?

Imagine the receptionist is unable to read information written by another staff member in the appointment book. How might that affect the receptionist's work?

Offices that use paper appointment books should choose books that support their number of physicians and patients. In multiple-physician practices, appointment books might be color coded by provider (Figure 6-3).

Even in one-physician practices, different columns of the appointment book may be used for different procedures. For example, all new patients might be scheduled in the far left-hand column and all follow-up appointments in the far right-hand one. In some offices, appointment types are highlighted in different colors to indicate type of patient or procedure. For example, patients undergoing laboratory work might be highlighted in orange, whereas patients having x-rays might be highlighted in blue. Each office will devise a system that works for it.

Types of Appointment Scheduling

cluster scheduling
a scheduling system in which several patients are booked around the same block of time

Medical practices use several different methods for scheduling patient appointments. Practice type and physician preference determine which method is used.

Cluster scheduling is a system of booking several patients around the same block of time. This method is typically used when the patients all need the same type of service, such as laboratory work or consultations. By clustering similar appointments, the office can serve patients most efficiently.

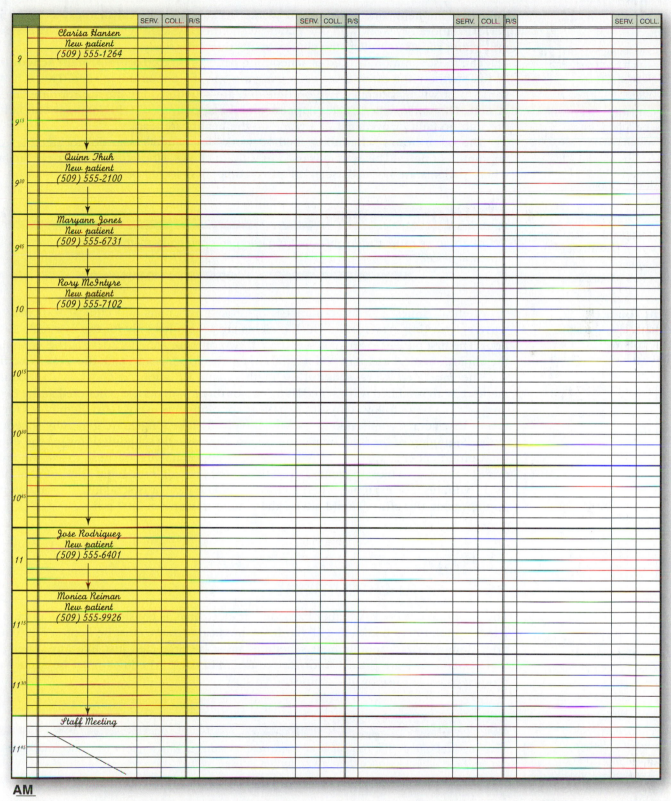

		SERV.	COLL.	R/S		SERV.	COLL.	R/S		SERV.	COLL.	R/S		SERV.	COLL.
9	*Clarisa Hansen* *New patient* *(509) 555-1264*														
9¹⁵															
9³⁰	*Quinn Thuh* *New patient* *(509) 555-2100*														
9⁴⁵	*Maryann Jones* *New patient* *(509) 555-6731*														
10	*Rory McIntyre* *New patient* *(509) 555-7102*														
10¹⁵															
10³⁰															
10⁴⁵															
11	*Jose Rodriguez* *New patient* *(509) 555-6401*														
11¹⁵	*Monica Reiman* *New patient* *(509) 555-9926*														
11³⁰															
11⁴⁵	*Staff Meeting*														

AM

FIGURE ■ 6-3 A color-coded appointment book that shows where the receptionist would schedule new patient appointments.

Double booking is done when two or more patients are scheduled to see the same healthcare provider at the same time. This method is used when an emergency patient must be seen that day, or it may be used to accommodate patients who need added services while in the office. For example, if the medical office has two patients who are both going to need laboratory work, the receptionist might schedule both patients for the

double booking
when two or more patients are scheduled to see the same healthcare provider at the same time

fixed appointment scheduling
a scheduling system in which each patient is given a specific appointment time

open hours scheduling
a scheduling system in which patients are normally seen on a first-come, first-served basis, with no appointment necessary

wave scheduling
a scheduling system in which patients are scheduled only for the first half of each hour

modified wave scheduling
a scheduling system in which two or three patients are scheduled at the beginning of each hour, followed by single patient appointments every 10 to 20 minutes for the rest of that hour

same appointment time. This option works because the clinical medical assistant can perform laboratory work with one patient while the physician sees the other. This system uses exam rooms as well as the clinical staff's time effectively.

The most common method of scheduling patients is **fixed appointment scheduling**. In this method, the office gives each patient a specific appointment time. This schedule works best when patients arrive on time and are scheduled for the appropriate amount of time. Of course, emergencies happen, and the appointment schedule may run behind through no fault or oversight of anyone on the healthcare team.

The **open hours scheduling** method works for patients who do not need specific appointment times. This system is used in walk-in clinics, laboratories, and x-ray facilities where patients are normally seen on a first-come, first-served basis.

Critical Thinking 6.7 ?

What are some issues that might arise from using an open hours method of scheduling in a medical office?

Medical clinics with large numbers of procedure rooms and clinical staff may use **wave scheduling**, a system in which patients are scheduled only for the first half of each hour. The first patient to arrive is seen first. If two or more patients arrive at the same time, the clinical medical assistant will need to triage the patients and take the sicker one first.

The **modified wave scheduling** method is a variation on the wave scheduling method. With modified wave scheduling, two or three patients are scheduled at the beginning of each hour, followed by single patient appointments every 10 to 20 minutes for the rest of that hour. Complicated cases, which typically take longer, are generally scheduled at the beginning of the hour, while minor cases are usually scheduled toward the end.

Certain patients are habitually late for their appointments. In these cases, the receptionist should give those patients arrival times that precede scheduled appointment times by 15 minutes. For example, when a chronically late patient is scheduled for a 2:15 p.m. appointment, the office should advise the patient to arrive at 2:00 p.m.

The Appointment Schedule as a Legal Document

slack time
a system for leaving certain times of day open to accommodate situations such as patients who call for same-day appointments

buffer time
a scheduling system for leaving certain times of day open to accommodate situations such as patients calling for same-day appointments

The appointment book, whether hardcopy or electronic, is considered a legal document. Paper appointment books, like all hardcopy medical records, must be kept in a safe location. Computerized appointment schedules must be protected just like any other item that contains private patient information. Computerized schedules must be secure and require password use by all administrative staff.

Critical Thinking 6.8 ?

For medical offices that use paper appointment schedules, where might the office manager keep these schedules once they are no longer in use?

Allowing for Unforeseen Appointments

Most medical offices that use scheduling systems for patient appointments leave certain times of day open to accommodate situations such as patients who call for same-day appointments or physicians who need to catch up on charting. Such open periods, called **slack time** or **buffer time**, are generally 15- to 30-minute slots at the end of the morning and the end of the afternoon or evening.

Triage and Appointment Scheduling

Patients with medical emergencies will sometimes call their physicians' offices for assistance. When they do, receptionists should have clearly written protocols for handling the situations. A triage notebook, detailed in Chapter 5, outlines these protocols and provides questions to ask patients who call with possible medical emergencies. Such a notebook, which should be clear, concise, and written under the physicians' direction, should reside near the telephone where patient calls are answered.

Appointment Reminder Systems

Typically, patients are given **appointment reminder cards** as they leave the office (Figure 6-4). These reminder cards are usually the size of a business card and contain the date, day, and time of the patient's next appointment, as well as the office's name and telephone number.

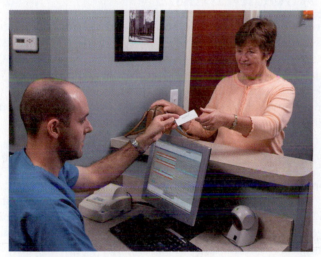

FIGURE ■ **6-4** Typically, patients are given appointment reminder cards when they leave the office.
Source: Michal Heron/Pearson Education.

> **appointment reminder cards**
> usually the size of a business card and contain the date, day, and time of the patient's next appointment, as well as the office's name and telephone number

Even with reminder cards, patients may forget their appointments. For this reason, many offices choose to call patients the day before their appointments to remind them. As with all calls, such calls must remain confidential. When leaving messages, staff should disclose no healthcare information. Instead, the receptionist can leave a message like "This is Michelle calling from Dr. Hecker's office to remind Gloria of her appointment tomorrow at 2 p.m. If you have questions, please call me back at 425-555-3410."

For patients who schedule follow-up appointments a month or more in the future, many offices choose to send reminder cards. Postcards can be used for this purpose only when they contain no personal patient information. If the name of the office discloses the reason for the patient's visit, the office should not use postcard reminders. For example, if the office is called "Vickland Oncology Center," anyone who sees a postcard with this name may assume the patient has cancer. Offices like these should either mail appointment reminders in envelopes or call patients with reminders. The use of some form of reminder card or call has been proven to dramatically reduce the number of no-show appointments.

Many medical offices today use automated telephone reminder systems to remind patients of their upcoming appointments. These systems, which are typically paired with computerized appointment systems, automatically dial patients' contact telephone numbers and play recorded reminder messages.

Making Corrections to the Appointment Schedule

White correction fluid should never be used in a paper appointment book. When an appointment is changed in the appointment book, it should not be obliterated or erased or blacked out with a marker. Instead, the receptionist should draw one line through the patient's name and note why the patient failed to keep the appointment (Figure 6-5).

Some medical offices use color-coded systems to indicate schedule changes. For example, a red "X" next to a patient's name might indicate an appointment cancellation. Electronic appointment schedules accept notations, cancellations, and rescheduled or missed appointments, while retaining a tracking system for the user to see the original appointment data.

No-Show Appointments

Patients who fail to arrive for their appointments and do not call to reschedule are considered "no shows." The medical office must try to reach all no shows. Typically, this is done via telephone 15 to 30 minutes after a patient's appointed time. When receptionists reach such patients, they should try to reschedule the appointments. When they cannot reach patients, they should leave messages requesting return calls to reschedule. When receptionists can neither reach patients nor leave messages, they may mail notes requesting rescheduling.

FOLLOW-UP FOR NO-SHOW APPOINTMENTS

Missed patient appointments must be documented in the patients' medical records. Any steps staff take to try to reschedule those patients must be documented as well. When patients refuse to reschedule or remain unreachable, medical staff must make notes in those patients' medical records and alert the physician regarding the no show.

Well-documented patient medical records become particularly important when patients experience adverse outcomes due to missed appointments. Medical offices with clear, comprehensive patient records are better able to defend against malpractice suits. Some offices take the extra step of sending patients certified letters when they miss important follow-up appointments, such as postoperative appointments. Proof of the patients' receipt of such letters demonstrates the office took every step possible to encourage patients to obtain needed care.

Achieving the Most Efficient Scheduling System

All medical offices at some point realize that their appointment scheduling procedures could be improved. Physicians may routinely be exceeding scheduled appointment times or extended delays may regularly be irritating patients. When flaws like these become apparent, it is important for the healthcare team as a whole to reevaluate how the office schedules appointments. Every member of the team should participate in improvement efforts, because scheduling affects every staff member.

Managing the Physician's Professional and Travel Schedule

Many physicians attend professional meetings outside the office. These range from lunches with colleagues to traveling to out-of-state seminars. In many medical offices,

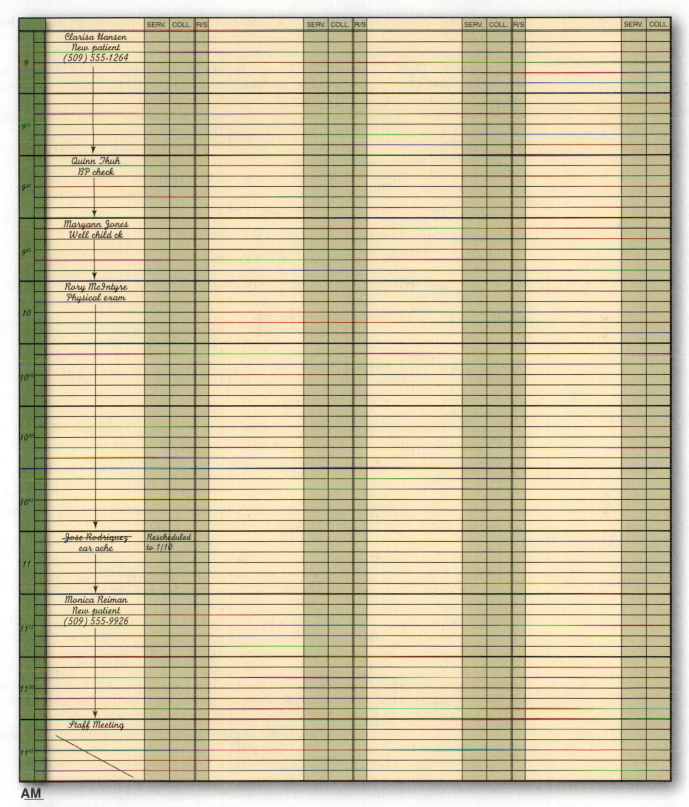

	SERV.	COLL.	R/S		SERV.	COLL.	R/S		SERV.	COLL.	R/S		SERV.	COLL.
9	Clarisa Hansen New patient (509) 555-1264													
9¹⁵														
9³⁰	Quinn Thuh BP check													
9⁴⁵	Maryann Jones Well child ck													
10	Rory McIntyre Physical exam													
10¹⁵														
10³⁰														
10⁴⁵														
11	Jose Rodriquez ear ache	Rescheduled to 1/10												
11¹⁵	Monica Reiman New patient (509) 555-9926													
11³⁰														
11⁴⁵	Staff Meeting													

AM

FIGURE ■ 6-5 Sample appointment book indicating patient who has changed his appointment.

the receptionist, medical assistant, or medical office manager manages the physician's professional schedule. At a minimum, this task includes blocking out times in the appointment schedule when the physician is unavailable for patient appointments. The medical staff member may also be asked to book airline flights or hotel rooms or reserve seats at conferences.

To ensure accuracy and efficiency, medical staff should clearly write all information on the physician's travel plans, including any confirmation numbers (Figure 6-6). A copy of all such information should remain in the office to keep the rest of the healthcare team apprised of the physician's schedule. The physician can retain any original documents. When the physician attends a seminar or conference that awards continuing-education credits, the medical staff should track that information as well.

- Leaving on Delta Airlines Flight #29 at 6:10 p.m. Thursday night.

- Arriving in Minneapolis at 9:30pm.

- Reservations with Avis car rental, Confirmation #980098.

- Reservations at the Hilton hotel, Confirmation #HIU998.

- Seminar starts in the Venetian Boardroom at 9 a.m. Friday.

- Return flight on Delta Airlines Flight #54 at 6:10 a.m. Sunday morning.

FIGURE ■ 6-6　Sample physician's travel schedule.

Scheduling Hospital Services and Admissions

Many physicians care for or perform procedures on patients in hospital settings as well as in the medical clinic. For this reason, medical office staff must be well versed in the procedures for scheduling patients for hospital services. In larger medical offices, staff members may be hired to perform only the scheduling task. In smaller facilities or departments, the hospital scheduling task may be performed by the receptionists, medical assistants, or nurses.

To facilitate the hospital scheduling process, the medical office should keep all hospital and related telephone numbers near the telephone or program them into a speed dialer. Most health insurance plans require physicians to obtain preapprovals for surgical procedures. Unless the procedure is an emergency, the medical staff should call the patient's insurance carrier to obtain authorization for the procedure before scheduling the patient. Whenever possible, medical staff should schedule patients for hospital services while those patients are in the office. With patients present, staff are better able to coordinate patients' schedules.

Every office should have guidelines for scheduling patients for hospital services. Such guidelines should list the type of procedure, the physician, the time the physician needs, and any information that must be relayed to the patient, such as fasting prior to the surgery. The medical office should also have preprinted informational forms from the hospital or outpatient facility that gives such specifics as directions to the facility and check-in procedures. Patients should receive such forms before they leave the office.

It is important to keep in mind that medical procedures make many patients nervous. Medical staff can help make patients' experiences positive ones by letting them know exactly what to expect before, during, and after their procedures. Staff should include any dietary or activity restrictions before or after procedures, specify how long the procedures are expected to take, and provide information on warning signs.

Critical Thinking 6.9 ?

Imagine you are a patient being scheduled for a medical procedure in the hospital. What information would you like to have provided to make you feel more at ease with the upcoming hospitalization?

Arranging Transportation for Patients

Many medical offices treat patients who cannot drive themselves to the offices. Patients may have disabilities or offices may be in challenging locations. As a courtesy to patients, receptionists should keep telephone lists of transportation services. Such lists should include taxicab services as well as local services for those who are elderly or have a disability.

Case Study Questions

Refer to the case study presented at the beginning of this chapter to answer the following questions:

1. How should Tully proceed in designing a system that will work with the pediatricians in this office?
2. Which of the tools presented in this chapter would be best suited to the task?

Chapter Review

Summary

- Scheduling new patients to the medical office will differ from scheduling those patients who have already established care in that office.

- There are distinct differences between a new patient (one who has never been seen or has not been seen in the past 3 years) and an established patient.

- Guidelines for scheduling patient appointments are invaluable tools for medical offices intent on providing effective, efficient patient service. Scheduling the appropriate amount of time is imperative to proper patient flow in the office.

- Medical offices often have systems in place for scheduling patients so that the use of equipment and staff is maximized.

- Today, medical offices can choose between paper and electronic scheduling systems. Most medical offices today use an electronic schedule.

- Both paper and electronic scheduling systems should be capable of documenting no-show situations. Proper documenting of no-show patients is required for legal and other purposes. The appointment book (whether electronic or paper) is a legal document.

- Many medical offices allow time in the schedule each day for those patients who need to be seen for an urgent matter. This scheduling practice keeps the physician and staff on time when unforeseen delays occur.

- Triage of patients is the process of determining the patient's need for care, and the urgency of that request.

- Reminder systems for patient appointments will vary from manual processes, such as staff calling patients to remind them of appointments, to automated processes, such as computer-generated reminder telephone calls.

- Corrections to the appointment schedule must be done in a way that follows laws regarding medical records. This is the case because the appointment book is a legal document.

- When patients miss their appointments, the medical staff should attempt to reschedule them.

- Achieving an efficient appointment scheduling system consists of studying the schedule to determine the amount of time the physician requires for a particular appointment type. With this information, templating of the schedule may occur to maximize staff and equipment in a manner that allows for the best patient flow in the office.

- The physician's professional schedule, which includes travel, is often part of the medical staff's tasks.

- Like the physician's travel, the medical staff must be able to accommodate patients' hospital appointments in the office's scheduling system.

- Medical office receptionists commonly arrange appropriate transportation services for patients in need.

Multiple Choice

Choose the letter that best answers each question or completes each statement.

1. At _____ minutes after a patient has missed an appointment, the receptionist should call to reschedule.
   a. 5
   b. 10
   c. 15
   d. 60

2. A new patient is defined as someone who has:
   a. not been seen in the medical office for more than 1 year.
   b. not been seen by any physician in the office for more than 3 years.
   c. been seen by another physician in the office within the past year but is now seeing a new provider in the office.
   d. all of the above.

3. Which of the following scheduling methods books several patients around the same time?
   a. Cluster booking
   b. Stream scheduling
   c. Set appointment time scheduling
   d. None of the above

4. Which of the following messages would be appropriate to leave on a patient's home voicemail?
   a. "This is Vicki from Gleason Oncology Center calling for Maria."
   b. "This is Vicki from Dr. Green's office calling for Maria."
   c. "This is Vicki from Dr. Green's office calling with Maria's recent lab work. Your cell count is showing as normal. It looks like the cancer is in remission."
   d. "This is Vicki calling from Dr. Green's office for Maria. I want to remind you of your appointment tomorrow for the bone scan."

5. Which of the following is a benefit of an electronic appointment book over a paper appointment book?
   a. Users do not have to discern someone's handwriting.
   b. More than one person can be in the appointment book at the same time.
   c. There is no chance of losing the book.
   d. All of the above.

6. Maria is working in a same-day access clinic. There are no set appointment times. Which of the following is the likely method used in this clinic for scheduling?
   a. Open hours
   b. Cluster booking
   c. Double booking
   d. Wave scheduling

7. Which of the following medical staff members may be asked to arrange for the physician's professional travel plans for an upcoming seminar?
   a. The receptionist
   b. The medical assistant
   c. The office manager
   d. All of the above

8. Which of the following is a reason for designing an appointment matrix?
   a. Scheduling in time for the physician to perform hospital rounds
   b. Allowing for double booking of patients
   c. Offering patients open hours for scheduling
   d. None of the above

9. Barney Williams is a patient who is chronically late for his appointments. How might the receptionist get Mr. Williams to come to his appointments on time?
   a. Ask the physician to stress the importance of arriving on time.
   b. Threaten to dismiss Mr. Williams from care in the office if he does not arrive on time.
   c. Call Mr. Williams 20 minutes before his appointment to remind him to get in his car.
   d. Tell Mr. Williams his appointment is 15 minutes earlier than it actually is scheduled.

10. Which method of scheduling might be used for patient appointments where the patients all need to have the same type of service performed, such as lab work?
    a. Double booking
    b. Wave scheduling
    c. Modified wave scheduling
    d. Cluster booking

True/False

Determine if each of the following statements is true or false.

_____ 1. The time allowed for patient appointments remains constant from one provider to another.

_____ 2. The appointment book is a legal document.

_____ 3. Double booking is the process of allowing patients to arrive for appointments at their leisure.

_____ 4. It is appropriate to tell chronically late patients that their appointments are 15 minutes before the times scheduled in the appointment book.

_____ 5. It is unnecessary to chart a no-show appointment in a patient's chart.

_____ 6. Medical offices that chart patients' missed appointments can help avoid losing malpractice lawsuits.

_____ 7. When scheduling patients for procedures, it is important to disclose everything the patient should expect.

_____ 8. Receptionists do not arrange transportation services.

_____ 9. A medical office's appointment scheduling system should be reviewed periodically to determine its efficiency.

_____ 10. Fixed appointment scheduling is a system in which each patient is given a specific time to come to the office for care.

Matching

Match each of the following terms with its definition.

a. cluster scheduling

b. double booking

c. fixed appointment scheduling

d. matrix

e. new patient

f. established patient

g. office brochure

h. triage notebook

i. open office hours

j. accidental injury claims

1. Scheduling more than one patient for the same appointment time

2. Scheduling system that assigns every patient a specific appointment time

3. A patient whom the medical office has seen previously

4. Scheduling method that groups patients with similar appointments around the same time of day

5. A pamphlet outlining an office's staff and services

6. A scheduling method that allows patients to seek treatment without appointment times

7. The process of blocking out times in the appointment schedule when the provider is unavailable or out of the office

8. A reason for a patient to have two medical records

9. A patient whom no provider in the office has seen for the past 3 years

10. A notebook that outlines questions and steps to follow in the event callers have potentially life-threatening conditions

Chapter Resources

MedStar medical appointment scheduling software: www.medstarsystems.com

MicroWiz medical appointment scheduling software: www.microwize.com/ohpro.htm

ScheduleView medical appointment software: www.scheduleview.com/

CHAPTER 7

Medical Records Management

CHAPTER OUTLINE

- Information Contained in the Medical Record
- Purpose of the Medical Record
- Signing Off on the Medical Record
- Keeping Chart Notes Professional
- Forms of Charting
- Using Abbreviations in Charting
- Charting Communications with Patients
- Filing and Filing Systems
- Cross-Referencing Medical Records
- Locating Misfiled Medical Records
- File Storage Systems
- Retention of Medical Records
- Active, Inactive, and Closed Patient Files
- Converting Paper Records to Electronic Storage
- Properly Disposing of Medical Records
- Medicare Guidelines Regarding Retention of Medical Records
- Making Corrections or Additions to Medical Records
- Charting Conflicting Orders
- Ownership of the Medical Record
- Electronic Medical Records
- Releasing Medical Records
- Mandatory Reporting Requirements
- Documenting Advance Directives
- Faxing Medical Records
- Improper Disclosure of Medical Records
- Online Medical Records
- Documentation of Prescription Refill Requests
- Medical Records in Research

LEARNING OBJECTIVES

Upon completion of this chapter, you should be able to:

- Spell and define the key terms in this chapter.
- Describe the purpose and the various types of information found within the medical record.
- Understand how to keep professional notes in the medical record.
- Define the various forms of medical charting techniques, including the importance of standardizing the abbreviations used in charting.
- Understand why charting communications with patients in the medical chart is important.
- Understand how to cross-reference medical records and how to locate a missing medical record.
- Describe the types of filing systems and file storage systems used in medical offices.
- Understand how to determine the length of time for retaining medical records.
- Define active, inactive, and closed patient files.
- Outline the process of converting paper records to electronic storage and how to properly dispose of medical records once converted.
- Discuss Medicare guidelines for the retention of medical records.

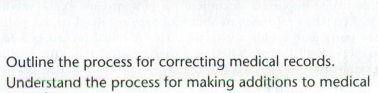

- Outline the process for correcting medical records.
- Understand the process for making additions to medical records.
- Understand what to chart when charting conflicts occur.
- Define ownership of the medical record.
- Describe the role of the electronic medical record in today's medical office environment.
- Describe the process for releasing medical records.
- Outline the process to follow in mandatory reporting situations.
- Document advance directives in the medical chart.
- Understand when it is appropriate to fax medical records.
- Describe the impact of improper disclosure of the medical record on the medical office.
- Describe the use of online medical records.
- Document prescription refill requests in the medical record.
- Understand the importance of documenting patient participation in medical research.

KEY TERMS

active patient file
advance directive
chief complaint
chronologic
clear
closed patient file
complete
concise
correct
cross-referencing
discovery rule

electronic signature
financial information
flowchart
inactive patient file
indecipherable
medical information
medical record
medical research program
narrative chart note
nontherapeutic research
obliterated

personal information
problem-oriented medical record (POMR) charting
progress notes
purge
shingling
SOAP note charting
social information
standard of care
statute of limitations
subpoena

Case Study

Take note of the following scenario and answer the case study questions that appear at the end of this chapter.

Corey Shephard is the medical office manager in a large multispecialty medical practice. The physicians have just purchased an electronic medical record program and are beginning the process of converting the paper medical records to electronic format.

Introduction

The medical record is the most important document on patient care in the medical office. The medical record contains information about all care received by the patient while under care in any particular healthcare facility. The medical record is a legal document and must be kept confidential. Whether paper or electronic, the medical record is the most important tool to be used to defend against malpractice lawsuits, should they occur.

Information Contained in the Medical Record

medical record
a record of the patient's healthcare

personal information
information pertaining to the patient, such as address and telephone number

financial information
items in the medical record pertaining to the patient's insurance coverage or account status

medical information
information in the patient's medical record pertaining to his medical history or condition

social information
information in a patient's chart relating to his social status, such as smoking or participating in high-risk behaviors

Medical records have four types of patient information: **personal information**, **financial information**, **medical information**, and **social information**. Personal information is the information patients supply when first seeing physicians for care. Such information includes the patient's name, birth date, gender, marital status, occupation, next of kin, and any other items collected for personal identification. Personal information may also include any comments the medical staff might write in the patient's file regarding the patient's language or cultural background, if such information pertains to the patient's healthcare.

Patients sometimes refuse to divulge such private information as Social Security number or birth date or such lifestyle information as smoking, drinking, or drug habits. Medical office staff should let such patients know that anything in their medical records is confidential and cannot be released to anyone without the patient's written consent or a court order. If a patient remains uneasy, medical staff should notify the physician. Notification gives physicians an opportunity to discuss issues with patients and decide if they wish to treat those patients in the event those patients continue to refuse to provide the requested information.

Critical Thinking 7.1 ?

Think about the reasons why patients may be uneasy revealing information such as their Social Security number or date of birth. Once you have some reasons in mind, what might you say to a patient who is having just that concern?

A patient's financial information includes a patient's insurance information, which includes policy and identification numbers; insurance plan contact information; and any other information needed to bill the insurance company for the patient's care. In many medical offices using either paper or electronic medical charts, some portion of the patient's financial information is kept in a separate file from medical information. Because any information kept in the patient's medical record must be released upon request or court order, financial information is often kept separate so that it does not have to be disclosed. Financial information also includes account information, copies of insurance company correspondence, and signed authorizations from the patient allowing the medical provider to release information to the insurance company.

chief complaint
the main reason the patient sought care today

Medical information includes the patient's **chief complaint** (the main reason for today's visit); any family medical history; the patient's medical history; the results of examinations; data collected during the physical examination; the prescribed course of treatment, including any medications or referrals; and the patient's diagnoses, progress notes, operative reports, radiology reports, laboratory reports, and any other reports or information that pertains to the patient's healthcare.

Social information is any personal information on the patient, such as race and ethnicity, hobbies, and regular sports participation. Social information also includes such lifestyle choices as smoking, alcohol consumption, drug use, and sexual habits.

In addition to personal, financial, medical, and social information, other documents are routinely part of the patient's medical record. These documents include the HIPAA acknowledgment form (Figure ■ 7-1), which indicates that the patient has been notified of the office's privacy policies; the information release form (Figure ■ 7-2), which authorizes the medical provider to discuss the patient's care with other designated parties; documents from hospitalizations; and any items the patient brings to the appointment, such as a list of current medications or copies of information from other medical providers' files.

All notes entered into the medical chart must adhere to the following "five Cs rule," which means patient charts must be:

- **Concise**—Patient charts must be to the point and contain no entries that fail to relate to the patient's healthcare in some way.

- **Complete**—Medical records must be complete and objective. All pertinent information must be included and opinions and judgments must be excluded.

- **Clear**—When handwritten, patient information should be printed, not written in cursive, and delivered in a clear, easy-to-read manner. Whether handwritten, typed, or electronic, information should be easy for the reader to understand.

- **Correct**—Medical records must be error free. Errors include both improper additions and omissions. When errors are made, their creators must correct them as soon as possible.

- **Chronologic**—Medical records should be in chronologic order, with the newest entries on top.

concise
containing only the necessary information, nothing more

complete
containing all necessary information

clear
to the point and easily understood

correct
accurate

chronologic
the order in which events occur in time, from oldest to newest

Purpose of the Medical Record

A patient's medical record documents the patient's treatment plan and goals in paper or electronic form. The medical record must contain a full account of all patient treatment, including what treatment was given and why it was given or withheld.

In whatever form, medical records must be complete, accurate, organized, concise, timely, and factual. They should never contain opinions or judgments about patients. Whenever medical records are the subject of a **subpoena** for trial, physicians may have to explain notations. A jury who thinks a physician is judgmental or unkind could hand down an unfavorable verdict for the physician. In addition, unprofessional notations may predispose other healthcare professionals to treat patients differently. The best way to keep medical charting professional is to always write as if the patient will be reading the comments. Anything the medical staff would not say to the patient should remain out of the patient's medical record.

subpoena
a court order received by the medical office for all or a portion of a patient's medical record

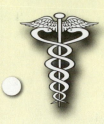

Martin Country Medical Clinic
2413 NW Greenlake Ave.
Westford, CA 12745

ACKNOWLEDGMENT OF RECEIPT of the Notice of Privacy Practices of the Martin County Medical Clinic (MCMC)

I acknowledge that I have received or been offered the Notice of Privacy Practices of the Martin County Medical Clinic. I understand that the Notice describes the uses and disclosures of my protected health information by the Covered Entities and informs me of my rights with respect to my protected health information.

_____
Name of Patient

_____
Patient Date of Birth

_____
Signature of Patient or Personal Representative

_____
Printed Name of Patient or Personal Representative

_____
Date

If Personal Representative, indicate relationship:

_____

Declinations

_____   The Individual declined to accept a copy of the Notice of Privacy Practices.

_____   The Individual received a copy of the Notice of Privacy Practices but declined to sign an Acknowledgment of Receipt.

_____
Signature of MCMC Healthcare Representative

_____
Name of MCMC HealthCare Representative

FIGURE ■ 7-1   HIPAA acknowledgment form.

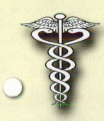

Martin County Medical Clinic
2413 NW Greenlake Ave.
Westford, CA 12745

AUTHORIZATION TO RELEASE HEALTHCARE INFORMATION

Patient's Name:		Date of Birth:	

Previous Name:		Social Security #:	

I request and authorize _____ to release healthcare information of the patient named above to:

	Name:	
	Address:	
	City:	State:	Zip Code:

This request and authorization applies to:

• Healthcare information relating to the following treatment, condition, or dates:

• All healthcare information

• Other: _____

• Yes • No	I authorize the release of my STD results, HIV/AIDS testing, whether negative or positive, to the person(s) listed above. I understand that the person(s) listed above will be notified that I must give specific written permission before disclosure of these test results to anyone.

• Yes • No	I authorize the release of any records regarding drug, alcohol, or mental health treatment to the person(s) listed above.

Patient Signature:		Date Signed:	

THIS AUTHORIZATION EXPIRES NINETY DAYS AFTER IT IS SIGNED.

FIGURE ■ 7-2 Sample information release form.

standard of care
the care that is expected from a clinician with a certain level of training and resources available

Risk management departments use medical records to determine if the **standard of care** has been met. The standard of care states that a healthcare provider must use reasonable and necessary skill when caring for patients and provide the same care another provider with the same training would use in the same circumstances. The best defense against malpractice claims is well-kept, accurate medical records. Some civil cases have held healthcare providers liable for their failure to maintain proper records. Chapter 8 provides more detail on medical malpractice.

A pertinent phrase in healthcare is "If it wasn't charted, it wasn't done." This means anything that is not documented in a patient's medical record did not happen as far as the law is concerned. Similarly, anything that is charted in a record did happen from a legal standpoint. Therefore, medical staff must ensure that medical records are comprehensive and accurate, because even the smallest omission or incorrect statement can cause a host of problems, including malpractice lawsuits, incorrect patient care, patient injury, and miscommunication between healthcare providers.

Some healthcare providers may review patient medical records as part of consultation visits, second opinions, or insurance audits. Others will review medical records when patients transfer to other offices. It can be difficult for providers to understand records created by another provider if those records are not complete and clear.

Critical Thinking 7.4 ?

How might incomplete or unclear patient records affect a provider who is asked for a consultation on a patient's condition? As the office manager, how might the lack of complete information in the patient's medical record affect your ability to do your job?

Signing Off On the Medical Record

electronic signature
an electronic version of a person's signature, used in the electronic medical record

Any entry in a patient's medical record must have an identifying mark indicating the person who made the entry. Policies on this will vary from one medical office to the next, but the minimum should be no less than the initials and credentials of the person making the entry. Some medical offices require a complete signature along with credentials; others allow a first initial, last name, and credentials. An office that uses electronic medical records may use an **electronic signature**. In offices where medical notes are dictated and printed for patient files, an electronic signature or rubber-stamp signature may replace handwritten signatures.

Keeping Chart Notes Professional

Any time a member of the medical office staff places a note in a patient's medical record, attention must be paid to keeping the note professional. This means the notes should always be objective and never contain conjecture or the opinion of the author. Only facts as stated or observed are to be placed in the medical record. It is important to remember that a copy of the medical record may be requested by the patient, his insurance company, or his attorney, at any time. If information contained within the record is not professional, the medical office staff and providers may not be seen as the highly competent medical professionals they are. This type of charting includes attention paid to proper spelling and grammar as well.

Critical Thinking 7.5 ?

Why do you think the lack of proper spelling and grammar on behalf of the medical office staff may be seen as problematic?

Forms of Charting

Just as medical offices vary, so do the methods of charting information into medical records. **Narrative chart notes** in the medical record are simply written descriptions of patients' visits. As one of the oldest forms of medical charting, narratives are chronologic. Findings of the visit appear with the doctor's instructions or prescriptions. Many physicians dictate their narrative notes about patient care, have their notes transcribed, and place their typewritten notes in the patients' files, although narratives can be manual or electronic. In some offices, physicians underline or outline certain terms in narrative notes to add emphasis.

narrative chart note written descriptions of patients' visits; the oldest form of medical note taking

SOAP NOTE CHARTING

SOAP note charting is a method that tracks the subjective, objective, assessment, and plan (SOAP) for a patient's visit. Subjective findings include patient verbal statements, including any information about the chief complaint. Subjective findings are symptoms that are imprecise in measurement. Objective findings are observations by the medical assistant, examination findings, and patient vital signs. Objective findings are those that can be objectively observed. The assessment of the patient is the doctor's diagnosis, possible diagnosis, or the diagnosis the physician wishes to rule out for that visit. The assessment is what the physician believes is the cause of the patient's complaint or the reason for that visit. The plan is the doctor's prescribed plan of action, which includes any prescriptions, tests, instructions, or referrals. The plan is anything the physician is recommending the patient do for her condition.

SOAP note charting subjective, objective, assessment, and plan; a common form of charting in the medical record where clinicians chart information in an easy-to-find format

The SOAP method of charting is extremely popular and easy to use. By clearly identifying the four areas in the SOAP format, anyone reading the notes can easily locate information. For example, assume Mildred Anderson arrives for an initial appointment with Dr. Gomez. When Ms. Anderson arrives, she mentions she has had trouble with shoulder pain for the past year or so. She also states that she has been diagnosed as mildly hypertensive. The chief complaint for today's visit, however, is Ms. Anderson's problems with depression and fatigue. Under the subjective findings, the medical assistant, nurse, and physician will chart what the patient states about her condition. Under the objective findings, any positive or negative examination findings will be charted. The assessment section for Ms. Anderson will include the physician's immediate assessment of her condition, including what he believes is the cause of her symptoms. The plan for her care will include any medications or follow-up care the physician recommends Ms. Anderson undergo.

PROBLEM-ORIENTED MEDICAL RECORD CHARTING

Problem-oriented medical record (POMR) charting tracks a patient's problems throughout medical care. Each problem is assigned a number, and that number is referenced when the patient comes in for care. Advocates for POMR charting believe that charting according to patients' problems renders healthcare providers less likely to overlook previous problems. For example, use the same scenario with Mildred Anderson arriving for an initial appointment with Dr. Gomez. When Ms. Anderson arrives, she mentions she has had trouble with shoulder pain for the past year or so. She also states that she has been diagnosed as mildly hypertensive. The chief complaint for today's visit, however, is Ms. Anderson's problems with depression and fatigue.

problem-oriented medical record (POMR) charting a charting process that allows providers to assign a number to each medical problem and chart each item each time the patient is seen for care

Using the POMR method of charting, Dr. Gomez would assign a number to each of the problems Mildred mentioned. He might assign the main reason for the visit, depression and fatigue, the number 1; Ms. Anderson's shoulder pain number 2; and hypertension number 3. Each of these problems would have its own page in the medical chart so Dr. Gomez can easily reference the problems at each visit. Once a condition is resolved, a notation is made so the doctor need not reference the problem on subsequent visits.

As new problems arise, new numbers are assigned, and new pages are allotted for tracking the problems.

USE OF FLOWCHARTS IN THE MEDICAL RECORD

flowchart
chart used in the medical record to chart the progress of growth, such as child height, weight, and head circumference

Flowcharts are visual tools that help track certain information in patients' medical records. An example is the growth progress of children (Figure ■ 7-3). Each time the physician sees an infant, the medical assistant or nurse will measure the child's weight, length, and head circumference and make notations on a flowchart that the physician can then use when discussing any concerns with the child's parent or guardian.

PROGRESS NOTES

progress notes
the daily chart notes taken at the time of a patient's visit to a clinic

Progress notes are daily chart notes made during patient visits to document a patient's progress or status with certain conditions. As an example, assume a patient arrives for an appointment complaining of weight gain. On the patient's subsequent visits, progress notes would outline the patient's current weight, any treatment recommendations, and outcomes. Depending on the office, progress notes may be made in SOAP, POMR, or narrative format. The notes may also be handwritten or electronic.

Using Abbreviations in Charting

Given that abbreviations can lead to confusion in healthcare or even errors in patient care, medical staff must be extremely careful when using abbreviations in patients' charts and ensure that the abbreviations are accepted by their facilities. Because different facilities may use different abbreviations for medical terms, when in doubt medical staff should write out rather than abbreviate words. For example, one office may use the abbreviation "cx" to mean appointment cancellation. Another office may use the same abbreviation to indicate a cancer diagnosis. Confusion among abbreviations can be avoided if facilities agree to use a standard list of abbreviations. To avoid confusion about medical abbreviations, The Joint Commission has published a list of abbreviations that should never be used. This will be discussed in further detail later in the chapter.

Charting Communications with Patients

Staff will sometimes need to document communications with patients in the patients' charts. Such communications include telephone calls or e-mails from patients that relate to their medical care, missed or cancelled appointments, or pharmacy requests to refill prescriptions. It is important to accurately chart all such exchanges in patients' medical records so as to avoid potential errors in communicating the information. Each office should have a policy regarding the type of communication that requires charting, and all members of the healthcare team should closely follow that policy. Such chart notes help to safeguard the medical office from malpractice claims. Although thoroughness is important, not all patient conversations need to be charted in the patient's medical record. Medical staff should use their best judgment to determine if conversations are medically relevant.

Critical Thinking 7.6 ?

Think of the types of calls the office manager takes from patients in the medical office. How would you determine which calls need to be charted in the patient's medical record?

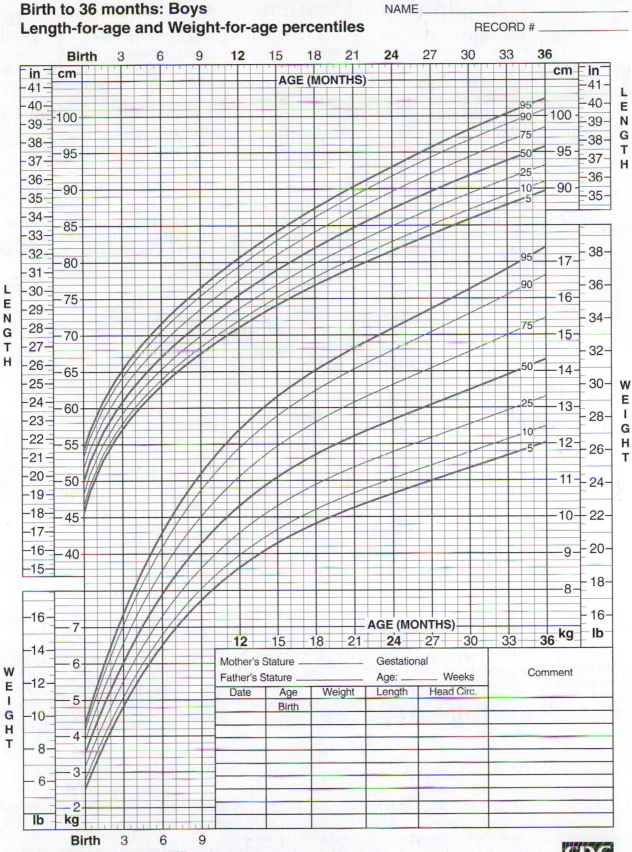

FIGURE ■ 7-3   Sample child growth chart.
Source: www.cdc.gov.

Filing and Filing Systems

Most medical offices use one of two types of filing systems when using paper medical charts: alphabetic or numeric. While alphabetic is far more common overall, numeric filing is often used in facilities where patient treatment records must be kept extremely confidential, such as in facilities specializing in mental health, human immunodeficiency virus (HIV) or acquired immune deficiency syndrome (AIDS) treatment, or reproductive healthcare.

ALPHABETIC FILING

With alphabetic filing, patient information is filed alphabetically by the patient's last name. Offices that use alphabetic filing place color-coded alphabetic stickers on the outside of patients' charts (Figure ■ 7-4). Color-coding causes misplaced charts to stand out when charts are filed. Some offices color code using the first two letters of the patient's last name; others use the patient's first and last name initials. Still others use a portion of the patient's last name and the first initial of the first name.

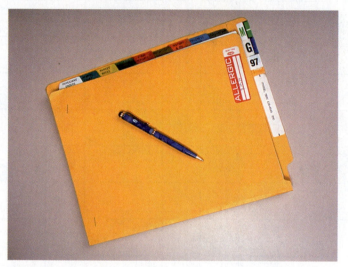

FIGURE ■ 7-4 A color-coded chart.
Source: Michal Heron/Pearson Education.

SHINGLING ITEMS FOR MEDICAL RECORDS

shingling
the process of taping small pieces of paper to a full size sheet of paper so that small items are not lost in the chart

Small items, such as written telephone messages or half-size sheets containing patient progress notes, often need to be filed in patients' paper medical records. To keep these small items from being lost in the records, offices employ **shingling**, which is the process of simply taping the small items to an 8½″ × 11″ sheet of paper and then filing the paper in the patient's chart (Figure ■ 7-5).

NUMERICAL FILING

Some paper patient medical records, such as those in offices devoted to HIV or AIDS-related care, mental health, pregnancy or family planning, or alcohol and drug rehabilitation, may require a high level of security. So in these types of offices, numeric filing is often used. Because the numeric system masks the identity of patients, it is difficult to retrieve filed information without the proper codes. In offices that file with numeric systems, lists of patient names and corresponding codes must be kept in a secure location for the system to work.

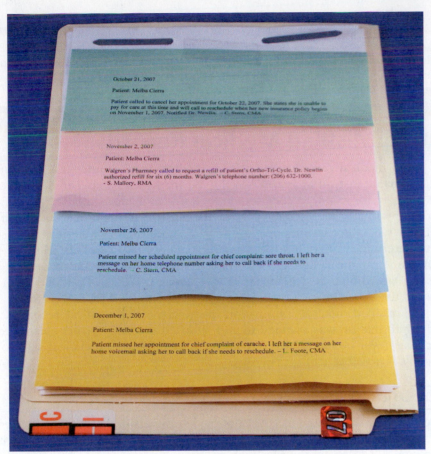

FIGURE ■ 7-5   An example of a shingled chart note.
Source: Dylan Malone/Pearson Education.

Cross-Referencing Medical Records

Patients with hyphenated last names can cause confusion in medical offices. When a patient's last name is Morris-Davidson, for example, some staff may file the patient's chart under the first part of the hyphenated name, Morris, whereas other staff may file according to the latter part of the name, Davidson. To avoid confusion, medical offices should have clear policies for filing the charts of patients with hyphenated names and strictly follow those policies. This same policy may be applied to families where more than one last name is used. As an example, the parents in a household may have a different last name than one or more of the children.

Unfortunately, even with clear policies, hyphenated names can still be confusing. A patient with the last name of Morris-Davidson may go by Morris on some occasions yet use Morris-Davidson or even Davidson on others. **Cross-referencing** files with cards that direct staff to proper files can help address such variations. In the case of Morris-Davidson, for example, the patient's original paper medical record would be filed under the correct full name of Morris-Davidson and blank patient files, one labeled Morris and one Davidson, would be filed under those alternative names. Under this system, if the patient called and identified herself as "Mrs. Ann Davidson," the medical staff member would look in the "Davidson" file and find a blank file that says "Ann Davidson's file is under Morris-Davidson." With an electronic medical record system, the patient would be asked for her birth date as an identifier. Once the name and birth date have been entered, the correct electronic file will be found.

cross-referencing
a process for locating files when a patient may go by one or more last names

Locating Misfiled Medical Records

When a paper medical record is misplaced, medical staff should look first under the patient's first name instead of last. When the file for Krystle Shawger is not filed under "S" for "Shawger," for example, staff should look under "K" for "Krystle." If the file is not there, the staff will next determine when Krystle was last in the office. By identifying the other patients who were in the office at the same time Krystle was there last, staff may be able to determine if Krystle's file was accidentally filed with one of those patients' files. Staff can apply the same method to find misfiled medical information. If, for example, Krystle's lab results are missing, staff may check the files of patients who had lab work around the same time to see if the information was filed there in error.

Locating misfiled medical information in the electronic medical record is no easy task. If the information was scanned in and attached to the incorrect electronic patient record, it may never be found again, requiring a member of the clinical staff to request another copy, if possible.

File Storage Systems

Most medical office filing systems consist of metal cabinets that hold paper patient charts in alphabetical order. Old-style filing cabinets were designed in a tower shape, with drawers that pulled out to reveal the files within. Other styles of freestanding filing cabinets have drawers that pull out to reveal the sides of files. These cabinets are useful for identifying files by their color-coded alphabetic or numeric tabs (Figure ■ 7-6).

Large medical offices often require large file storage systems for paper medical charts. These offices may use filing systems that allow the entire filing cabinet to move to access files (Figure ■ 7-7). These types of filing systems take up less space than stationary models and are ideal for large facilities that must accommodate large numbers of paper files.

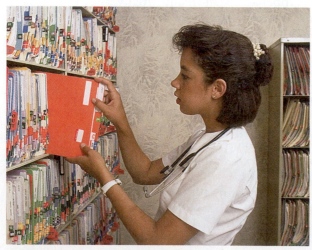

FIGURE ■ **7-6** A medical office filing cabinet.
Source: Michal Heron/Pearson Education.

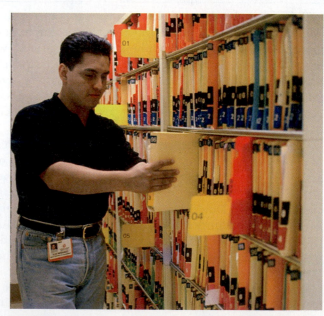

FIGURE ■ **7-7** A space-saving filing system allows the user to move the entire cabinet to access files.
Source: Michael Newman/PhotoEdit, Inc.

Retention of Medical Records

State and federal regulations dictate how long medical records must be kept. To comply with those regulations, a medical office manager should know the statutes of limitations in the state where her practice is located and arrange for the office to keep medical records at least as long as those statutes require. Patients can bring malpractice lawsuits during the **statute of limitations**, which typically begins when the injury occurs. In many states, however, the **discovery rule** can greatly alter the statute of limitations. The discovery rule states that the statute of limitations starts on the day an injury is discovered or should have been discovered, rather than when the injury actually occurred. As an example, imagine a patient who has had surgery during which the surgeon leaves a surgical sponge in the surgical site. This patient may fail to realize the medical error for some time. In states where the discovery rule applies, the statute of limitations would begin when the injury, the sponge in this case, is discovered, even if it is many years later. This rule can also apply to minors by beginning the statute of limitations on the day the minor child turns 18.

statute of limitations
the period of time provided by law for a patient to file a malpractice lawsuit from the date of the injury

discovery rule
relates to when an injury was discovered, rather than when the injury occurred

Active, Inactive, and Closed Patient Files

Paper medical charts take up a lot of space, especially in large offices or offices where physicians have been practicing for long periods.

Most offices would agree that files for patients who actively have appointments or who have been in to see the physician recently are considered **active patient files**. **Inactive patient files** are typically those assigned to patients who have not been in to see the physician for a period between 2 and 5 years depending on the type of practice, the number of files the practice must store, and the office policy. Removing inactive patient files leaves room for new patient files and makes it easier to find active patient files.

The term *closed* is typically reserved for the files of patients who have moved and will not be seen by the physician any longer. It is also used to describe files for patients who are deceased or for patients who have stated that they will be discontinuing treatment in that facility. **Closed patient files** are typically moved to other storage facilities, leaving the available space for active patient files.

Patient files may fluctuate between active, inactive, and closed status. A file that is considered active today may be closed tomorrow if the patient contacts the office to report an out-of-state move. That same file may return to active status if the patient moves back and resumes care in the medical office.

active patient file
medical record for a patient who is actively treated in the medical office

inactive patient file
patient file for a patient who has not been seen in a certain period of time, but who will likely return one day

closed patient file
medical record for a patient who has moved out of the area, is deceased, or has indicated that he will not be returning for care

Converting Paper Records to Electronic Storage

Keeping all patient charts in the same filing system can be overwhelming and increases the time it takes to find patient files. For these reasons, most clinics **purge** inactive or closed patient files. This process entails moving medical files to other locations, or perhaps scanning the documents in the files and then digitally storing the data on microfilm, microfiche, CD, DVD, or other electronic storage system. Once this process is done, the paper medical records can be destroyed by shredding the paper medical file. To purge properly, however, a clear policy on what constitutes a closed or inactive file must be written.

purge
to go through files and remove the items or charts that are old or no longer needed

Properly Disposing of Medical Records

Paper records can be converted to an electronic format for long-term storage. When this happens, the paper records are typically no longer needed. Paper records that are no longer needed must be destroyed so their information cannot be related to patients. Typically, paper records are shredded after they have been copied or scanned (Figure ■ 7-8). All medical offices should use paper shredders to destroy confidential information. Shredding companies may be contracted to complete large projects. Such companies will shred documents and provide certifying notices. Many large healthcare facilities have shredding companies who take care of shredding documents on a regular scheduled basis.

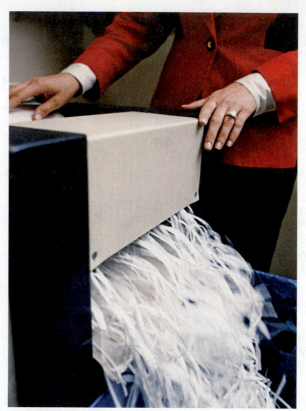

FIGURE ■ 7-8 Using a paper shredder ensures patient confidentiality.
Source: Michael Malyszko/Getty Images.

HIPAA states that medical records must be kept confidential. A medical record can only be disclosed with a patient's consent or a court order. When it is determined appropriate to destroy a medical record, HIPAA dictates that the record must be shredded beyond recognition. It cannot be in a condition such that it can be put back together to reveal personal patient information.

Medicare Guidelines Regarding Retention of Medical Records

Medicare guidelines state that medical records must be retained for at least 5 years. Because the statute of limitations may exceed 5 years in some states, and because medical records are an extremely important part of defending any claim of medical negligence, it is a good idea to keep medical records for as long as possible. Once an office has run out of room for storing medical record files, records can be scanned and kept on CDs, DVDs, microfilm, or any other safe electronic format. In all forms, medical records must be stored in a secure environment, safe from any water or fire damage, and easily accessible by the healthcare team as needed.

Making Corrections or Additions to Medical Records

Medical records must be corrected lawfully, or it may appear the medical office is trying to conceal an error in patient care. When errors do happen, they must be corrected as soon as possible. The correct way to address an error in a paper record is to draw one line through the error, initial and date the correction, and write the correct information above or beside the inserted line (Figure ■ 7-9).

> 1/10/13 CMJ, CMA (AAMA)
> 1/10/13 Patient complains of pain in her ~~left~~ right hand, constant for the past 2 days.
> C. Jones, CMA (AAMA)

FIGURE ■ 7-9 A corrected paper medical record.

When an error is an entire line or several lines in the patient chart, the entire portion of the entry that is in error should be struck with a single line. When an entire entry is in error, which can happen if the medical assistant, nurse, or physician accidentally charts in the wrong patient's chart, the author should draw a single line through the entire entry, make a notation such as "wrong patient's chart," and include the date and the author's initials and credentials. The person who made the error should be the one to correct the medical chart; this is a task that should not be delegated or requested of another member of the medical office team.

Errors in medical charts should never be **obliterated**, scribbled out, or covered with correction fluid, because records with such changes may be viewed as attempts to hide the truth or cover wrongdoing. One line through an incorrect entry leaves no doubt as to the information being corrected.

When an error in a medical chart is one of omission, information may be added to the medical record after the fact by beginning the entry with the date the addition is being added, followed by the words "Late Entry," the date of the visit the late entry pertains to, the notes that were originally omitted, and the signature of the person making the entry. When a correction exceeds the space where the error is, the medical assistant can insert an addendum to the medical record. This insertion should read "ADDENDUM to [date of the visit]" at the beginning of the entry.

Additions and corrections may be made to electronic medical records. These changes will reflect the date of entry and will not overwrite the original error in the record.

obliterated
completely marked out so that the original is unrecognizable

Charting Conflicting Orders

Every member of the healthcare team is obligated to take reasonable action to ensure patient safety. Medical assistants and nurses should not follow orders that they feel may harm patients. Instead, they should consult the physicians out of patients' hearing range. When physicians insist that their orders be followed according to their instructions and they explain the risks and benefits of the treatment, the medical assistants and nurses should chart the events, including the fact that they questioned the doctor as to the accuracy of the orders. They should also include the physicians' responses.

Ownership of the Medical Record

Medical records belong to the physician or facilities where they are created. The information inside, however, belongs to the patients. Patients have a right to access their medical records and to correct those records when they feel errors have been made. When patients request corrections to their medical records, the healthcare team must determine whether errors exist. If the physician agrees an error has been made, the correction should be made as described earlier. If the physician feels the entry was not in error, the physician cannot be forced to treat the entry as an error. In this case, patients must be allowed to create their own versions of the event, and copies of those written statements must be placed in the medical records (Figure ■ 7-10). Such statements become a permanent part of patients' medical records.

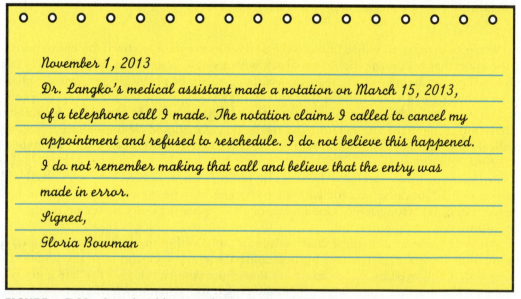

November 1, 2013

Dr. Langko's medical assistant made a notation on March 15, 2013, of a telephone call I made. The notation claims I called to cancel my appointment and refused to reschedule. I do not believe this happened. I do not remember making that call and believe that the entry was made in error.

Signed,

Gloria Bowman

FIGURE ■ 7-10 Sample addition to the medical record from a patient.

Electronic Medical Records

Electronic medical records (EMRs), sometimes called electronic health records (EHRs), are part of healthcare's future. Although electronic medical records have been around since the Mayo Clinic began using them in the 1960s, the technology has been slow to move into ambulatory care. As today's healthcare providers strive to make healthcare safer and allow for efficient team communication, electronic records are playing a more prominent role.

In his 2004 State of the Union address, President George W. Bush stated, "By computerizing health records, we can avoid dangerous medical mistakes, reduce costs, and improve care." Shortly after this speech, President Bush outlined a plan to ensure that most Americans have electronic health records by 2014.

Electronic medical records are simply the portions of patients' medical records that are kept via computer rather than on paper. While physicians must physically retrieve paper files, electronic records are easily accessible. In large offices where patients may see several different providers, electronic medical records allow physicians to easily locate patients' laboratory results, consultations, x-rays, and examination findings from other providers. With an electronic medical record, a patient's file may be accessed by more than one provider or medical staff member at the same time.

Critical Thinking 7.10 ?

Why do you think it may be useful for more than one provider or medical staff member to access the same patient's file at the same time?

Depending on the program, electronic records are accessible via a keyboard connected to a computer system or stylus tapped on a notebook computer (Figure ■ 7-11). Most electronic medical records systems can be configured to work according to an office's specific needs. The following is a list of some of the functions many of these systems provide:

- Time-stamp recordings in the EMR/EHR
- Prescriptions printed or faxed to the pharmacy
- Printed patient education information that directly relates to the patient's care
- Search for a certain type of condition or certain age or geographic location of a group of patients
- Digital photos attached in the patient's EMR/EHR
- Electronically ordered lab results, imaging items, or medical tests
- Electronic graphs of lab results or height, weight, or blood pressure data
- Letters to or about patients
- Electronic data transmission to other healthcare providers.

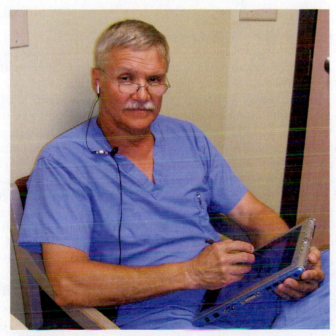

FIGURE ■ 7-11 A physician uses a TabletPC to enter patient data while in the examination room.
Source: Richard Gartee.

One of the many benefits of such systems is the ability to access medical record information from many locations in the healthcare facility and to quickly search for and retrieve information in the patient's medical record.

USING ELECTRONIC RECORDS TO AVOID MEDICAL MISTAKES

Electronic medical records can be used to alert healthcare providers to possible medication reactions. This is especially helpful when patients are treated by several specialists at the same time. EMRs also allow medical staff to easily transmit patient information to patients' health insurance companies when requested, rather than having to photocopy the paper records and send them via the postal service.

One of the most convincing arguments for converting paper medical records to an electronic format is based on patient safety. In 1999, the Institute of Medicine (IOM) published a report called "To Err Is Human: Building a Safer Health System." This report stated, "At least 44,000 people, and perhaps as many as 98,000 people, die in hospitals every year as a result of medical errors that could have been prevented." One of the IOM's recommendations was to move to electronic medical records. Their conclusions suggested that some medical errors are caused by **indecipherable** handwriting, a problem that would be eliminated if providers made their entries electronically rather than in handwritten form.

indecipherable
unreadable

Some states have enacted legislation to address the issue of bad handwriting and medical errors. In March 2006, Washington State passed a law that requires all prescriptions issued by physicians to be electronically submitted to pharmacists or to be printed rather than written in cursive handwriting.

SAVING TIME WITH ELECTRONIC MEDICAL RECORDS

The time saved by using electronic medical records may be better invested in patient care. Many healthcare providers believe they spend a great deal of time charting, far more time than they spend on actual patient care. With the cost of healthcare rising, it makes sense to free up the healthcare provider's time while decreasing avoidable patient injuries.

Releasing Medical Records

Because medical staff members are patient advocates, they must keep patients' best interests, notably patient confidentiality, at the forefront of their work. Medical staff must never reveal patient information without a patient's signed consent or a court order. As a result, when patients' family members call the office, medical staff can tell them nothing about the patients. Similarly, medical staff is forbidden from releasing information to insurance companies, even bills for services, without a patient's consent.

Requests for patients' medical records are common. Patients may need to see specialists, obtain second opinions, or seek care at different facilities. Any request for copies of a patient's medical record must be accompanied by the patient's signed authorization. The medical staff member must be certain the authorization is directed to the correct facility and that it contains a date indicating when the signature was made. In addition to verifying the authorization, the medical staff member must also be completely clear about the nature of the request. Patients may authorize the release of their entire records, or they may authorize the release of information for one date of service only. Some physicians require their staff to alert them to any requests for records. In these offices, the medical staff member pulls the patient's paper file, attaches the request for copies, and gives the file to the physician for review. In an office that uses EMRs, the medical staff member would simply give the request to the physician to review prior to making copies of the requested documents.

Before sending any copies of medical records, however, the medical staff member must review the file to ensure that it is complete and that it contains only information about that patient. Some facilities provide counseling services to patients and their family members. For these records, the medical staff member must obliterate any non–patient-specific information before sending copies.

SUBPOENAED MEDICAL RECORDS

Occasionally, medical offices may receive subpoenas for patients' medical records. Subpoenas may arise from lawsuits due to injury, such as from a car accident. A judge must sign a subpoena, which authorizes the physician to release the information without the patient's signature. Medical facilities are not required to notify the patient of the subpoena or the release of the information, but many will as a courtesy. HIPAA legislation requires medical facilities to keep records of all patient-record disclosures and to make those records available to patients upon request.

SITUATIONS WHEN ORIGINAL MEDICAL RECORDS MAY BE RELEASED

In rare cases, medical offices may release original patient records. These requests are most often received via subpoena for court cases in which the judge or attorneys wish to see original material. When original medical records are required, the medical staff member should make a complete copy of every item and keep the copies in the office as proof of the contents at the time of release.

RELEASING INFORMATION WHEN THE PHYSICIAN LEAVES THE PRACTICE

When a medical practice closes and no other facility takes responsibility for the patients' medical records, notices must be sent to all patients with medical files at the facility. Such notices should give patients a reasonable timeline within which to contact the office to request file transfers. Whether transfer requests are made or not, the physician or the physician's estate will be responsible for the original files (whether electronic or in paper format) for the period outlined by the state's statue of limitations.

DISCLOSURE OF A MINOR'S MEDICAL INFORMATION

In most states, children under 18 years of age may receive certain types of medical treatment without their parents' consent. Such treatments are limited to those for family planning (i.e., birth control or abortion), sexually transmitted infections (STIs), mental health, HIV/AIDS, and alcohol or drug rehabilitation. Because laws for releasing minors' information vary from state to state, medical office managers must be very clear about the laws in the states where they work and be sure all staff members are aware of the requirements.

Minors may receive copies of only those documents their parents cannot see. For example, minors could request and receive copies of their STI treatments, but they could not receive copies of the vaccines they received. Parents, in contrast, could receive only copies of their children's vaccinations, not their STI treatments.

SUPER-PROTECTED MEDICAL INFORMATION

A few areas of medical information are considered *super-protected*. Although the definition varies from state to state, super-protected information is usually any material pertaining to family planning; STIs; mental illness; HIV or AIDS treatment, diagnosis, or testing; and alcohol or drug rehabilitation. Super-protected information typically requires a separate authorization before it can be released to a third party. As a result, the medical office requires written and signed requests from patients, or a subpoena to be able to release super-protected information.

Mandatory Reporting Requirements

According to the 1986 National Childhood Vaccine Injury Act, vaccine injuries must be reported by physicians' offices to alert other physicians to possibly contaminated batches of vaccine. To report a vaccine injury, the medical staff member should obtain the patient's name and age, as well as the name and lot number of the vaccine. The call must be documented in the patient's file.

REPORTING CASES OF ABUSE

Any incapacitated person, elderly person, or child who shows signs of suspected abuse or neglect must be protected. To that end, physicians are required to report all cases of suspected child abuse to the proper authorities. After accidents, abuse is thought to be the second leading cause of death in children under age 5. When patients of any age sustain violent injuries, including injuries from gunshots or knives or criminal acts like assault, attempted suicide, or rape, those injuries must be reported. The law protects healthcare workers from being sued for reporting suspected abuse.

REPORTING CERTAIN ILLNESSES AND INJURIES

All states have a department of health that oversees information regarding illnesses and injuries, among other tasks. Each state determines the types of illnesses and injuries that must be reported by healthcare providers when patients present for care. Examples of illnesses and injuries that must be reported include anthrax, certain STIs, and dog bites. Each state determines the maximum length of time that can elapse from the time when a healthcare provider sees a patient to when the provider must file a report. Some illnesses and injuries must be reported the same day they are seen; others must be reported within 2 weeks.

Critical Thinking 7.11 ?

Why do you think some illnesses and injuries must be reported sooner than others?

Documenting Advance Directives

advance directive
a legal document that outlines a patient's desire regarding life-sustaining treatment or names a guardian to speak for the patient

Today, many patients use **advance directives** to outline their wishes should they be unable to speak for themselves. Advance directives consist of living wills, orders outlining patients' desire to not be resuscitated, and a durable power of attorney for healthcare. Any do-not-resuscitate (DNR) order must be written and signed by the patient's doctor. A copy should be kept in the patient's file. Concealing or altering an advance directive is a misdemeanor. Creating an advance directive falsely is a felony. Living wills, which are legal in every state, state patients' desires should those patients become incapacitated (Figure ■ 7-12). Instructions address patients' desire concerning life-support procedures.

Patients may sometimes give durable power of attorney to other people. The power of attorney names people who can speak or act for the patient in the event the patient cannot speak for himself. Power-of-attorney documents typically address patients' desires concerning life support, but authorized parties may do such things as sign contracts or access bank accounts.

LIVING WILL OF _____

I, _____, a resident of the City of _____,

_____ County, State of _____, being of sound and dispos-
ing mind, memory and understanding, do hereby willfully and voluntarily make, publish, and declare this to
be my LIVING WILL, making known my desire that my life shall not be artificially prolonged under the
circumstances set forth below, and do hereby declare:

1. This instrument is directed to my family, my physician(s), my attorney, my clergyman, any medical facility in
   whose care I happen to be, and to any individual who may become responsible for my health, welfare, or
   affairs.

2. Death is as much a reality as birth, growth, maturity, and old age. It is the one certainty of life. Let this
   statement stand as an expression of my wishes now that I am still of sound mind, for the time when I may
   no longer take part in decisions for my own future.

3. If at any time I should have a terminal condition and my attending physician has determined that there can
   be no recovery from such condition and my death is imminent, where the application of life-prolonging
   procedures and "heroic measures" would serve only to artificially prolong the dying process, I direct that
   such procedures be withheld or withdrawn, and that I be permitted to die naturally. I do not fear death
   itself as much as the indignities of deterioration, dependence, and hopeless pain. I therefore ask that
   medication be mercifully administered to me and that any medical procedures be performed on me which
   are deemed necessary to provide me with comfort or care or to alleviate pain.

4. In the absence of my ability to give directions regarding the use of such life-prolonging procedures, it is my
   intention that this declaration shall be honored by my family and physician as the final expression of my
   legal right to refuse medical or surgical treatment and accept the consequences for such refusal.

5. In the event that I am diagnosed as comatose, incompetent, or otherwise mentally or physically incapable of
   communication, I appoint _____ to
   make binding decisions concerning my medical treatment.

6. If I have been diagnosed as pregnant and my physician knows that diagnosis, this declaration shall have no
   force or effect during the course of my pregnancy.

7. I understand the full import of this declaration and I am emotionally and mentally competent to make this
   declaration. I hope you, who care for me, will feel morally bound to follow its mandate. I recognize that this
   appears to place a heavy responsibility on you, but it is with the intention of relieving you of such responsibility and of placing it on myself, in accordance with my strong convictions, that this statement is made.

IN WITNESS WHEREOF, I have hereunto subscribed my name and affixed my seal at _____,

_____, this _____ day of _____, 20 _____, in the presence of the
subscribing witnesses whom I have requested to become attesting witnesses hereto. _____

                                                                                    Declarant

The declarant is known to me and I believe him/her to be of sound mind.

_____

_____ Witness   Address

_____

_____ Witness   Address

Subscribed and acknowledged, before me by _____, and subscribed and sworn
   to before the witnesses, on the _____ day of _____, 20_____.

_____

(SEAL)

NOTARY PUBLIC State of _____ My Commission
   Expires:_____

Copies of this instrument have been given to:

Receipt and acknowledged & date:

FIGURE ■ 7-12   Sample living will.

Faxing Medical Records

Medical records should be faxed only when no other method of data transfer is available, because the risk of unintended recipients seeing the fax is very high. The American Health Information Management Association recommends fax use for confidential patient information only when sending copies via postal service or messenger does not suffice. Medical offices should use a HIPAA-compliant fax cover sheet like the one shown in Figure ■ 7-13 any time patient information must be faxed.

Anne Wager, MD

Quan Lee, MD
8282 Arlington Way
Arlington, WA 12345
360-555-4545

Facsimile transmittal

To: _____   Fax number: _____

From: _____   Date: _____

Re: _____   No. of pages, including cover sheet: _____

___ Urgent   ___ For Review   ___ Please Comment   ___ Please Reply

Comments:

CONFIDENTIAL INFORMATION

The information in this facsimile message and any accompanying documents is confidential. This information is intended for use only by the individual or entity named above. If you are not the intended recipient of this information, you are hereby notified that any disclosure, copying, or distribution of this information is strictly prohibited. Please notify the sender immediately by telephone. Thank you.

FIGURE ■ 7-13   Sample HIPAA-compliant fax cover sheet.

Improper Disclosure of Medical Records

Disclosing confidential patient information without proper authorization or a subpoena is cause for a lawsuit. Patients who feel they have been harmed by improper disclosure may sue a medical office for defamation of character, invasion of privacy, or breach of confidentiality. When information is disclosed improperly, the office is responsible for reporting the event to the Office of Civil Rights.

Patients who believe medical offices have inappropriately disclosed medical information may contact the Office of Civil Rights directly. Every medical office must have the complaint forms on file and help patients file the proper paperwork. Normally, the Office of Civil Rights will only issue fines or written warnings when violations were intentional or offices have logged a number of violations.

The fines for HIPAA violations range from $100 to $25,000. Criminal penalties may also apply if it is determined that an individual knowingly obtained or disclosed personal health information without the proper authority. The most severe penalties under HIPAA legislation apply to anyone who commits an offense with the intent to sell, transfer, or use another person's health information. Figure ■ 7-14 outlines the penalties for HIPAA violations.

General penalty for the failure to comply with requirements and standards:

■ Not more than $100 for each violation up to a $25,000 for all violations of an identical requirement during a calendar year.

Wrongful disclosure of protected health information:

■ A person who knowingly and in violation of HIPAA regulations:
  ■ Uses or causes to be used a unique health identifier
  ■ Obtains private health information relating to an individual
  ■ Discloses individually identifiable health information to another person

Shall be punished by:

  ■ A fine of not more than $50,000, imprisoned for not more than 1 year, or both
  ■ If the offense is committed under false pretenses, be fined not more than $100,000, imprisoned for not more than 5 years, or both
  ■ If the offense is done with the intent to sell, transfer, or use private health information for commercial purposes or to cause harm, be fined not more than $250,000, imprisoned not more than 10 years, or both

FIGURE ■ **7-14**   Penalties for HIPAA violations.

Online Medical Records

Some clinics, like the Everett Clinic in Washington State, allow patients to look up portions of their electronic medical records via the Internet. Using this password-protected system, patients can access their lab results or medication dosages, which can help when patients travel or need to seek emergency care with someone other than their primary care providers. Several Internet-based businesses now offer individuals online storage of medical information, such as immunizations, medications, and surgeries.

Critical Thinking 7.12 ?

As a patient yourself, would you like the opportunity to access some or all of your own medical record online? What portions would you find useful?

Documentation of Prescription Refill Requests

Pharmacies will frequently fax or call in prescription refill requests to the medical office. Each medical office should have a policy that requires at least 24 hours for refill requests so physicians have time to review patients' files.

When a pharmacy calls with or faxes a prescription request, the medical assistant or nurse must pull the patient's file and place the request and patient file on the physician's desk for review. If the medical office uses electronic medical records, the medical assistant or nurse will enter the prescription request into the EMR and forward the request to the prescribing physician. If the physician feels the patient should be seen in the office before a prescription refill, the medical assistant or nurse should first call the pharmacy to alert them to the delay and then call the patient to schedule an appointment. If the physician authorizes the refill request, the medical assistant or nurse should call the pharmacy or fax the approval with the appropriate information. All information about the refill request, authorized or not, must be charted in the patient's medical record.

Medical Records in Research

medical research program
medical program geared toward researching a particular condition or treatment

nontherapeutic research
medical research that does not have therapeutic value to the patient

When patients participate in **medical research programs**, their medical records must be kept on file indefinitely. If adverse affects arise, even in future generations, the medical office must be able to prove the physician had the patient's consent to participate in the research. Medical research involves patients taking experimental medication or patients involved in **nontherapeutic research**.

In nontherapeutic research, a pharmaceutical company develops a new drug to combat a certain disease or disorder. Before that company can market the drug, however, it must receive approval from the Food and Drug Administration (FDA). The FDA requires extensive testing before drugs are considered safe and effective enough to be released. Part of FDA testing usually includes a nontherapeutic research trial in which companies pay physicians to dispense the drug to healthy patients who do not have the disease or disorder the drug is targeting so as to identify any side effects. Patients in these types of research programs must be fully aware of the risks and must sign consent forms to that effect.

Case Study Questions

Refer to the case study presented at the beginning of this chapter to answer the following questions:

1. How should Corey lead the group into the change from paper medical records to electronic?
2. Would it be best to begin with the active patient files? Why or why not?
3. What should Corey do with the paper medical records once the conversion has taken place?

Chapter Review

Summary

- The information contained within the medical record may be personal, financial, medical, or social.

- The medical record is used for various purposes, from accurate care of the patient to the defense of a lawsuit.

- Charting in the medical record must be done with extreme care for accuracy. Notes made in the medical record must be professional in nature because these notes may be viewed by outside sources. Unprofessional notes may be seen as a sign of incompetence on the part of the medical team.

- The oldest form of medical charting is the narrative format. This type of chart takes a narrative form, with notations listed in a running order. SOAP (subjective, objective, assessment and plan) note taking is the most commonly used format in medical records today. This format allows users to quickly see information contained in the medical record. POMR (problem-oriented medical record) note taking is not commonly used. Advocates for this form of charting appreciate the ability to retire patient complaints once resolved. Flowcharts and progress notes are commonly used to chart patient progress toward treatment goals.

- Use of abbreviations in charting should only be done with accepted medical abbreviations. Each medical office or facility should have a list of accepted abbreviations. When a medical staff member is in doubt, he should spell the word out, rather than use an abbreviation.

- Communications between the patient and members of the healthcare team are charted in the patient's medical record when those communications are related to the patient's medical care.

- Alphabetic filing of paper medical records is the most common method used in the medical office. With this method, charts are filed alphabetically by the patients' last names. Numerical filing is a system used in clinics where a higher level of security is needed to protect patient information. With this system, patient files are given a number and filed numerically. The list of patient names and assigned numbers is kept in a secure location. The process of shingling items in the medical chart is done when items are smaller than a standard size sheet of paper.

- Cross-referencing of medical records is used in clinics that use paper medical records. Patients who have hyphenated last names or who sometimes use two different last names may have their files misfiled. Using cross-referencing, the medical office staff will be better able to find these charts.

- Locating misfiled paper medical records can sometimes be done by looking for the chart under the patient's first name, or by looking for those patient charts that were pulled at the same time to see if the lost chart is located there.

- Medical offices that use paper charts store them in physical file storage systems. These systems vary from horizontal to vertical systems and medical charts must be kept in an area free from patient view.

- The retention time for medical records depends on the statute of limitations in the state where the medical practice operates. Medicare guidelines dictate that medical records remain stored for a period of no less than 5 years after the patient's last visit to the clinic.

- In medical practices where paper medical records are used, storage space may necessitate the removal of charts for inactive patients. By creating a policy of when to consider the charts inactive or closed, an office may remove those charts to an offsite location, thereby creating more space for storage in the clinic of current patients' files.

- Once a paper chart has been scanned into an electronic medical record, the original chart may be disposed of. This must be done via shredding of the chart so that the original document cannot be read.

- Corrections must be made in the medical record following a clear process. The original entry must not be obliterated. Correction fluid is not to be used in a paper medical record. Additions may be made to the medical record following a clear process as well. It must never appear as if the medical office staff attempted to alter the record in any way.

- In the event a nurse or medical assistant is asked to perform a procedure with a patient that seems to conflict with the nurse or assistant's training, the nurse or medical assistant should check with the physician on the orders, and chart the resulting conversation in the patient's chart.

- The actual medical chart, whether paper or electronic, belongs to the medical facility where the patient was seen for care. The information within the chart belongs to the patient. Patients have the right to see what is in their medical record and to make corrections and additions if they feel they are needed. This must be done according to office policy.

- Electronic medical records are what all medical offices and facilities will be moving toward in the future. It is easier to find items in an electronic record, and more than one person may access an electronic medical record at any given time.

- When releasing medical records, the medical office must make certain the process is done following the law and HIPAA guidelines. Only those items requested are to be released. When the patient is involved is some form of legal action, the court may subpoena a copy of the medical record. When this is done, a signature from the patient is not required prior to the release. On rare occasions, the medical office may be asked to release the original patient medical record. When this occurs, the office must make a copy of all items in the record before releasing the original. This enables the office to have an exact record of what is contained within the original record.

- When physicians retire, or leave their practice for another reason, the patients seen must be given the opportunity to have their records released to another facility.

- Children under the age of 18 are considered minors by law. Minors are not able to receive copies of their medical records; this must be done by the parent. For some information, such as family planning and drug counseling, however, the minor is able to receive copies of the information and the parent is not.

- Super-protected information is that information in the medical record that pertains to family planning, HIV/AIDS testing or treatment, drug counseling, or mental health treatment. A separate signed order must be received before this type of information may be released.

- Various situations must be reported to the authorities. These include suspected child or elder abuse, violent crimes, and the presence of certain illnesses and injuries.

- Patients may request that advance directives be placed within their medical record. These directives are items such as a DNR order or a durable power of attorney for healthcare.

- Using the fax machine to send medical records should be done only when another transfer method is not available. When faxing items from the medical record, the medical office must use a HIPAA-compliant cover letter.

- If information from the medical chart is disclosed inappropriately, the result may be a violation of HIPAA law. When this occurs, all effort must be made to retrieve the improperly disclosed item, and the patient whose privacy was violated must be notified.

- Many healthcare organizations today are allowing patients to access all or a portion of their medical record online.

- Any prescription refill request that comes into the medical office must be recorded in the patient's medical record, even if the provider denies the refill.

- When patients participate in medical research programs, their medical records must be kept on file indefinitely so that if adverse affects arise, the medical office can prove the patient's consent to participate in the research.

Multiple Choice

Choose the letter that best answers each question or completes each statement.

1. Which of the following determines how long a patient has to file a lawsuit after an injury occurs?
   a. Malpractice
   b. Statute of limitations
   c. Records retention
   d. HIPAA

2. Patients' medical records cannot be released without which of the following?
   a. The patient's signed consent
   b. The spouse's signed consent
   c. The physician's signed consent
   d. The office manager's signed consent

3. Who discussed the use of electronic medical records in his 2004 State of the Union address?
   a. Al Gore
   b. Bill Clinton
   c. Ronald Reagan
   d. George W. Bush

4. By what year did the person from Question 3 state electronic records should be in use in all medical facilities?
   a. 2010
   b. 2014
   c. 2018
   d. 2022

5. Dr. Jones is being paid to perform nontherapeutic research for a new blood pressure–lowering medication. Which of the following patients would be eligible to participate?
   a. A 65-year-old man with elevated blood pressure
   b. A 25-year-old woman with low blood pressure
   c. An 80-year-old man with no known health conditions
   d. None of the above

6. Online medical records are useful to which of the following?
   a. Patients who want to look up their own lab results
   b. Employers who want to see when their employee's next appointment is scheduled
   c. Spouses who want to know what their spouse was seen for
   d. All of the above

7. Which of the following patients does the medical provider have to file a report with the authorities about?
   a. A 2-year-old child with a bad diaper rash
   b. A 45-year-old woman with a bruise on her back from falling on the stairs
   c. A 10-year-old child with a positive test for an STI
   d. An 80-year-old man who has a sore knee

8. From an act passed in 1986, which of the following injuries must be reported?
   a. Vaccine injuries
   b. Injuries caused by automobile collisions
   c. Injuries caused by drug abuse
   d. Injuries that happen in the home

9. Which of the following is a reason to add an addendum to a patient's medical record?
   a. The day after the patient is seen, she calls back to say she is having an allergic reaction to the medication prescribed.
   b. Two hours after the patient is seen in the office, the medical assistant realizes she forgot to list the patient's complaint of arm pain when she made her entries during the visit.
   c. The physician reads the patient's lab results 2 days after the patient is seen.
   d. The office manager receives a call from a patient with a complaint about the amount of time the patient waited in the exam room that day.

10. Linnea Edwards is a 16-year-old. She comes into the clinic alone today asking for copies of her medical records. What portion of her records can she be given without her parent's signature?
    a. Immunization records
    b. Copy of her x-ray report
    c. Lab results for STI screening
    d. All of the above

True/False

Determine if each of the following statements is true or false.

_____ 1. The proper way to completely destroy a patient's paper medical record is to burn it.
_____ 2. The best way to send patient medical records from one healthcare facility to another is via fax.
_____ 3. Drug companies must receive approval from the FDA before they can market new drugs.
_____ 4. One of the many uses of the electronic medical record is the ability to date and time-stamp entries in the chart.
_____ 5. Prescription refill requests must be documented, even if the physician denies the refill.
_____ 6. The oldest form of charting is the POMR method.
_____ 7. The shortest form of charting is the narrative method.
_____ 8. In SOAP note charting, the S stands for subjective.
_____ 9. Intentional violation of HIPAA legislation may result in prison time.
_____ 10. A durable power of attorney for healthcare names people who can speak for a patient if she is unable to speak for herself.

Matching

Match each of the following terms with its definition:

a. complete
b. advance directive
c. clear
d. chief complaint
e. concise
f. chronologic
g. correct
h. discovery rule
i. closed patient files
j. cross-referencing

1. The main reason the patient sought care today
2. A legal document that outlines a patient's desire regarding life-sustaining treatment
3. To the point and easily understood
4. In order of when events occur in time
5. Accurate
6. Containing all necessary information
7. Medical record for a patient who has moved out of the area
8. Containing only the necessary information, nothing more
9. Relates to when an injury was discovered, rather than when the injury occurred
10. A system for locating files when a patient may go by one or more last names

Chapter Resources

American Health Information Management Association: www.ahima.org

Department of Health and Human Services for information on HIPAA legislation: www.hhs.gov/ocr/hipaa/

PEARSON myhealthprofessionskit™

Additional interactive resources for this chapter can be found at **www.myhealthprofessionskit. com.** Choose "Medical Assisting" from the discipline menu and then click on the book cover for *Medical Office Management.*

CHAPTER 8

Regulatory Compliance in the Healthcare Setting

CHAPTER OUTLINE

- The Impact of HIPAA Legislation on Patient Care
- The Business Associate Agreement and HIPAA Legislation
- The Red Flags Rule
- Developing a Corporate Compliance Plan
- The Health Information Technology for Economic and Clinical Health Act
- The Joint Commission and Ambulatory Care
- OSHA and Ambulatory Care
- CLIA and Ambulatory Care
- Fraud and Abuse
- Healthcare Reform

LEARNING OBJECTIVES

Upon completion of this chapter, you should be able to:

- Spell and define the key terms in this chapter.
- Describe the impact of HIPAA legislation in the medical office and on patient care.
- Describe the function of the HIPAA business associate agreement and its use in the medical office.
- Understand how the Red Flags rule applies to the medical office.
- Describe the purpose and content of a corporate compliance plan.
- Outline the various ways HIPAA legislation affects computer privacy.
- Describe how the medical office staff must work to remain in compliance with laws associated with The Joint Commission, OSHA, and CLIA.
- Define fraud and abuse as they pertain to the practice of healthcare.
- Understand the Healthcare Reform Act as it pertains to the medical office.

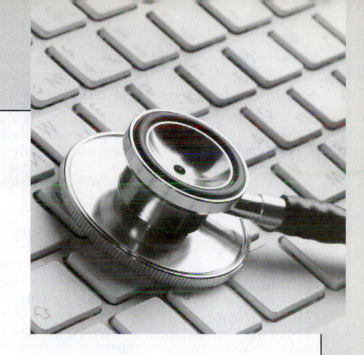

KEY TERMS

abuse

bloodborne pathogens

Clinical Laboratory
Improvement Amendments
(CLIA) Act

electronic billing

encrypt

false claim

firewall

fraud

Health Information Technology
for Economic and Clinical
Health (HITECH) Act

Health Insurance Portability
and Accountability Act (HIPAA)

The Joint Commission

Material Safety Data Sheet
(MSDS)

Occupational Safety and
Health Act

preexisting condition

privacy officer

protected health information
(PHI)

Red Flags rule

sentinel event

unbundling

unique identifier

upcoding

Case Study

Take note of the following scenario and answer the case study questions that appear at the end of this chapter.

Janeen Colbert is the HIPAA privacy officer in a large ambulatory healthcare center. As part of her job, she is responsible for the training of staff on HIPAA regulations and for responding to complaints about breach of privacy. Janeen has been faced with multiple complaints of breach of privacy during the past few months, most of them coming from patients who have been to a particular provider in the facility.

Introduction

Given the number of regulatory compliance organizations involved with the healthcare industry, the medical office manager needs to stay abreast of changing legislation, on both the state and federal level. Although regulations differ in a facility that is certified by The Joint Commission from one that has not sought this certification, it is still vital for the medical office to understand the laws and how to operate within legal boundaries.

The Impact of HIPAA Legislation on Patient Care

Health Insurance Portability and Accountability Act (HIPAA)
passed by Congress in 1996, this law addresses patient privacy and insurance carrier rules

Congress passed the **Health Insurance Portability and Accountability Act (HIPAA)** in 1996. Title I of HIPAA legislation was designed to provide protections for healthcare consumers who are covered by private medical insurance carriers. This portion of HIPAA addressed the issue of portability of health insurance benefits. At issue was the concern that employees, upon leaving their employment with one company and going to another company, might encounter difficulty obtaining coverage for their health needs with the new company's insurance carrier. This was of particular concern to those patients with preexisting conditions. The following sections discuss HIPAA legislation as it pertains to the ambulatory setting.

PREEXISTING CONDITIONS

preexisting condition
a condition that existed prior to coverage with a new insurance carrier

A **preexisting condition** is any healthcare condition that existed prior to coverage with a new insurance carrier. An example would be a chronic condition, such as diabetes. Prior to the passage of HIPAA legislation in 1996, healthcare consumers would often find themselves without coverage for certain conditions when they would move from one job (and insurance carrier) to another. Although HIPAA legislation did not entirely remove the ability of insurance carriers to impose preexisting condition periods, it limited them to no more than 12 to 18 months, depending on the type of insurance plan. Patients who have proof of insurance coverage that was not interrupted by a period of 63 days or more may be able to avoid preexisting condition clauses with their new insurance plan. If patients have had a full year of health insurance coverage at a previous job, and enroll in new coverage in less than 63 days, the new health plan cannot subject the patient to preexisting condition clauses.

Critical Thinking 8.1 ?

How might a patient be affected by the imposing of a preexisting condition period after changing insurance policies? What might the medical office manager tell the patient to prepare him for this possibility?

TITLE II OF HIPAA LEGISLATION

protected health information (PHI)
any patient information that includes identifiers that could be used to identify the patient

Title II of HIPAA legislation pertains to the prevention of healthcare fraud and abuse and to the simplification of administrative processes in the deliverance of healthcare. This is the section of HIPAA that caused the most concern and confusion when the privacy rule portion was enacted in 2003. The privacy rule regulates how **protected health information (PHI)** may be transmitted from one place to another.

DISCLOSURE OF INFORMATION TO THE PATIENT

HIPAA legislation requires healthcare providers and facilities to disclose patient information to the patient within 30 days of a request for that information. Patient information must also be disclosed to others under certain circumstances. This may happen with the patient's written consent in the case of the transfer of records from one provider to another (Figure ■ 8-1). Disclosing patient information may also happen without the patient's consent or knowledge in some cases. An example would be in the case of child abuse. If a healthcare provider is aware of abuse, she must report it to the local governing authorities and does not need patient or parental permission to do so.

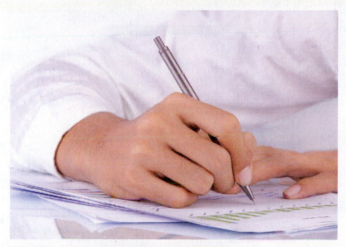

FIGURE ■ 8-1 Patients need to sign a transfer of records request to have records transferred.
Source: © Robbiverte/Dreamstime.com.

THE MINIMUM NECESSARY RULE

When disclosing information about a patient, HIPAA requires providers to use the minimum necessary rule. This rule states that only the minimum amount of information necessary is to be shared. As an example, if a patient's insurance carrier requests information about a patient visit to a physician, the physician's office may release information about that particular visit. Release of all information in that patient's file is not necessary to complete the request.

Critical Thinking 8.2 ?

How might a patient be adversely affected if more information were disclosed than the minimum necessary? What are some techniques the medical office manager could employ to keep these types of HIPAA violations from happening?

ALLOWING PATIENTS TO MAKE CORRECTIONS TO THEIR HEALTH RECORD

The privacy rule enables patients to request that corrections be made to their health record if the patient feels an error in charting has been made. This does not mean that the patient's request to remove information from the record or add information that was not documented prior must be granted. In some cases, patients may disagree with what is in their health record, even though the healthcare provider believes the information is accurate. When this happens, the patient may submit a written statement pertaining to the reason he wants the change made. That written document becomes part of the patient's medical record, but the original information also remains. In the case of electronic medical records, the patient's statement is scanned into the medical record (Figure ■ 8-2).

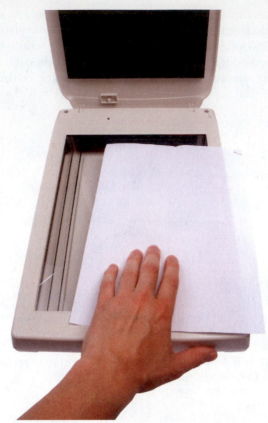

FIGURE ■ 8-2 A scanner is used to copy documents into an electronic medical record. *Source:* © Scramblerd/Dreamstime.com.

Critical Thinking 8.3 ?

Why might a patient object to information that is contained in her medical record? What could the medical office manager do if the patient insists on having objectionable information removed from her file?

OUTLINING DISCLOSURES TO THE PATIENT

Under the privacy rule, HIPAA requires healthcare providers to disclose to the patient information about the release of PHI. In other words, upon request, the patient may have the healthcare provider provide a list of all occasions when information about the patient was shared, including details on the information that was shared and to whom the information was provided. In the event of an improper disclosure (a disclosure of patient information that was accidental or unintended), the patient must be notified with details of the information disclosed and to whom it was released.

Any individual who feels his or her healthcare provider has violated the privacy rule may file a complaint with the Department of Health and Human Services, Office of Civil Rights.

THE HIPAA PRIVACY OFFICER

privacy officer
an employee in a healthcare facility charged with the duty of educating others on HIPAA compliance

The HIPAA privacy rule dictates that all healthcare facilities must employ a **privacy officer**. This person is the contact source for patients who feel their privacy has been violated in some way. The privacy officer is also the person responsible for training staff on HIPAA regulations, as well as maintaining a log of any improper disclosures of patient information. Depending on the size of the practice or facility, the privacy officer may be an individual who performs this job as his sole occupation, or it may be only a portion of the entire job performed by that person.

THE USE OF ELECTRONIC BILLING

Part of the simplification of administrative processes outlined in HIPAA legislation is the use of electronic means for transmitting medical claims from healthcare providers to insurance carriers. This is called **electronic billing**, or e-billing. Prior to the use of electronic billing, all insurance claims were billed on paper. With the use of electronic billing, data on the patient's visit is entered into the computer system and the claim is sent electronically to the insurance carrier. In many cases, payment is made electronically from the insurance carrier to the medical provider, making the process entirely paperless. Aside from saving time and money by not printing and mailing paper claims, electronic billing creates a faster process for submitting claims and obtaining reimbursement. See Chapter 13 for more on medical insurance billing.

electronic billing
the process of sending medical claims to insurance carriers electronically

THE HIPAA SECURITY RULE

The security rule portion of HIPAA legislation went into effect in 2005. This rule pertains to the safekeeping of electronic information within the healthcare facility. The security rule has three parts, each pertaining to a separate type of safeguard for keeping medical records secure: administrative, physical, and technical.

ADMINISTRATIVE SAFEGUARDS UNDER THE SECURITY RULE

The first part of the security rule is the administrative safeguards. These rules require healthcare providers or facilities to properly disclose to patients the privacy practices used in that facility. The privacy practices must be written and given to patients upon request. Because the privacy practices document is typically several pages in length, most providers and facilities have chosen to use a shorter form, which is signed by each patient. The statement simply alerts patients to the existence of the privacy practices document and informs patients of their right to receive a copy upon request.

Access to Records

Under the HIPAA security rule, providers and facilities are required to have a policy outlining the employee type that should be permitted access to patients' personal information. This is another area where the minimum necessary rule comes into play. Only those employees who must have access to patients' personal information should have that access. Of those employees, each should have access only to the information he needs to properly perform his job. In other words, if a patient is coming in to the office to see Dr. Brown, there is no valid reason for Dr. Smith or her medical staff to see that patient's medical information.

Proper Training Regarding Protected Health Information

The security rule requires healthcare providers and facilities to have written policies regarding training of personnel on the handling and care of PHI. These policies must include information on the ramifications involved for misuse of information or improper disclosure. All employees must be made aware of these policies, and in many facilities, the employee's signature is required as proof that this information has been provided to the employee.

PHYSICAL SAFEGUARDS UNDER THE SECURITY RULE

The second part of the security rule is the physical safeguards that must be in place to control access to patient information and data. This section of HIPAA legislation addresses the need to properly erase and dispose of old computer equipment, or any other electronic

encrypt
to mathematically scramble information in a way that keeps unauthorized persons from viewing it

firewall
a software program or hardware device designed to work with the computer to add a layer of security between the data on the computer and the network to which it is connected

system that houses patient information. All access to computers or other electronic systems must be safeguarded against improper use. This involves the use of password protection, as well as systems to block access to those without authority. Part of the physical safeguards that must be in place include storage of patient information in areas that are not easily accessible to the patient, and ensuring that patient information is kept out of view of those who do not have authority to see it.

TECHNICAL SAFEGUARDS UNDER THE SECURITY RULE

The third part of the HIPAA security rule relates to the technical safeguards that must be in place to protect patient information. HIPAA legislation demands that any patient information that is sent electronically be **encrypted** and only sent over protected networks. By encrypting the data, as well as using passwords to access any computer systems, patient data is kept safe from unauthorized eyes when transmitted. Use of **firewalls** and other forms of protection of computer equipment is also necessary.

Critical Thinking 8.4 ?

How might a medical office manager answer a patient who asks if her personal information is secure once the information has been entered into the electronic medical record?

THE UNIQUE IDENTIFIER RULE

unique identifier
a unique number issued by Medicare to each individual provider

Another HIPAA aspect of simplifying the administrative processes associated with sending patient data between physicians and health insurance payers relates to the use of the **unique identifier** (or National Provider Identifier). Prior to HIPAA legislation, every physician had at least one identifying provider number. Physicians who dealt with numerous insurance payers had numerous identifying numbers, with each number being issued by a particular insurance company, for example, Medicare and Medicaid. The numbers were used to pay the provider for claims. HIPAA's unique identifier rule dictates that each provider will have only one identifying number, and that number is to be used for all insurance payers. Much like a person's Social Security number, the unique identifier number is individual to the provider and follows that provider throughout his or her career. The unique identifier number does not take the place of the provider's drug enforcement agency number, state license number, or federal tax identifier number used for correspondence with the Internal Revenue Service.

HIPAA ENFORCEMENT RULE

Violations of HIPAA legislation may result in fines or even jail time in some cases. The HIPAA civil penalties were updated in February 2009. See Table ■ 8-1 for the penalties associated with particular violations.

HIPAA violations carry criminal penalties in rare instances. The U.S. Department of Justice clarified this section of the HIPAA enforcement rule in 2005 when they stated that any individual or organization that knowingly obtains or discloses protected patient information in violation of HIPAA regulations may face a fine of $50,000 as well as imprisonment of up to 1 year. Any individual found to be in violation of HIPAA regulations under false pretenses, such as an individual claiming to be doing research when he is not involved with any such research, may be subject to a fine of $100,000 and up to 5 years in prison. Last, any individual found to be in violation of HIPAA regulations with the intent to sell or transfer the information obtained may be subject to a fine of $250,000 and up to 10 years in prison.

Critical Thinking 8.5 ?

How might a HIPAA privacy officer educate staff on the importance of following HIPAA legislation and protecting patient privacy? What part does a medical office manager play in this education?

TABLE ■ 8-1   HIPAA Violations and Associated Penalties

Violation	Minimum Penalty	Maximum Penalty
Unintentional violation	$100 per violation, with annual maximum of $25,000 for repeat violations	$50,000 per violation, with an annual maximum of $1.5 million
Violation due to reasonable cause, but not due to willful neglect	$1,000 per violation, with an annual maximum of $100,000 for repeat violations	$50,000 per violation, with an annual maximum of $1.5 million
Violation due to willful neglect, but violation is corrected within the required time period	$10,000 per violation, with an annual maximum of $250,000 for repeat violations	$50,000 per violation, with an annual maximum of $1.5 million
Violation due to willful neglect that is not corrected within the required time period	$50,000 per violation, with an annual maximum of $1.5 million	$50,000 per violation, with an annual maximum of $1.5 million

The Business Associate Agreement and HIPAA Legislation

Under HIPAA legislation, employees of the physician or healthcare organization are covered by the rules and regulations outlined in HIPAA. Anyone who may come into contact with patient information, but is not an employee of the organization or physician, is not typically covered (Figure ■ 8-3). It is in these situations when a business associate agreement must be signed and kept on file. The business associate agreement is a written form that outlines the

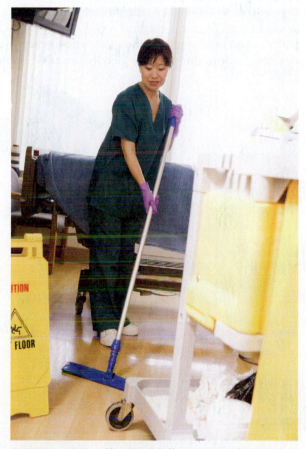

FIGURE ■ 8-3   Cleaning staff may come into contact with protected patient information.
Source: © Monkeybusiness/Dreamstime.com.

expectations of the healthcare provider or organization with regard to the business associate. The following individuals may need to sign a business associate agreement:

- Janitorial staff who are not employees of the healthcare provider or organization
- Transcription employees who are not employees of the healthcare provider or organization
- Healthcare students who are performing an externship or internship in the healthcare organization
- Equipment manufacturers or sales staff who come in to demonstrate or service medical equipment
- Computer repairpersons who are not employees of the healthcare provider or organization
- Students performing an externship in a healthcare facility.

Critical Thinking 8.6 ?

What other entities can you think of that would require a business associate agreement when working with the medical office? In what ways might someone use patient information illegally? What could a medical office manager do to help stave off these risks?

The Red Flags Rule

Red Flags rule
government legislation that requires all healthcare facilities to implement a written Identity Theft Prevention Program to detect the warning signs of identity theft in their day-to-day operations

The Federal Trade Commission (FTC) compiled a set of regulations in 2007. These regulations are known as the **Red Flags rule**. The purpose of these regulations is to combat identity theft. Although the implementation of the Red Flags rule was originally planned for November 1, 2008, this was pushed back a number of times and finally went into effect on December 31, 2010. To comply with the FTC's Red Flags rule, medical facilities must have "reasonable policies and procedures in place" to prevent identity theft. For most medical practices, this practice consists of requiring patients to show photo identification upon checking in for a medical appointment. With the use of the electronic medical record, many medical practices are taking a photograph of patients and attaching it to the electronic medical record (Figure ■ 8-4). This practice alerts front desk staff to the patient's identity on subsequent visits.

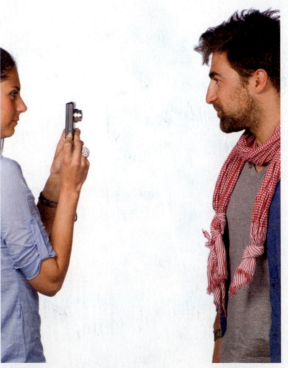

FIGURE ■ 8-4 Many clinics that use electronic medical records have the ability to store a photo of the patient with the record.
Source: © Heroskop/Dreamstime.com.

Chapter 8   Regulatory Compliance in the Healthcare Setting   **173**

Critical Thinking 8.7 ?

How might a medical office manager prepare and educate his staff on how to abide by the Red Flags rule in the medical office?

Developing a Corporate Compliance Plan

Regardless of the size of a medical organization, every facility needs to develop and enact a corporate compliance program. Corporate compliance programs are designed to keep organizations in compliance with all federal and state laws, particularly with HIPAA legislation. In larger facilities, this task may be an employee's sole function. In smaller facilities this task may be done by an employee in addition to his other tasks. The purpose of a corporate compliance plan is to establish how the organization will comply with federal, state, and local requirements. The corporate compliance plan outlines the policies and procedures the employees within the facility will follow, along with the standards of conduct.

A corporate compliance plan addresses these topics:

- Employees are not to read other employee's medical records, unless that employee is a patient under care with that particular employee.
- Employees are not to share computer passwords.
- Employees are not to discuss patient care with anyone without the patient's permission.
- Employees are to be trained in the proper disposal of sensitive medical records.

The Health Information Technology for Economic and Clinical Health Act

As part of the American Recovery and Reinvestment Act of 2009, Congress passed the **Health Information Technology for Economic and Clinical Health Act (HITECH) Act**. This legislation addresses the electronic transmission of patient data and goes beyond what was originally written into HIPAA legislation. The HITECH Act extended the possible penalties for HIPAA legislation to business associates of covered providers or organizations. As part of the HITECH act, healthcare organizations are required to notify patients of any potential breach of information and to create new rules for keeping track of disclosures and disclosing requirements.

Health Information Technology for Economic and Clinical Health (HITECH) Act federal legislation that addresses the privacy and security concerns associated with the electronic transmission of health information

The Joint Commission and Ambulatory Care

The Joint Commission, formerly known as the Joint Commission for the Accreditation of Healthcare Organizations, is a not-for-profit organization that accredits and certifies more than 19,000 healthcare organizations within the United States. The accreditation and certification offered by The Joint Commission is recognized as a symbol of quality and signifies that the organization is committed to meeting certain performance standards.

Accreditation from The Joint Commission may be earned by many types of healthcare organizations, including ambulatory settings. As of 2012, more than 1,900 ambulatory care facilities were certified by The Joint Commission. The performance areas reviewed by The Joint Commission in ambulatory care settings are:

- Environment of care
- Emergency management
- Human resources
- Infection prevention and control
- Information management
- Leadership

The Joint Commission Federal organization that bestows accreditation status to healthcare facilities after a thorough inspection and passage of safety and quality measures

- Life safety
- Medication management
- National patient safety goals
- Performance improvement
- Provision of care, treatment, and services
- Record of care, treatment, and services
- Reporting of sentinel events
- Rights and responsibilities of the individual
- Transplant safety
- Waived testing.

sentinel event
any incident in a healthcare facility in which a patient is injured or could have been injured

To achieve accreditation, ambulatory organizations must apply for accreditation with the commission. The entire process is funded by the healthcare organization and the expense associated with accreditation depends on the size of the healthcare facility. A **sentinel event** is defined as any incident in which harm came to the patient or could have resulted in harm to the patient. Sentinel events must be reported to The Joint Commission as part of the accreditation standards.

Critical Thinking 8.8 ?

Why might a physician practice choose to seek Joint Commission accreditation? How might this benefit the patients seen by that physician?

OSHA and Ambulatory Care

Occupational Safety and Health Act
legislation that affects safety for employees in all occupational settings

The **Occupational Safety and Health Act** was passed by Congress in 1970. The law enacted rules and regulations that pertain to all employers, not just those in healthcare. It also created the Occupational Safety and Health Administration (OSHA). OSHA laws regulate working conditions to ensure a safe and healthy environment in the workplace. OSHA is part of the U.S. Department of Labor, and the administrator for OSHA is the Assistant Secretary of Labor for Occupational Safety and Health.

As a federal law, the Occupational Safety and Health Act must be followed in all states. This legislation pertains to the materials employees are exposed to, and the protections that must be in place if anything in the workplace may be harmful to the employee. OSHA inspectors have the right to inspect any private or public healthcare facility.

BLOODBORNE PATHOGENS AND OSHA

bloodborne pathogens
any infectious material in blood that can cause disease in humans

In 1983, OSHA added an additional layer of employee safety with its **bloodborne pathogens** rules. This occurred after the discovery of the HIV virus, as well as the increased exposure to hepatitis B that healthcare employees were reporting. OSHA defines bloodborne pathogens as any infectious material in blood that can cause disease in humans. This includes hepatitis B and C and HIV. As of 1992, the bloodborne pathogens regulations were enacted into law, and what was originally voluntary protections were then required of healthcare employers. To be in compliance with the Bloodborne Pathogens Act, healthcare employers must do the following:

- Have an exposure control plan in place. This must consist of a written plan that outlines how to minimize or eliminate any employee exposure. The plan must be updated each year and employers must demonstrate that they have looked for ways to reduce possible exposures throughout the year.
- Use controls for reducing exposure. These consist of sharps containers for disposing of needles (Figure ■ 8-5), and retracting needles for injections and blood draws.
- Provide appropriate measures for reducing exposures. These include training for adequate hand washing, sharps disposal, and the handling of laundry as well as lab specimens.

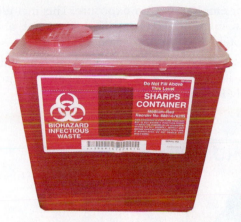

FIGURE ■ 8-5   A sharps container.
Source: © Emgallaghe/
Dreamstime.com.

■ Provide employees with necessary protective equipment, including gloves, gowns, protective eyewear and masks. Employers are responsible for the cleaning, repairing, and replacement of this equipment as needed (Figure ■ 8-6).

■ Provide hepatitis B vaccinations to all employees who become exposed to a blood-borne pathogen. This must be done within 10 days of the exposure.

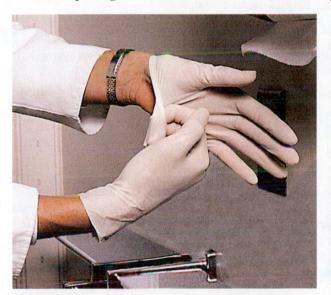

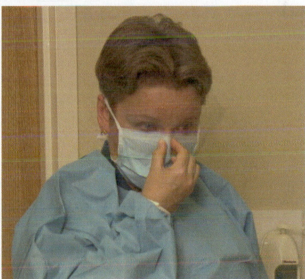

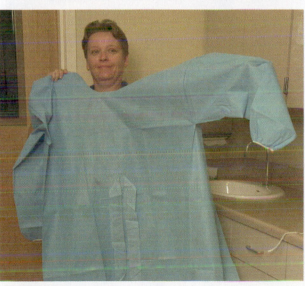

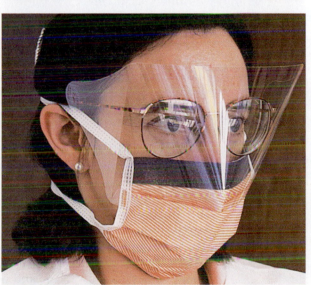

FIGURE ■ 8-6   Personal protective equipment: gloves, gown, mask, and protective eyewear.
Source: Michal Heron/Pearson Education.

- Provide any needed follow-up for employees after exposure. This includes, but is not limited to, providing laboratory testing, providing medical treatment, and testing the source person, if possible, for potential contagious bloodborne diseases.

- Label any items that contain hazardous materials. These include containers for soiled laundry as well as garbage. Any item used for healthcare related purposes, such as blood products, must be properly labeled as well (Figure ■ 8-7).

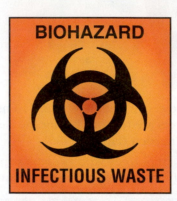

FIGURE ■ 8-7 Biohazard symbol.
Source: © Brilt/Fotolia.

- Provide proper training on possible hazards in the workplace to all employees. This includes the use of equipment and protective gear.

- Maintain a record of all training. This must be available for review if the healthcare employer is inspected by an OSHA representative.

THE MATERIAL SAFETY DATA SHEET

Material Safety Data Sheet (MSDS)

a sheet that outlines the potential risks associated with a chemical; required by OSHA for any potentially dangerous chemical

OSHA requires employers to maintain a hazard communication plan for employees. This includes labeling all chemicals in the clinic that have a potential for harm to an employee, such as cleaning supplies. Each potentially dangerous supply must have a **Material Safety Data Sheet (MSDS)**. This sheet outlines the risks associated with exposure to the chemical. MSDS forms are often available from manufacturers, or they may be created by the healthcare employer. All MSDS forms should be kept together in a binder, or in an online format, readily available to all employees.

Critical Thinking 8.9 ?

What are some benefits for the employee to having access to the MSDS in a medical office? What are the benefits to the employer of having employees properly trained on the use of hazardous materials? How might a medical office manager set up such a training process for employees?

THE OSHA EXPOSURE CONTROL PLAN

OSHA requires all healthcare employers to have a plan in place for preventing exposure to bloodborne pathogens. All employees must have access to this plan, and it must be updated each year. The plan must also be available for OSHA inspection, if requested. The exposure control plan must outline OSHA regulations pertaining to bloodborne pathogens, the ways in which the employer is working to protect its employees, the availability of hepatitis B vaccine and needed evaluation and medical care to employees who are exposed, communication about any hazards that exist in the medical facility, and the requirements for record keeping OSHA requires of the employer.

Part of the exposure control plan should be a list of policies and procedures pertaining to the labeling of biohazards in the medical facility, how exposure is determined, what the employee may expect if exposed, and the proper handling of potentially hazardous bodily fluids. The plan should also contain information on the proper use of protective equipment, including fitting for masks.

OSHA requires the medical facility to have a procedure for any situation where the employee may come into contact with potentially infectious material. Examples of policies the OSHA exposure control plan must contain are:

- Proper handling and disposal of needles
- Proper use of masks, as well as when different types of masks are needed
- Appropriate procedure for donning and disposing of gloves and gowns
- Proper procedure for sterile hand-washing technique.

LABELING BIOHAZARDS

Any biohazard must be properly labeled (see Figure ■ 8-7) using red bags or containers. The purpose of the labeling is to warn employees of the possible danger. These labels must be used on any container that may contain biohazardous waste, such as refrigerators that may contain specimens, laundry hampers for soiled linens, containers for used sharps, and waste bins if they are used for disposal of biohazards. OSHA requires that containers for biohazardous materials, such as sharps containers, be readily available to employees. For example, an employee should not be expected to walk from one room to another with a used needle after giving an injection to a patient. Instead, a sharps container should be available in any room where the employee is asked to give injections, so that the needle may be disposed of with little travel.

PERSONAL PROTECTIVE EQUIPMENT

Medical office personnel must wear personal protective equipment when there is an occasion to come into contact with body fluids (Figure ■ 8-8). This includes tasks such as drawing a patient's blood and administering a vaccination. The employee must be provided with gloves to use for this purpose. For those employees allergic to latex, the employer must provide a latex-free alternative. Whenever there is a potential for blood, or other potentially infectious material, to spray or splatter, employees must be provided with face and eye protection, as well as a gown to protect any exposed skin. All of this equipment must be provided to the employee at the expense of the employer. The employer must keep appropriate sizes on hand, so that employees have the proper size to wear when needed.

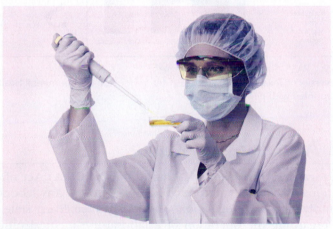

FIGURE ■ 8-8   Persons performing lab work should be wearing full protective gear.
Source: © Cemark/Dreamstime.com.

Critical Thinking 8.10 ?

What are some examples of situations where the medical staff member should don some form of personal protective equipment? Are there situations where only part of the protective gear should be donned, as opposed to donning all of it? What information should a medical office manager include in a policy on the use of personal protective equipment?

OTHER OSHA-MANDATED SAFETY PRECAUTIONS

Because OSHA oversees all areas of safety in the workplace, the agency dictates the need for the medical office to have a fire safety plan in the event of a fire. This safety plan includes the need for exit signs in the facility, the existence of fire alarm pull stations, emergency lighting in the event of a power outage, regular fire drills held during patient hours, posted floor plans throughout the building, testing of emergency response processes, and appropriate employee training (Figure ■ 8-9).

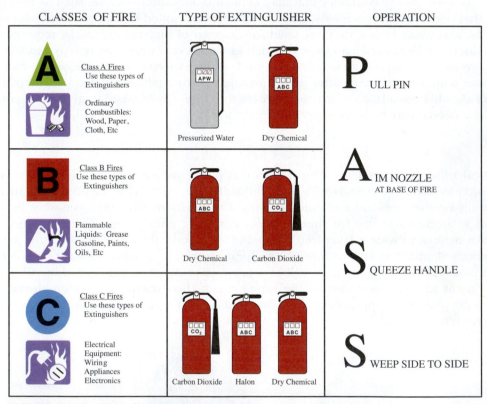

FIGURE ■ 8-9   PASS diagram.
Source: The University of Texas Health Science Center at Houston Environmental Health and Safety Department. Reprinted with permission.

CLIA and Ambulatory Care

Clinical Laboratory Improvement Amendments (CLIA) Act
passed in 1988, this legislation guides policies and procedures for laboratories

The **Clinical Laboratory Improvement Amendments (CLIA) Act** of 1988 guides the rules and regulations associated with operating a laboratory. Any laboratory, of any size, is required to comply with CLIA regulations and to pay a fee. Every state has its own rules and regulations regarding the operation of a laboratory; medical offices must comply with these as well.

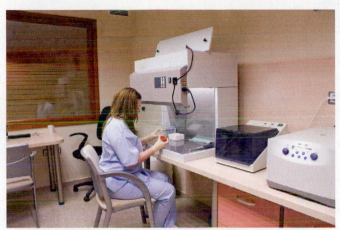

FIGURE ■ 8-10 Laboratory office in a small medical office.
Source: © Lemonadv/Dreamstime.com.

Prior to the enactment of CLIA in 1992, most physician offices operated a laboratory (see Figure ■ 8-10). The tests offered varied, as did the quality of the testing. The enactment of CLIA changed this scenario, and many tests previously performed in physician office locations were no longer processed there. Instead, more complicated laboratory testing began to be sent to outside, professional laboratories (Figure ■ 8-11). CLIA categorizes laboratory testing into tests that are of low, medium, or high complexity. The more complex the laboratory test, the more restrictions in place to ensure safety and high quality, as well as accuracy in results. In essence, CLIA has standardized the way laboratory testing is done, so that the patient receives the same results regardless of where the test is performed.

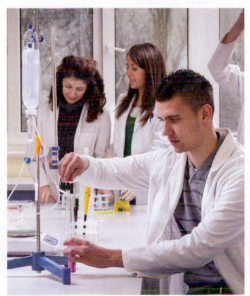

FIGURE ■ 8-11 Laboratory in a large medical facility.
Source: © Fotokostic/Dreamstime.com.

Critical Thinking 8.11 ?

Why would the passage of CLIA matter to the patient? How might CLIA affect the medical office? Do you believe CLIA rules make the laboratory tests more standardized? If so, in what way?

Fraud and Abuse

fraud
intentional deception or misrepresentation

abuse
charging for a higher level of service

upcoding
choosing to use a higher level of service code than is appropriate for the actual level of service provided

unbundling
billing for services (typically, lab services) separately, instead of as a bundled group

false claim
billing for services that were not provided to the patient, billing for services that were different from what was actually rendered, and providing services to the patient that were not medically necessary

Fraud in the healthcare facility is an intentional deception or misrepresentation made by a person with the knowledge that the deception could result in a benefit to himself or another. Laws governing fraud exist on both the state and federal levels. **Abuse** in the healthcare facility is defined as a practice that is inconsistent with sound fiscal, business, or medical practices, and results in unnecessary costs to the Medicaid or Medicare program or in reimbursement of services that are not medically necessary.

EXAMPLES OF FRAUD AND ABUSE

Examples of fraud and abuse in the healthcare setting include providing patients with treatments or services that are unnecessary; billing for services that were not rendered; misrepresenting credentials; providing narcotics to drug-seeking patients; **upcoding** (choosing to use a higher level of service code than is appropriate for the actual level of service provided); submitting duplicate claims in order to receive double payment; offering or soliciting bribes; and unbundling codes for services, such as laboratory testing. **Unbundling** is the practice of billing for services separately, instead of as a bundled group.

PENALTIES ASSOCIATED WITH FRAUD AND ABUSE

Physicians who are found guilty of fraud and abuse within the Medicare or Medicaid programs can be excluded from those programs. According to a 2009 report, Medicaid and Medicare fraud costs $60 billion each year. This is 10 percent of the program's total cost nationwide. These fraudulent activities consist of billing for services not rendered, upcoding of services, and pharmacies filling prescriptions for patients who are no longer living. These costs are passed on in the form of increased premiums and costs to physicians, healthcare facilities, and consumers alike.

Simply having a billing error on a claim does not translate to a penalty. Medicare officials believe that most payment errors are simple mistakes, and not the result of intentional fraud and abuse. Patients who are covered by Medicare are encouraged by their plan to report any possible fraud and abuse in healthcare. Medicare maintains a reporting telephone hotline for Medicare recipients to use to report suspected abuse.

Physicians who intentionally file a **false claim** for medical services could be subject to 5 years in prison, a $250,000 fine as an individual (double that figure for a corporation), or both. False claims are defined as billing services that were not provided to the patient, billing for services that were different from what was actually rendered, and providing services to the patient that were not medically necessary. Physicians who make false statements or intentionally cover up the facts in a case, with the intent of deceiving Medicare or Medicaid, may be subject to a $10,000 fine and/or 5 years in prison.

AVOIDING FRAUD AND ABUSE

Training of all medical office staff on the proper use of billing codes is essential to avoiding accusations of fraud from insurance carriers (Figure ■ 8-12). Typically, it is the physician who assigns the procedure codes in clinic settings today. These are passed on to the staff who perform the billing process. It is at this step that a check should be done to ensure that the proper code has been used.

When medical office staff members feel a physician is intentionally attempting to defraud an insurance carrier by billing incorrectly, the staff member should bring this to the attention of his or her supervisor. In some criminal cases, staff who were aware of the

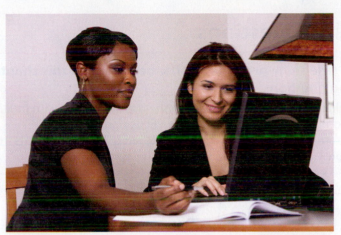

FIGURE ■ 8-12   All members of the medical billing team must be properly trained and up to date on coding laws. *Source:* © Camptown/Dreamstime.com.

abuse, but did nothing to stop the fraudulent activities, have been convicted of fraud and abuse along with the physician.

Medicare and Medicaid have telephone hotlines for medical office staff to use to report suspected cases of fraud and abuse. These are often handled anonymously, with investigations leaving out the identity of the reporter.

Critical Thinking 8.12 ?

What are some checks a medical office manager might put into place to avoid the accusation of fraudulent billing activity? How might the medical office manager stress the importance of avoiding fraudulent billing to the medical office staff?

Healthcare Reform

On March 23, 2010, President Barack Obama signed the Patient Protection and Affordable Care Act into law. This healthcare reform act made sweeping changes to the healthcare system and to the way in which healthcare services are paid. The major changes that came with this reform were the elimination of lifetime monetary limits on healthcare, the removal of preexisting care clauses, and the provision of care to more American children. With this legislation, insured Americans have access to preventive services, such as mammograms and colonoscopies, without copayments. This legislation expands Medicaid eligibility and picks up coverage for many Americans whose income was too high to qualify for Medicaid, while too low to afford purchasing private insurance benefits. To expand the risk pool to include as many Americans as possible, this legislation includes tax penalties for citizens who do not obtain health insurance. Those without health insurance coverage will pay a tax penalty that will range from $695 to $2085 per family. There will be exemptions granted for financial hardship, or religious objections, among other reasons. Dependants will be covered on their parents' health insurance plans up to age 26, regardless of enrollment in college.

Critical Thinking 8.13 ?

What benefits does the Patient Protection and Affordable Care Act offer to families who were unable to afford healthcare coverage prior to the act?

Case Study Questions

Refer to the case study presented at the beginning of this chapter to answer the following questions:

1. How should Janeen address the problem she is encountering with multiple complaints coming from patients who have seen a particular provider?

2. What are some methods Janeen could use to keep these complaints from happening in the future?

Chapter Review

Summary

- HIPAA legislation contains many rules and regulations pertaining to the medical office. Medical offices that do not comply with HIPAA regulations may be subject to fees and penalties.

- HIPAA regulates not only privacy, but also the protection of electronic data. HIPAA regulations must be enforced regardless of the size of the medical facility.

- To be compliant with HIPAA legislation, every healthcare facility or department must have a privacy officer. The privacy officer may hold this job as her sole task, or may perform the functions of the privacy officer in addition to other duties.

- The Red Flags rule was implemented on December 31, 2010. This rule requires medical facilities to verify a patient's identity prior to receiving medical care. This is most commonly done by asking to see photo identification.

- Medical facilities must develop a corporate compliance plan to ensure that federal and state regulations are followed according to the law. This reduces the likelihood of fines and penalties for inadvertent actions.

- The HITECH Act is a recent addition to HIPAA legislation that outlines further rules for patient privacy. This act pertains to the use of computers and increased security in the medical office.

- The Joint Commission offers accreditation to facilities, either on a voluntary or mandatory basis. Accreditation by the commission signifies that a healthcare facility is offering excellent quality of care.

- OSHA is a federal organization that outlines safety rules and regulations for all workplaces. Although OSHA applies to all workplaces, this organization also has special regulations that pertain only to healthcare. One of OSHA's additional rules for healthcare organizations is the Bloodborne Pathogens Act. This act applies to any employee who comes into contact with bodily fluids in the workplace.

- CLIA regulates laboratories in healthcare facilities. These regulations vary according to the complexity of the test. Certain laboratory tests are waived by CLIA. More complicated procedures require a higher level of regulation and monitoring.

- Fraud and abuse in healthcare costs have contributed to the high costs associated with healthcare. Severe penalties are associated with Medicare and Medicaid fraud and abuse.

- Healthcare reform legislation has enacted many changes in healthcare, from the ability of lower middle class families to purchase health insurance to the retention of young adult children on parents' insurance policies.

Multiple Choice

Choose the letter that best answers each question or completes each statement.

1. An employee would find a list of the potential hazards associated with a cleaning supply in the medical office by consulting:

a. the MSDS.
b. the privacy officer.
c. the patient's PHI.
d. None of the above

2. Which of the following individuals would likely need to sign a HIPAA business associate agreement?
   a. The janitor who cleans the clinic after hours
   b. The receptionist who works in the afternoons
   c. The nurse who works only one day each week
   d. The physician

3. Mrs. Jones is coming in to see Dr. Black. Melissa is the medical assistant working with Dr. Black. Gordon is the medical office manager. Under the minimum necessary rule, which of the following staff members in the medical office should review Mrs. Jones' medical chart today?
   a. Melissa the medical assistant
   b. Gordon the medical office manager
   c. The front desk receptionist
   d. All of the above

4. If a patient believes an error has been made in his medical chart, which of the following is true?
   a. The patient should be given his original chart and asked to remove the erroneous material.
   b. The medical assistant or nurse should redact the erroneous material from the medical chart.
   c. The patient may supply a written statement outlining his belief that the chart contains erroneous material. That statement would then become part of the permanent medical record.
   d. None of the above

5. Under the OSHA Bloodborne Pathogens Act, which of the following is true?
   a. The medical office must provide needed protective medical equipment.
   b. The medical office manager must observe each employee when performing blood draws.
   c. The patient may request the staff wear protective equipment, even when potentially hazardous materials will not be present.
   d. All of the above

6. Which of the following is essential to avoid accusations of fraud and abuse in healthcare?
   a. Provide the staff with proper training on billing and coding.
   b. Ask patients to report to the office manager any suspected fraud or abuse.
   c. Ask the physician to meet with the office manager monthly to discuss fraud and abuse.
   d. None of the above

7. Which of the following are governed by CLIA legislation?
   a. Small laboratories located within physicians' offices
   b. Large, freestanding laboratories
   c. Laboratories located within hospitals
   d. All of the above

8. Violation of HIPAA legislation may result in:
   a. fines and a possible prison sentence.
   b. revocation of the physician's license.
   c. confiscation of the physician's medical equipment.
   d. closure of the physician's practice.

9. Which of the following is a duty of the HIPAA privacy officer?
   a. To suggest changes to the legislation to Congress
   b. To receive complaints from patients who believe their privacy has been violated
   c. To meet weekly with the office manager to discuss potential privacy violations
   d. None of the above

10. Which of the following would be considered a sentinel event?
    a. The patient is late for her appointment.
    b. The physician charts in the wrong patient's chart.
    c. The patient is given the wrong medication.
    d. The physician is called away for a hospital emergency and patients must be rescheduled in the clinic.

True/False

Determine if each of the following statements is true or false.

_____ 1. In the event of an improper disclosure of patient health information, the patient must be notified with details of the information disclosed and to whom it was released.

_____ 2. Any patient health information that is to be sent electronically must be encrypted.

_____ 3. Unbundling is the term used when a physician intentionally uses a higher code in order to receive a higher payment.

_____ 4. Any biohazardous waste must be disposed of using green bags or containers.

_____ 5. The medical office must have an MSDS on any potentially hazardous substance used in the facility.

_____ 6. The unique identifier number takes the place of a physician's medical license number.

_____ 7. Medicare encourages its recipients to report suspected cases of fraud and abuse in healthcare.

_____ 8. The business associate agreement is a voluntary part of HIPAA legislation; small physician offices are not required to comply.

_____ 9. As part of the Bloodborne Pathogens Act, all employees must be properly trained on the use of personal protective equipment.

_____ 10. If an employee does not fit into the personal protective equipment purchased by the employer, the employee must provide their own.

Matching

Match each of the following terms with its definition

a. encrypt

b. electronic billing

c. bloodborne pathogens

d. CLIA

e. firewall

f. Material Safety Data Sheet (MSDS)

g. sentinel events

h. PHI

i. upcoding

j. HITECH act

1. Any infectious material in blood that can cause disease in humans

2. The process of sending medical claims to insurance carriers electronically

3. Legislation that guides policies and procedures for laboratories

4. To mathematically scramble information in a way that keeps unauthorized persons from viewing it

5. A software program or hardware device designed to work with the computer to add a layer of security

6. The law addressing patient privacy and insurance carrier rules

7. A sheet that outlines the potential risks associated with a chemical

8. Any patient information that includes identifiers that could be used to identify the patient

9. Any incident in a healthcare facility in which a patient is injured or could have been injured

10. Choosing to use a higher level of service code than is appropriate for the actual level of service provided

Chapter Resources

CLIA: www.cms.gov/clia/

The Joint Commission: www.jointcommission.org/

Occupational Safety and Health Act (OSHA): www.osha.gov

PEARSON myhealthprofessionskit

Additional interactive resources for this chapter can be found at **www.myhealthprofessionskit. com.** Choose "Medical Assisting" from the discipline menu and then click on the book cover for *Medical Office Management.*

CHAPTER 9

Duties of the Medical Office Manager

CHAPTER OUTLINE

- Different Management Theories
- Management versus Supervision
- Delegating Authority to Others
- Coaching and Mentoring Staff
- Motivating Employees
- Characteristics of the Medical Office Manager
- Responsibilities of the Medical Office Manager
- Different Leadership Styles
- Effective Staff Meetings
- The Medical Office Manager's Role with Supplies
- Negotiating Service Contracts
- Employee Theft

LEARNING OBJECTIVES

Upon completion of this chapter, you should be able to:

- Spell and define the key terms in this chapter.
- Define various management theories and the characteristics associated with each.
- Discuss the difference between management and supervision.
- Understand the importance of delegating authority to others.
- Describe the concepts of coaching and mentoring staff.
- Understand how to motivate employees.
- Describe the characteristics of the medical office manager.
- List the responsibilities of the medical office manager.
- Describe various leadership styles and the characteristics associated with each.
- Manage effective staff meetings, and compose the staff meeting agenda and staff meeting minutes.
- Understand the concept of contracting with suppliers and service providers, and outline the process of ordering and receiving supplies in the medical office.
- List techniques for responding to and discouraging employee theft.

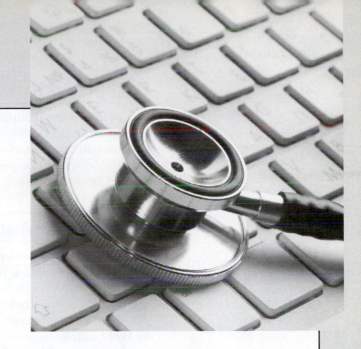

KEY TERMS

agenda	humanistic	service contract
authoritarian	intimidate	staff meeting
autonomy	leading	supervisor
catalystic	motivating	Theory X
coaching	multitask	Theory Y
coordinating	negotiate	visionary
delegation	organizing	warranty
democratic	participative	working supervisors
feedback	performance evaluation	
front-line staff	planning	

Case Study

Take note of the following scenario and answer the case study questions that appear at the end of this chapter.

Barb Totem has been managing a busy pediatric clinic for the past 10 years. She is friendly with her employees and considers many of them to be her friends. When conflict occurs in the workplace, Barb sometimes finds it difficult to separate her personal feelings for her employees from her job of disciplining them. Barb feels uncomfortable when she needs to speak to some employees about performance because she worries the employees will think she does not like them.

Introduction

The duties of the medical office manager differ depending on the size and type of practice. In a smaller facility, the office manager may work as a nurse, receptionist, or medical assistant, in addition to managing the medical office. Many of the core duties the office manager does will be present in the job description of both small and large-size offices' managers.

Different Management Theories

Theory X
a management theory that states employees cannot be trusted to think for themselves

Theory Y
a management theory that states employees want to do well and will perform well if given the opportunity

authoritarian
a leadership style in which the manager is always in charge and control of the employees

The management of people has long been the subject of study, both in the United States and around the world. In his book *The Human Side of Enterprise*, published in 1960, Douglas McGregor discussed the concepts of **Theory X** and **Theory Y** as they relate to managing people. Theory X is considered an **authoritarian** management style. Under this theory, the manager assumes that those being managed dislike the work and will try to avoid doing the work when possible. Theory X managers believe staff must be managed by fear and intimidation (Figure ■ 9-1).

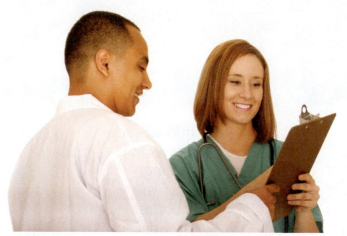

FIGURE ■ 9-1 The medical office manager will often oversee the work of staff members.
Source: © Pemotret/Dreamstime.com.

participative
a management style in which the manager seeks out the opinions of those they manage

Theory Y is considered a **participative** management style. Under this theory, the manager believes that staff will work best when they feel good about their work. Theory Y managers believe that staff will seek out responsibility and that they will use their skills to solve problems independently of the manager. Although these theories are more than 50 years old, they are still commonly referred to in the field of management.

Critical Thinking 9.1 ?

Between Theory X and Theory Y, which one do you think would be best used in an office where the manager makes all of the decisions without gathering input from staff members?

Management Versus Supervision

planning
the process of setting goals for a group

Management theories and styles have been studied since the early 1900s. Management basically consists of four main functions. The first function is that of **planning**. Part of planning consists of setting goals for the group and determining how those goals will be reached and the dates by which they should be accomplished. Examples of planning include strategic planning (determining when to bring on new physicians or begin a new product line), marketing endeavors (determining the products that are best for marketing and the demographic to target), and staffing (determining the number and type of staff to bring into the practice to support the providers).

The second function of management is that of **organizing** the resources under the manager's control. An example of this function would be the medical office manager determining the need for equipment in the facility and how best to use that equipment to get the most benefit from it.

The third function of management is that of **leading** others. This is where the manager sets the vision for the practice, or individual person. Another example of leading others would be that of helping staff in setting their own personal and professional goals or career planning.

The fourth function of management is that of **coordinating** the staff and resources of the practice. This involves financial areas, such as setting up a budget for the practice or determining when particular equipment should be replaced. The coordinating function is also where the task of risk management lies, and where the medical office manager seeks to discover and reduce or eliminate risks to patients, as well as staff.

Supervision of employees typically consists of management of the **front-line staff**. **Supervisors** carry out the instructions of the managers to whom they report. Supervisors may be full time in the supervisory role, or they may be **working supervisors**, spending a portion of their time working in a clinical or administrative role in the office and the rest of their time supervising others. Supervisors typically set staff schedules and approve and arrange for staff vacation days. The supervisor often hires and trains new employees, conducts performance evaluations, and handles disciplinary actions (Figure ■ 9-2).

organizing
the process of gathering the necessary tools, staff, and resources to accomplish set goals

leading
the process of showing others how a task should be done; setting the vision or tone for the group

coordinating
the process of setting up separate functions so that a team is able to perform

front-line staff
employees who have direct contact with patients, such as a receptionist, medical assistant, or nurse

supervisor
the person who oversees staff and their work

working supervisors
supervisors who spend a portion of their time working in the same role as the employees they supervise

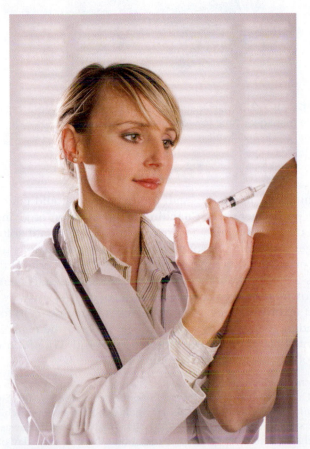

FIGURE ■ **9-2** A performance evaluation will include a review of performance in administrative and clinical areas.
Source: © Dušan Zidar/Fotolia.com.

Delegating Authority to Others

delegation
the process of taking one's tasks and giving them to another

Former President Ronald Reagan is quoted as saying "Surround yourself with the best people you can find, delegate authority, and don't interfere." The successful medical office manager will follow that advice. **Delegation** is the process of taking tasks from one person's responsibility and moving it to another's. For the medical office manager, this can take any of a number of forms, though typically it entails moving the daily functions to other members of the healthcare team. As an example, the medical office manager may be given a task from upper level administration in an organization, such as data collection. If the manager feels she has a staff member who is capable of this task, the manager may delegate the task to another. By delegating, the manager frees up her time to perform other tasks in the medical office. It is important for the medical office manager to realize that not all functions can be performed by the same person and therefore the manager will need to delegate tasks to various members of the healthcare team (Figure ■ 9-3). Delegating tasks to other members of the healthcare team is one way to mentor staff and build their skills.

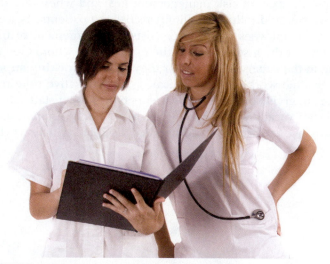

FIGURE ■ 9-3 Delegating tasks to other employees frees up the manager's time to work on other tasks.
Source: © Josetandem/Dreamstime.com.

Coaching and Mentoring Staff

coaching
the process of giving advice to employees to help them find their own solutions to problems and encouraging employees to do their best

feedback
opinions provided to an individual about what they have done or said

The tasks of coaching and mentoring staff are ones that should take up a large portion of the medical office manager's day. **Coaching** is the function of giving advice to staff in a way that allows the staff member to arrive at the appropriate solution to a problem without the manager providing the solution. By making suggestions to the staff member, the medical office manager allows that person to develop his critical thinking skills. This creates and fosters a more productive work environment as staff members learn to find solutions on their own, instead of coming to the manager for answers.

Mentoring staff involves setting an example for staff members to follow. This function also involves providing **feedback** to staff members on how the manager feels a situation was handled or how it could have been handled differently. The following is an example of how a medical office manager may mentor a staff member.

> Carlene King is the medical office manager in a busy family practice office. Steve Monroe is a lead medical assistant in the department; he reports to Carlene. After Steve put together a staffing schedule for the upcoming holiday weekend, he was approached by one of the medical assistants assigned to work the holiday. The medical assistant was not happy with Steve's proposed schedule and argued that she should be given the day off. Steve worked through the schedule with the assistant, explaining that she was given the day off for that holiday in the past year. After the conversation, Steve goes to Carlene for advice on how he handled the situation. Carlene tells Steve she agrees with what he said to the assistant, but she would suggest he hold similar future conversations in private, rather than in front of other members of the team.

Critical Thinking 9.2 ?

What do you think the benefits are for the manager when he or she provides consistent feedback to employees? Do you think this method makes the medical office manager's job easier or more difficult?

Motivating Employees

Motivating employees to perform at their highest level can be challenging to many medical office managers. It has been proven in many studies that staff members who are satisfied with their job perform at a higher level than those who are not satisfied. Creating a supportive and enriching work environment is key to motivating employees to perform at their best.

The medical office manager needs to set clear expectations of staff in the department and also provide regular feedback on how well the team is performing. Setting expectations starts with a clear and concise job description. Feedback may be done in formal **performance evaluations**, though it is most beneficial to provide feedback on a regular basis.

When an employee is not performing at his best, the manager should take him aside in private and discuss the performance. Discussions about performance should never take place in front of other employees or patients. This gives the employee privacy as well as dignity, and allows the discussion to include information the employee would not want coworkers to hear. To motivate this employee, the manager needs to determine what may be at the root of the performance issue. If the employee is having personal problems, the manager may need to refer that employee to assistance. By showing the employee that the manager cares about him as a person, the employee is far more likely to be motivated to perform at a higher level. The same is true when dealing with conflict between two staff members. The medical office manager will want to speak with the employees apart from other members of the staff.

The best way to motivate employees is to recognize and encourage desired behaviors. By showing employees that the manager cares about them, those employees will be more motivated to be high performers. Managers should look for opportunities to provide praise and encouragement on a weekly basis to all direct reports. During regular performance evaluations, managers should discuss with employees any opportunities that are available for advancement or to learn new skills.

motivating
the process of encouraging others to perform well; recognizing employees for a job well-done

performance evaluation
process by which a manager reviews job performance with an employee

Critical Thinking 9.3 ?

Think about the difference between showing staff you care about them and being "friends" with your staff. How do you think you could show staff you care about them without crossing the line of professional distance?

When an employee is performing at a high level, it is extremely important for the manager to recognize and praise that employee. While some people prefer to be recognized publicly, others prefer to be recognized in private. The successful medical office manager will take the time to find out what type and form of recognition the employee prefers upon hiring that employee. Figure ■ 9-4 shows an example of a tool the medical

> How do you like to be recognized (publicly or privately)?
>
> What is the best recognition you have received in your life?
>
> What form of recognition do you prefer (time off, cash bonus, gift)?

FIGURE ■ 9-4   How do you like to be recognized?

office manager might use to find out how employees would like to be recognized. The questions can be printed on a 3 × 5 card and given to all employees in the practice. By making recognition meaningful to the employee, the manager shows the employees that they are valued as individuals.

The medical office manager who spends time recognizing and praising the positive efforts of his employees will find that those employees are far more motivated to perform well than those who feel they are not noticed for the good work done (Figure ■ 9-5).

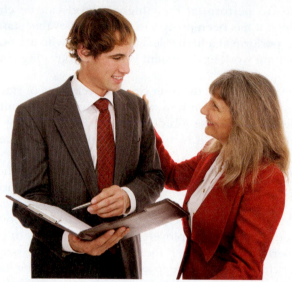

FIGURE ■ 9-5 Offering recognition and praise is the best way to keep employees motivated.
Source: © Lisafx/Dreamstime.com.

Characteristics of the Medical Office Manager

The most successful medical office managers are those who possess some core skills, as well as a host of other skills that may be needed for the job. The core skills for the position include the ability to **multitask**. The medical office manager often needs to perform multiple tasks at the same time often throughout the day. In doing so, the manager needs to be able to remain calm, no matter how hectic the day or how upset a patient or staff member may be. The most successful managers are very organized and able to recollect items from memory easily; they are able to communicate and to listen well. The medical office manager must be supportive of all office personnel and treat all staff members equally.

Successful medical office managers are able to manage multiple project deadlines at the same time. The manager must be able to handle conflict in a calm and quick manner, and be able to provide feedback—both positive and negative—in a professional way. Managers must delegate tasks to others, not only to free up the manager's time, but also to provide opportunities for professional growth to the employees. Knowledge of the financial part of the business, as well as the clinical and administrative functions, is essential for the successful manager.

multitask
the ability to handle more than one task at the same time

Critical Thinking 9.4 ?

If a manager forms personal relationships with his employees, do you think there is a potential for some employees to feel he is showing favoritism to certain members of the team? How do you think the manager could avoid this perception?

Responsibilities of the Medical Office Manager

Successful medical office managers know that being a leader involves more than simply telling others what to do. Good leaders lead by example and encourage those they manage to do the best jobs they can do. As the leader in the office, the medical office manager must have excellent communication skills and the ability to project confidence. See Figure ■ 9-6 for a list of responsibilities of the medical office manager.

- Supervision of employees
- Interviewing and hiring employees
- Scheduling staff
- Employee evaluations
- Disciplining and terminating employees
- Tracing the financial flow within the medical office
- Handling disputes between staff members
- Organizing and leading staff meetings
- Handling difficulties with patients
- Oversight of the inventory and equipment maintenance within the office
- Function as a buffer between the physicians and the staff
- Prepare quarterly financial reports
- Payroll

FIGURE ■ 9-6 Responsibilities of the medical office manager.

Different Leadership Styles

Most management theorists agree that there are six distinct management styles. Though most managers do not stay in one leadership style all of the time, every manager has a dominant style.

INTIMIDATING LEADERSHIP STYLE

The first leadership style is an **intimidating** style. The manager who uses this method uses fear as a motivator, demanding that employees do as they are told. While this method may work well in an emergent situation, when quick action is imperative, it does not work well as a primary leadership style. Employees under the manager using this style are not typically motivated to perform at the highest level. This type of manager does not usually spend time recognizing employees who are performing above and beyond in their tasks. Instead, this manager focuses on those employees who are not performing well.

intimidate
to lead others through fear

AUTHORITARIAN LEADERSHIP STYLE

The manager who uses the authoritarian leadership style is typically one who has years of experience and is therefore considered an expert by the employees. This manager may be one who has led other teams to success in an area and is therefore looked to for her **visionary** abilities. Like the intimidating style, the manager who leads in an authoritative style risks intimidating her employees. Also like the intimidating style, the authoritative style is one that works well at times when quick action is needed.

visionary
a leader who offers a vision for the future

humanistic
a leadership style in which employees are left alone to do their work as each employee believes is best

HUMANISTIC LEADERSHIP STYLE

The manager who uses the **humanistic** style of leadership is one who, after employees have been trained, leaves employees to do their jobs without interference. This manager

autonomy
the ability to work with little oversight or help

believes employees work best when they have **autonomy**, rather than oversight. Employees understand that they are allowed to do their jobs in the way they believe is best. Although high-performing employees may work well under this manager, employees who are not performing at their best are not motivated to change because this type of manager tends to forego disciplinary action. Because it is unlikely that all employees will be motivated to perform at their best, this style does not work well over time.

DEMOCRATIC LEADERSHIP STYLE

democratic
a leadership style in which employee opinions are used in the decision-making process

The leader using the **democratic** leadership style spends time gathering input from employees before making decisions. This manager believes that taking time to gain consensus from employees is the key to motivating and inspiring employees to perform at their best. Employees working under this manager will feel as if their opinions are important and valued—a key to keeping staff satisfaction high. One problem with this style is that it is time consuming. Often, a decision needs to be made quickly in healthcare management and gaining the input from all staff members is not practical.

CATALYSTIC LEADERSHIP STYLE

catalystic
a leadership style that consists of leading others by setting a fast pace for employees to follow

The manager using a **catalystic** style of leadership sets the example for employees by setting the pace. This manager is often a fast-paced person; a Type A personality. A person with a Type A personality is someone who tends to be competitive and work obsessed. By setting the pace, the manager is attempting to motivate employees to work as hard and as fast as she does. This manager tends to give feedback to employees only when they are not performing at the level the manager desires. This manager may be a *working manager*, one who not only manages employees, but also works alongside them in some function at times. An example would be a nurse manager who sometimes works with employees performing the nurse function in the office.

MENTORING LEADERSHIP STYLE

The manager who uses the mentoring style spends time coaching and mentoring her employees. This manager may use a combination of other leadership styles throughout the workday, while taking time to ensure that employees are motivated and encouraged to do well. The mentoring manager believes that employees should be encouraged to do their best and to learn from mistakes. This manager encourages employees to continue seeking educational opportunities. The mentoring leader understands that employees may not stay in their current role long term – the employee may seek higher-level positions within the organization. The manager using this style must possess a high level of self-confidence and security. He cannot fear being replaced by one of his employees. This manager understands that employees who are coached and mentored are typically happier, more satisfied employees (Figure ■ 9-7).

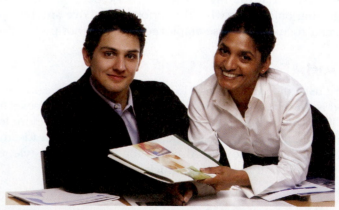

FIGURE ■ **9-7** Offering an employee guidance is one way to provide mentoring.
Source: © Orangeline/Dreamstime.com.

Critical Thinking 9.5 ?

Why do you think the mentoring leadership style works for employees? What benefit do you think it provides to employees?

Effective Staff Meetings

The key to the proper flow of communication in the medical office is frequent and effective **staff meetings** (Figure ■ 9-8). While the frequency and length of a staff meeting will vary with the size and type of medical practice, a minimum frequency is one meeting per month. In a larger office, smaller meetings may be held for certain groups of the team. An example would be all of the nurses or medical assistants meeting to discuss issues that pertain to their particular role in the office.

staff meeting
meeting attended by members of a department or office

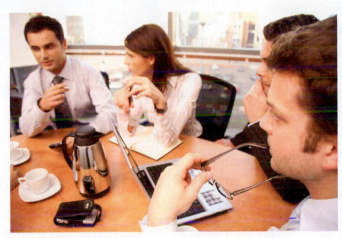

FIGURE ■ 9-8   A medial office staff meeting.
Source: © Endostock/Dreamstime.com.

Staff meetings should be held at a time of day that is convenient for the attendance of everyone within the office. This may not always be possible, especially in offices where physicians have staggered start and end times. Department meetings may or may not include the physicians. Those that include the physicians may be set up so that the entire department is together for a portion of the meeting, then the staff is excused so that the physicians are able to meet without the staff present.

Staff meetings should have a scheduled start and end time and should not go over the end time. This indicates to all persons present that their time is valuable. Staff who are paid on an hourly basis should be compensated for their time in the staff meeting. If the meeting is held over a meal period, such as lunch, many office managers will provide lunch for the attendees.

CREATING A STAFF MEETING AGENDA

Every scheduled meeting in the medical office should have a written **agenda**. The agenda contains a list of the items that will be covered during that meeting. Using the agenda, the manager, or person leading the meeting, is able to stay on task toward the purpose of the meeting. Often, items will arise in meetings that are not on the agenda. When this happens the manager needs to determine if the unscheduled item is more important than those on the agenda. If so, the new item should be discussed. If the new item can be deferred to the next meeting, the note-taker at the meeting should include that in the notes.

The staff meeting agenda should include the time allowed for each agenda item as well as the person who will take the lead on that item. See Figure ■ 9-9 for a sample staff meeting agenda.

agenda
a list of items to be discussed at a meeting

1. Upcoming holiday shifts—Melinda Jones, Manager—15 minutes
2. Storing medications—Thom Watson, RN—5 minutes
3. Scheduling patients for physical exams—Melinda Jones, Manager—10 minutes
4. Charting patient weight in the EMR—Nora Clark, MA—10 minutes
5. Raising patient satisfaction level in the office—All—20 minutes

FIGURE ■ 9-9   Sample staff meeting agenda.

COMPOSING STAFF MEETING MINUTES

All staff meetings should have a designated note-taker. Because it may not be possible for all members of the medical office to attend the meeting, the meeting minutes should be distributed to all members of the office after the meeting. Meeting minutes should contain the following information:

- Names of persons in attendance
- Names of persons not in attendance
- Date and time of the meeting
- Discussion items and results, including any action items or follow-up needed
- Items deferred to the next department meeting
- Date and time of the next department meeting
- Time the meeting ended

The Medical Office Manager's Role with Supplies

Managing the medical office requires a host of supplies, both administrative and clinical. The medical office manager may be the person in charge of inventory and ordering of supplies, or that task may be delegated to another member of the medical office staff.

CONTRACTING WITH SUPPLIERS

Given the variety of supplies needed in the medical office, the medical office manager may find it is cost effective to contract with various suppliers. This process consists of discussing with the supplier the type and number of supplies the medical office will need to order. The supplier will then propose a price for those supplies. The medical office manager may want to meet with more than one supplier to determine who can provide the best price. The manager may be able to **negotiate** the price of supplies, especially for a clinic that orders a large number of supplies. If the manager learns that the price of a certain supply is not negotiable, other services may be negotiable, such as the cost of shipping or the delivery time for the supplies to arrive.

negotiate
the process of asking for a lower price or other benefits when purchasing an item or service

ORDERING AND RECEIVING SUPPLIES

While the process of ordering and receiving supplies may be delegated to a member of the healthcare team other than the manager, the medical office manager will want to be apprised of the supplies that are ordered. In many offices, the task of ordering supplies is delegated to one particular person. That person keeps track of what is ordered and when it is received. In this type of practice, every member of the medical office needs to alert the person who handles the ordering of the need for new supplies.

Many clinical supplies in the medical office have expiration dates. Because it is illegal to use supplies beyond their expiration date, the medical office manager must have a system in place to ensure that supplies are used before they expire. Part of this system is making sure that only the required amount of supplies is ordered. As an example, the manager will need to determine how many syringes the office staff will use over the course of a year. The manager then needs to ensure that no more than that number of syringes is ordered, thereby reducing the likelihood of having to waste expired syringes.

Storage space must be considered when ordering supplies in the medical office. Though the manager may be able to negotiate a good price for a certain supply, if she orders a large number of that supply, and the supply cannot be stored due to space constrictions, the price of the supply may not be worth the cost of the space needed. An example would be sterile gloves. If the manager is able to negotiate a low price by ordering 100 boxes of sterile gloves, but there is no place to store those boxes of gloves, the order should not be placed.

Negotiating Service Contracts

Medical offices have equipment, both administrative and clinical, that requires service. Examples are the photocopier and the EKG machine. Although some minor maintenance may be performed by members of the medical office, most manufacturers have restrictions in the **warranty** for their equipment related to the type and frequency of the service received. As an example, the photocopier may be under warranty from the manufacturer for a period of 3 years after purchase. That warranty may be contingent on the purchaser proving that the photocopier has been serviced by a representative of the manufacturer at a frequency of once per year (Figure ■ 9-10).

warranty
the period of time within which the manufacturer is responsible for any repairs to equipment

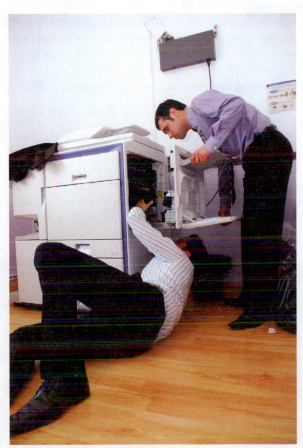

FIGURE ■ 9-10 When the photocopier malfunctions, a professional must be called to perform maintenance.
Source: © DURIS Guillaume.

service contract
a contract for maintenance and repair of equipment

Similar to negotiating for prices for supplies, the medical office manager may negotiate for the price or length of the **service contract**. This is best done at the time of purchase, when the manufacturer or salesperson is motivated to make the sale. The medical office manager may be able to negotiate a lower price for the service contract – even to the point of getting the contract for free. If the price of the contract cannot be negotiated, the manager should try to negotiate the length of the contract, adding a year or more at no additional cost.

Employee Theft

An unfortunate aspect of doing business for any type of organization is that of employee theft. In medical offices, employees may take small items, such as pens or note pads. In more severe cases, employees may take drugs or expensive supplies. The medical office manager should have a policy in place for what constitutes "theft" in the medical office. This policy should also outline the consequences for taking items from the office, including discharge.

To discourage employee theft of supplies, the person who takes inventory of supplies, the person who orders supplies, and the person who accepts receipt of supplies should be different staff members. The medical office manager should make it clear that employee theft will not be tolerated and by having different members of the team perform these integrated tasks, the medical office manager is better able to keep track of supplies in the office. This method makes it difficult for one member of the staff to take supplies without another member taking notice.

Critical Thinking 9.6 ?

How well do you think a manager who forms friendships with her staff would do if she had to have a conversation with employees about theft in the office? What suggestions would you make for this type of manager before she has this conversation?

In many medical offices, suppliers may drop off samples of items such as vitamins or medications (Figure ■ 9-11). If the physician does not choose to use these supplies, she may let the office manager know that the employees may take them, if they choose. This is the only example of when staff should be permitted to take home items from the medical office. This exception should be clearly spelled out in the policy pertaining to employee theft.

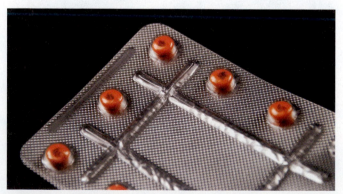

FIGURE ■ **9-11** Patients may be given sample medications by the medical team.
Source: © Albert Lozano-Nieto.

Case Study Questions

Refer to the case study presented at the beginning of this chapter to answer the following questions:

1. What type of management style do you think Barb falls under?
2. In what way do you think this style hampers Barb's ability with employees?
3. How does this style help Barb when interacting with employees?

Chapter Review

Summary

- There are a variety of different management styles, and rather than choosing just one of them, the successful medical office manager will use whichever style works best for a particular situation.

- The position of management is one where the manager sets the stage for employees to do their jobs well. The supervisor is the individual who actually oversees the employees at work and provides feedback regarding work performance.

- Delegating authority to others is the act of giving tasks to others to perform. The successful medical office manager needs to be good at delegating because it is not possible for one person to perform all of the tasks in a medical office.

- Coaching and mentoring of staff is the job of all medical office managers. This is done by allowing employees to see how the manager works and to offer the employee advice and feedback on tasks, rather than simply telling the employee what to do. Through coaching and mentoring, the medical office manager helps to build the skills of those employees she oversees.

- Employees need to be motivated to perform their jobs well. Motivation may take a number of forms, and the job of the medical office manager is to determine how to motivate each individual employee to perform at his or her best.

- The medical office manager possesses many characteristics. Some of the most important are excellent communication and time management skills.

- The responsibilities of the medical office manager will vary depending on the type and size of the medical practice. Most managers have core tasks in common, from oversight of the employees to management of the financial aspects of the clinic.

- There are six core leadership styles. The successful medical office manager will know when to use each of these because the style used depends on the situation in most cases.

- Effective medical office managers will use regular department staff meetings to communicate ideas and changes in person. These meetings should have a set start and end time and follow a preplanned agenda. Staff meeting agendas should include not only the name of the person who will lead the discussion of the item, but also the time allotted to that discussion item.

- Staff meeting minutes should be composed by the person designated to be the note-taker. These minutes should be distributed to all members of the medical office so that those who were not able to attend can stay abreast of discussion items.

- The medical office manager contracts with companies that sell supplies. This contracting often takes the form of negotiating for better prices or shorter delivery times.

- When ordering and receiving supplies, the medical office manager needs to determine how much of any individual supply is needed during a certain time frame. This keeps the office from keeping too much stock on hand, including those items that may expire before they are used.

- Much like negotiating with suppliers, the medical office manager may need to negotiate terms with companies providing service contracts. These are companies that provide service agreements for equipment in the office, such as a photocopier or EKG machine.

■ Employee theft may be minor or of more concern. Minor theft includes employees taking pens and paper, whereas major thefts consist of employees taking drugs or expensive office items. The medical office manager should have a policy in place regarding what employees can and cannot take from the medical office. This policy should include the consequences for employee theft, including termination of employment.

Multiple Choice

Choose the letter that best answers each question or completes each statement.

1. Margaret Rockas has been a medical office manager for over 30 years. She does not believe in letting her employees know why she is making the decisions she makes; Margaret leads by simply telling her team what they need to do. Which of the following best describes Margaret's leadership style?
   a. Mentoring
   b. Democratic
   c. Humanistic
   d. Authoritarian

2. Which of the following is true about staff meetings?
   a. Every meeting should have an agenda.
   b. Staff should be given the choice to attend or not.
   c. Physicians should not attend the same meeting as staff.
   d. The manager should not attend the staff meetings so that staff may discuss items openly.

3. Which of the following is **not** true about showing recognition to employees?
   a. Showing recognition increases employee performance.
   b. Showing recognition increases staff satisfaction.
   c. Showing recognition leads to the perception of favoritism in the medical office.
   d. Showing recognition lets employees know their manager cares about them as an individual.

4. Which of the following is **not** a reason a manager would want to delegate tasks to other members of the medical office team?
   a. Delegating tasks to others gives the manager time for other tasks.
   b. Delegating tasks to others allows the manager to mentor staff in learning new tasks.
   c. Delegating tasks to others means the manager will one day be unneeded.
   d. Delegating tasks to others allows the medical office manager to see that he does not have to perform all of the tasks in the office.

5. Which of the following is the first function in management theory?
   a. Planning
   b. Organizing
   c. Coordinating
   d. Leading

6. Which of the following would be considered employee theft?
   a. An employee who takes an additional 5 minutes for his lunch break
   b. An employee who uses the microwave in the break room
   c. An employee who takes home a roll of postage stamps for personal use
   d. An employee who takes his lab jacket home to be laundered

7. Which of the following would be the best time for a medical office manager to negotiate a service contract with a vendor or manufacturer?
   a. When the current contract is up for renewal
   b. When the equipment is originally purchased
   c. When the economy is down
   d. When the vendor or manufacturer is purchased by another company

8. Which of the following is included in staff meeting minutes?
   a. Names of persons in attendance
   b. Date and time of the staff meeting
   c. Items discussed
   d. All of the above

9. What is one reason why the manager should not discuss poor performance with an employee in front of others?
   a. The employee is entitled to keep this information private.
   b. The manager does not want other employees to know how she deals with poor performance.
   c. The employee may be inclined to become emotional if others are present.
   d. All of the above

10. What is one reason why the medical office manager will want to know how often and how many supplies are being ordered?
    a. To keep from purchasing more supplies than the office can use before they expire
    b. To keep from purchasing more supplies than the office can store
    c. To keep informed about the quantity of supplies so the manager can determine if there is a problem with employee theft
    d. All of the above

True/False

Determine if each of the following statements is true or false.

_____ 1. A working manager is one who watches his employees work.

_____ 2. The best way to mentor employees is for the manager to let the employees know they are considered close friends of the manager.

_____ 3. The humanistic leadership style is the best one to use in the event of an emergency in the medical office.

_____ 4. Part of providing feedback to an employee consists of the manager letting the employee know how well the employee handled a certain situation.

_____ 5. During a staff meeting, if an item is brought up that is not on the agenda, the medical office manager may need to defer that item to the next meeting.

_____ 6. Meaningful recognition from the manager starts with getting to know how each employee prefers to be recognized.

_____ 7. Staff should always be compensated for the time spent in staff meetings.

_____ 8. The catalystic style of leadership is the one that best motivates employees to perform at the highest level.

_____ 9. Employees are allowed to take home office supplies, such as pens and paper. This is not considered theft.

_____ 10. One function of the medical office manager is handling disputes between staff members.

Matching

Match each of the following terms with its definition.

a. democratic

b. Theory X

c. delegate

d. Theory Y

e. autonomy

f. planning

g. coaching

h. catalystic

i. authoritarian

j. organizing

1. A style of management where the manager is always in charge and control of the employees

2. The ability to work with little oversight or help

3. The management theory that states employees want to do well and will perform well if given the opportunity

4. The leadership style that consists of leading others by setting a fast pace for employees to follow

5. The management theory that states employees cannot be trusted to think for themselves

6. The process of giving advice to employees to help them find their own solutions to problems and encouraging employees to do their best

7. The process of taking one's tasks and giving them to another

8. The process of gathering the necessary tools, staff, and resources to accomplish set goals

9. The process of setting goals for the group

10. The leadership style where employee opinions are used in the decision process

Chapter Resources

American College of Healthcare Executives—website for medical practice executives: http://www.ache.org

American College of Medical Practice Executives—website for medical practice executives: http://www.mgma.com/acmpe

McGregor, D. (2006). *The human side of enterprise*. New York, NY: McGraw-Hill.

Sheldrake, J. (2003). *Management theory* (2nd ed.). London, UK: Thomson Learning.

PEARSON
myhealthprofessionskit™

Additional interactive resources for this chapter can be found at **www.myhealthprofessionskit.com.** Choose "Medical Assisting" from the discipline menu and then click on the book cover for *Medical Office Management*.

CHAPTER 10

Use of Computers in the Medical Office

CHAPTER OUTLINE

- Components of the Computer System
- Maintaining Computer Equipment
- Computer Software
- Computer Security

- Electronic Medical Records
- Using the Internet
- Prescription Management Software
- Ergonomics in the Medical Office

LEARNING OBJECTIVES

Upon completion of this chapter, you should be able to:

- Spell and define the key terms in this chapter.
- Understand the basic computer components and their functions.
- Outline the importance of maintaining computer equipment.
- Understand and describe the function of computer software used in the medical office.
- Outline steps for setting up training for staff on using software.
- Describe techniques for keeping computers and electronic information secure.
- Describe the benefits of using electronic medical records instead of paper medical charts.
- Describe how the Internet is useful in the medical office.
- Understand how prescription management software is used in the medical office.
- Discuss the importance of ergonomics in the medical office.

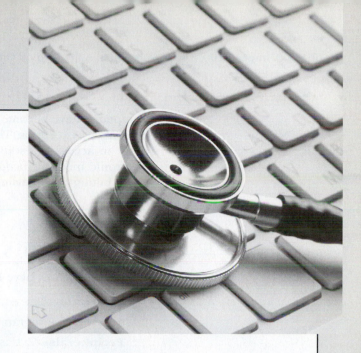

central processing unit (CPU)
computer virus
ergonomic

hacker
health-related calculators
Internet search engines

malware
medical management
software

Case Study

Take note of the following scenario and answer the case study questions that appear at the end of this chapter.

Nick Nowicki has just hired two new staff members into the family practice office he manages. One of the new hires has extensive experience in the use of computers in the medical office. The other new hire has been out of the medical field for several years and is new to the use of computers.

Introduction

Computers have become a mainstay in just about all parts of our lives. The medical office presents no exception. The medical office manager should be proficient at using the computer to access the software used by the practice. This software will typically include electronic medical record software, an electronic system for scheduling appointments, and a billing mechanism.

Components of the Computer System

Computer systems have three main components:

1. **Hardware**—The equipment itself, including the hard drive, monitor and keyboard

2. **Software**—Programs in the system

3. **Peripherals**—Extras that can attach to or be installed in the hardware, such as a scanner or printer.

Each computer component is intricately intertwined with the others. An office can have the most powerful hardware available yet be limited by its software. Similarly, an office can have top-of-the-line software that fails to work because it's being run on old, outdated hardware systems. Figure ■ 10-1 discusses main computer system types.

Supercomputers	Introduced in the 1960s; have the fastest processing capacity of today's computers.
Mainframe computers	Used for large-volume applications (e.g., government statistics).
Minicomputers	Multiuser computers that fall between mainframe computers (see preceding) and microcomputers (see following) in size and capabilities.
Microcomputers	Generally small, ranging from desktop models to handheld versions; commonly used in health care facilities.

FIGURE ■ 10-1   Main computer system types.

COMPONENTS OF COMPUTER HARDWARE

Computer hardware consists of several parts. For example, firewalls, which allow or deny computer access, may sometimes be hardware, but they can be software as well. All computers have a **central processing unit (CPU)**, which is the computer's brain. The CPU enables the computer to process data and run software. All CPUs function in the same basic way but differ in speed and capabilities. Generally, the faster the CPU, the higher the computer's cost. A CPU has several ports that accommodate a keyboard, monitor, mouse, printer, and often speakers (Figure ■ 10-2). Other ports may be used for such add-on items as scanners or backup drives.

The Keyboard

Computer keyboards may be standard or **ergonomic** (Figure ■ 10-3). Ergonomic keyboards reduce typing stress by supporting the hands and wrists comfortably. Keyboards typically attach to computers via cords, but many offices now have wireless models that work from any spot within the computers' ranges.

central processing unit (CPU)
the microchip inside the computer that processes the software program commands

ergonomic
designed to promote good posture and limit physical injuries

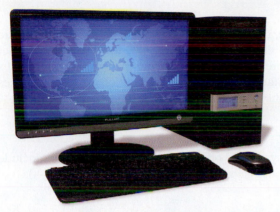

FIGURE ■ 10-2 Computer with monitor, keyboard, and mouse.
Source: Scanrail/Fotolia.com.

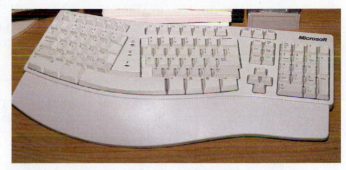

FIGURE ■ 10-3 An ergonomic keyboard.
Source: Michael Newman/PhotoEdit, Inc.

The Monitor

Computer monitors come in various sizes and qualities. To conserve desk space, many offices opt for flat-screen models. A monitor's display is based on the number of dots per square inch (DPI). The higher a monitor's DPI, the clearer its picture. Much like with the CPU just discussed, cost increases as DPI increases.

The Hard Drive

A computer's hard drive is a read/write device and houses the computer's files and programs. Because hard drives can fail, jeopardizing critical data, medical offices should back up their hard drives regularly. This is done by copying files from the main computer system to some form of backup system, such as a CD, DVD, or another computer. Again, the larger the hard drive, the more expensive the computer.

Various Computer Drives

Computers have varied types of drives. Most systems come with compact disc (CD) drives that allow computers to access files and programs on CDs. Digital versatile disc (DVD) drives, an option for most contemporary computers, provide access to files on DVDs. Floppy drives, for their part, provide a route to information stored on floppy disks. As technology advances, floppy disks are quickly becoming obsolete. Many computers, for example, no longer come with floppy disk drives.

Flash drives are small memory devices with no moving parts. These devices, sometimes called "thumb drives," vary in size from 8 megabytes to 64 gigabytes and are used to store files for transport between computer systems. These drives are small enough to carry in a pocket; many attach to neck chains for convenience. Flash drives usually connect to computers via a universal system bus (USB) port. Some flash drives are password protected, making them more secure in case the drive is lost. Just as with other computer components, the greater the storage capability the higher the price.

Like flash drives, Zip drives and Jaz drives store data. These devices are slightly larger than floppy drives and hold much more data. Because they are portable, Zip and Jaz drives can be used to transport data between computers. They are also often used for file backup.

Computer Memory

A computer's memory consists of read-only memory (ROM) and random access memory (RAM). The computer manufacturer writes permanent instructions on ROM chips, which are installed on the computer's motherboard. The amount of RAM, which varies according to users' needs, is also in chip form on the motherboard. Information stored in RAM disappears when the computer shuts down or experiences a power failure. When a computer's RAM is insufficient, the computer typically runs slower.

The Printer

When a printer is attached to a computer, the user can print information housed on the computer. Printers come in varied types, sizes, and speeds. Some printers, called inkjet printers, use liquid ink, whereas laser printers use toners to print. Offices may sometimes need to order printer supplies from manufacturers. Because the cost of printing supplies can vary greatly, offices should factor in these costs when selecting printers.

COMPUTER PERIPHERALS

Computer peripherals connect to computer systems to offer useful functions. Examples include scanners, digital cameras, bar-code readers, and electronic sign-in sheets (Figure ■ 10-4).

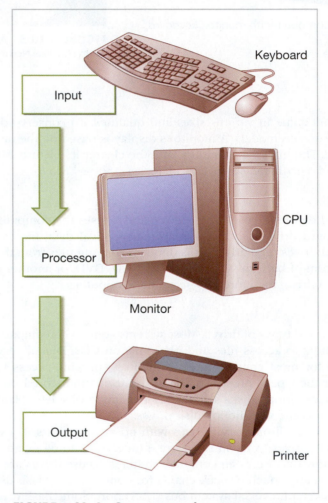

FIGURE ■ 10-4 Components of a computer system.

Scanners

Scanners are similar to photocopiers in that they copy documents. Unlike photocopiers, however, scanners can transfer electronic versions of documents or images to computers. Scanners look like small photocopiers and they work in much the same way. The document to be scanned is placed on the scanner and a photo is taken. The photo is then moved into the computer file.

Digital Cameras

Digital cameras take pictures without film. Images are stored electronically in the camera until the user downloads them to a computer. Digital cameras range from inexpensive models designed for home use to expensive models capable of producing high-quality images.

Bar-Code Readers

Many modern medical offices use bar coding to manage information. Some offices use bar codes to identify patient files or enter patient data in computers. Others use the technology to track inventory or supplies. Bar-code scanners vary in size and type. Some models work via trigger, similar to a gun, while others use what looks like an ink pen (Figure ■ 10-5).

FIGURE ■ **10-5** Bar-code scanner.
Source: Jeff Smith/Getty Images.

Electronic Sign-In Sheets

Electronic sign-in sheets, which work like the devices department stores use at checkout, arose because HIPAA deemed paper sign-in sheets insufficient for safeguarding patient information. With electronic sign-in sheets, patients enter their names electronically on tablets or pads, and the sheets display the resulting signatures on the receptionist's computer screen (Figure ■ 10-6).

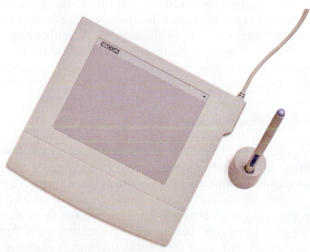

FIGURE ■ **10-6** Electronic sign-in sheet.
Source: Dorling Kindersley.

Maintaining Computer Equipment

Because computer equipment is expensive and fragile, the medical office should strive to maintain it. To start, office policies should disallow food and drink near computers. One liquid spill can irreversibly damage a computer or destroy a keyboard. In addition, computer systems, as well as CDs, DVDs, and other discs, should be kept in cool, dry places, out of direct sunlight and away from potentially damaging items. Discs should be handled carefully and cleaned only with static-free, soft cloths and appropriate chemicals (Figure ■ 10-7). All parts of the computer, including the keyboard and mouse, should be dusted regularly. A trained professional should perform any maintenance.

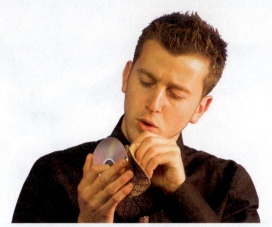

FIGURE ■ 10-7 CDs must be cleaned with a soft cloth to avoid damage.
Source: Andresr/Dreamstime.com.

SURGE PROTECTION

Computers should be protected against damage caused by power outages or electrical surges. All computers in the medical office should be connected to an uninterruptible power supply or battery backup systems. All computer power supplies should also have surge protection to prevent voltage surges, which can be very damaging to computer components.

BACKING UP THE COMPUTER SYSTEM

To avoid critical data loss, computers in the medical office should be backed up regularly. Offices can use the various tapes or drives discussed earlier in this chapter, or they can back up data from one computer system to another. Whatever backup system the medical office uses, the backup tape, drive, and computer should be housed in a location separate from the originating computer so fire, flood, or theft cannot threaten the data.

Computer Software

medical management software
computer software used in the medical office to assist in tasks such as billing, coding, and payroll

Most medical offices use some form of **medical management software** that performs such functions as appointment scheduling, patient charting, electronic medical record management, bookkeeping, insurance billing, and task and prescription managing. An office's needs determine which software it uses. Demonstrations can help medical offices ensure they buy programs that are appropriate for their needs. Following the trend in other areas of technology, feature-rich management software tends to cost more than simple programs. Figure ■ 10-8 lists common features in medical management software.

TRAINING STAFF ON MEDICAL SOFTWARE

Medical office management software should come with an onsite training option and also include telephone customer service support and manuals or demos for future training needs. All staff who will be working with the software should attend training. Because such training may incur costs, medical offices should explore that possibility before making any software purchases.

- **Patient accounting**—Enter patient charges and payments and track accounts receivables.

- **Coding**—Choose codes for patients' procedures and diagnoses.

- **Appointment scheduling**—Track patient appointment times and send reminder cards.

- **Insurance billing**—Print medical insurance claims.

- **Electronic billing**—Submit medical insurance claims electronically.

- **Verify insurance coverage**—Verify patients' insurance benefits via insurance companies' Web sites.

- **Credit card authorization**—Authorize patients' credit-card payments.

- **Accounts payable**—Track the medical office's finances and pay bills.

- **Payroll**—Process and track payroll functions and complete such tasks as printing paychecks and running quarterly reports.

- **Transcription**—Transcribe documents via dictation equipment or voice recognition.

FIGURE ■ 10-8   Common features in medical management software.

VARIOUS SOFTWARE PACKAGES

Most medical offices use word processing software, most commonly Microsoft Word. Medical office staff use this type of software to type patient letters, print mailing lists, format documents and brochures, and create charts and forms. Spreadsheet software, like Microsoft Excel, completes calculations, provides statistics, and creates corresponding graphs and charts. Medical office staff may use spreadsheet software to track statistics on patient care and personnel management. Presentation software like Microsoft PowerPoint helps when medical offices plan educational meetings or seminars for patients. Not only can presenters create slides for projection, they can print those slides as note-taking tools for attendees (Figure ■ 10-9).

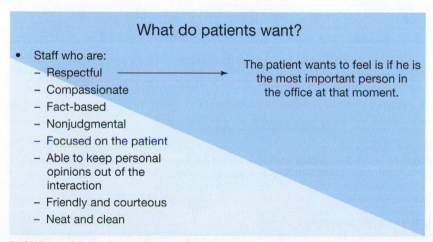

FIGURE ■ 10-9   Example of a slide from a PowerPoint presentation.

Several software programs currently on the market provide electronic calendars, which can be invaluable to medical offices trying to coordinate staff schedules. Many such programs send e-mail invitations that recipients can automatically add to their electronic calendars. They can also print daily, weekly, or monthly calendars.

CODING SOFTWARE

A number of software companies market programs that allow the medical provider to easily assign diagnosis or procedure codes to their patients. Figure ■ 10-10 lists several companies that offer this service. Using such software, the provider is able to insert certain parameters, such as the amount of time the provider spent with the patient or the symptoms the patient presented with, and obtain suggestions for proper coding. Because proper coding is the key to proper reimbursement, these programs may be something the medical office manager should look into for enhancing coding abilities in the medical office.

Speed eCoder http://www.speedecoder.com/

MB Guide http://www.mb-guide.org

FlashCode http://www.flashcode.com

CodoniX http://www.codonix.com/

White Plume http://www.whiteplume.com/

FIGURE ■ 10-10   Companies offering software for medical coding.

Computer Security

hacker
person who illegally obtains access to a computer network

To safeguard computer systems, staff members must be required to use passwords to access the computer systems. To thwart **hackers**, users should choose unobvious passwords, taking care to avoid using initials, birth dates, and telephone numbers. Users should also avoid sharing their passwords and leaving their passwords in plain view. It is good practice for users to log off whenever leaving their computer workstations unattended. Figure ■ 10-11 outlines HIPAA standards for safeguarding patient health information. (For more information about HIPAA compliance requirements, see Chapter 8.)

- Patient health information (PHI) must be backed up periodically.

- An audit trail must exist for backed up data that leaves the medical facility.

- Access to backed up data must be restricted to authorized parties.

- A backup plan and disaster recovery plan must be in place.

- Data must be a retrievable, exact copy.

- All computers must be password protected.

FIGURE ■ 10-11   HIPAA standards for safeguarding patient health information. *Source:* U.S. Department of Health and Human Services.

Critical Thinking 10.1 ?

Imagine a new hire comes to the practice with extensive experience using computers in the medical office. Do you think it is appropriate for the medical office manager to review the policies regarding computer privacy with the new hire? Why or why not?

computer virus
program designed to perform mischievous functions

malware
software designed to destroy portions of a computer; more malicious than a computer virus

COMPUTER VIRUSES

Computer viruses are programs designed to perform mischievous functions. **Malware**, a twist on the computer virus, is designed to damage or infiltrate computers. Malware includes spyware, adware, Trojan horses, and worms. These programs can damage or corrupt hard drives, as well as infect other computers without users' knowledge. Because of these types of programs, every computer in the medical office should be equipped with virus- and malware-protection software that is updated regularly.

Critical Thinking 10.2 ?

Imagine you have one new hire that has far more computer experience than another. Would you recommend both new employees attend the same training session? Or would you suggest the manager have the hire with computer experience attend an abbreviated program? Why or why not?

Electronic Medical Records

Electronic medical records, also called electronic health records, are part of healthcare's future. Although most large healthcare facilities have used some form of electronic medical record for many years, some smaller offices are still using paper charts. In his 2004 State of the Union address, President George W. Bush stated, "By computerizing health records, we can avoid dangerous medical mistakes, reduce costs, and improve care." Shortly after this speech, President Bush outlined a plan to ensure that most Americans have electronic health records by 2014. As of 2011, Medicare, at the direction of President Barack Obama, has enacted the Electronic Health Record Incentive Program. This program provides financial incentives to healthcare providers for demonstrating meaningful use of an electronic health record. "Meaningful use" is determined by three factors: (1) The medical provider must use the electronic medical record to prescribe medications electronically; (2) the electronic medical record must be used to exchange information electronically in order to improve the quality of care; and (3) the electronic medical record must be used to submit clinical quality measures. Eligible healthcare providers are eligible for up to $44,000 over 5 years under this incentive program. To obtain the maximum incentive, healthcare providers must have begun to use an electronic medical record by 2012. Those healthcare providers who do not implement an electronic medical record by 2015 will have their fees adjusted by Medicare to a lower rate than those who use an electronic record for their patients.

Electronic medical records are easier to access than a paper medical record. While physicians must retrieve paper files from separate and often large file rooms, electronic medical records are easily accessible on a computer. In large offices where patients may see several different providers, electronic medical records allow physicians to easily locate patients' laboratory results, consultation notes, x-rays, and examination findings from other providers.

Using electronic medical records, medical offices are able to access any one patient's file from more than one networked computer in the office. For example, the billing office might have the patient's medical record open on a computer screen while they are accessing information needed for coding a specific procedure. At the same time, the physician might have the same patient's file open on a separate computer screen while she inputs treatment notes (Figure ■ 10-12).

Charting patient information, such as telephone calls, is easily done within the electronic medical record. Typically, the software will contain a section for adding information, such as telephone calls or personal conversations that are related to a patient's medical care.

Many medical offices have computer terminals in each examination room, allowing the medical personnel to add information to the patient's electronic medical record, download test results, or research past medication records while the patient is in the room. In some cases, the medical provider will be able to access the patient's electronic medical record in another facility.

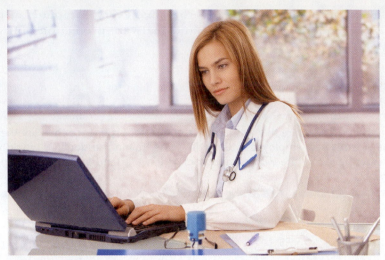

FIGURE ■ 10-12   A physician uses a computer to access a patient's electronic medical record.
Source: © nyul/Fotolia.

Using the Internet

Internet search engines
sites on the Internet used for locating needed information

Internet search engines use key words and phrases to retrieve information from the Internet. Popular search engines are Yahoo, Google, Dog Pile, and Ask.com. Contemporary healthcare providers often search the Internet for medical information. Medical offices often need source material for patient brochures or presentations, and the Internet provides a good resource for this material.

When newly diagnosed with conditions or illnesses, patients often have many questions for their healthcare providers. Many such providers find it helpful to give patients lists of reputable websites for further information; this is especially helpful when patients have long-term or chronic illnesses or conditions and may be seeking support groups. Before giving website information to patients, medical staff must be sure to obtain the physician's permission. Medical office staff should be instructed to give patients only information from reputable websites.

Professional medical websites are the sites physicians visit when seeking up-to-date information on conditions, illnesses, or pharmaceuticals. Figure ■ 10-13 lists some reputable examples. Generally, a site may be determined to be reputable if it is published by a college/university, a peer-reviewed journal, a healthcare agency such as The Joint Commission, a professional association such as the American Medical Association, or by a government agency. Many physicians subscribe to online journals that charge for access but offer the latest information on research, medications, and techniques. Seminars and conferences can be informative, but websites serve as ongoing resources as topics arise.

American Medical Association (AMA) (www.ama-assn.org)

The Joint Commission (TJC) (www.jointcommission.org)

Centers for Disease Control and Prevention (CDC) (www.cdc.gov)

Lancet (www.lancet.org)

Medical Association (JAMA) (www.jama.ama-assn.org)

New England Journal of Medicine (www.nejm.org)

FIGURE ■ 10-13   Reputable medical websites.

Many websites offer **health-related calculators** that aid both patients and healthcare staff. They are used to calculate health factors ranging from basal metabolic rate, body mass index, pregnancy and due date, ovulation, and target heart rate to children's adult height predictions, smoking costs, and seafood mercury intake.

Often, major health insurance carriers maintain their own, comprehensive websites that allow subscribers and physicians alike to access a wide span of information. Some sites even give physicians access to patients' benefit information, although direct contact with the insurance companies is often still needed, especially when authorizations are required. Such sites are particularly helpful for offices that need to verify that patients have active policies at the time of a visit.

> **health-related calculators**
> Internet sites that provide calculators for determining pregnancy due dates, body mass index, and other numbers

Prescription Management Software

As part of the Medicare-mandated meaningful use incentive, healthcare providers are using electronic means to send prescriptions more and more often. Though controlled substances (narcotics) continue to require a printed prescription and the actual signature of the provider, all other prescriptions may be sent electronically. This function may be done via a facsimile machine or via the electronic medical record. In using the electronic medical record to e-prescribe medications for patients, providers are immediately notified if the patient has already been prescribed a medication that is contraindicated by the new medication or if the dose appears out of range for a patient of this particular age or weight. The use of prescription management software allows providers to provide a higher level of safety to patients in the prescribing of medications. Prescriptions are sent immediately upon order of the physician, which means the prescription should be ready when the patient arrives at the designated pharmacy (Figure ■ 10-14).

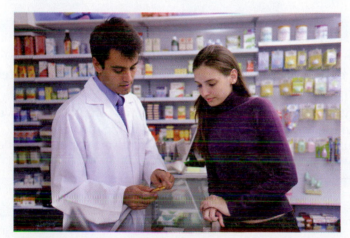

FIGURE ■ 10-14   A patient picks up her prescription at the pharmacy.
Source: Mangostock/Dreamstime.com.

Ergonomics in the Medical Office

Ergonomics is the study of workstations and employees' interactions with workstations to determine the proper posture or equipment needed to reduce the likelihood of injury in the workplace. Many healthcare employers today employ safety officers. Part of the job of the safety officer is to look at an employee's workstation to determine if any ergonomic adjustments need to be made to make the workplace more comfortable and free from possible injury for the employee.

Common areas assessed for ergonomic issues include the placement of the keyboard and mouse, as well as the height of the desk and chair. By ensuring proper alignment, employees are likely to be less susceptible to workplace repetitive stress injuries due to improper posture or improper placement of equipment in the workplace (Figure ■ 10-15).

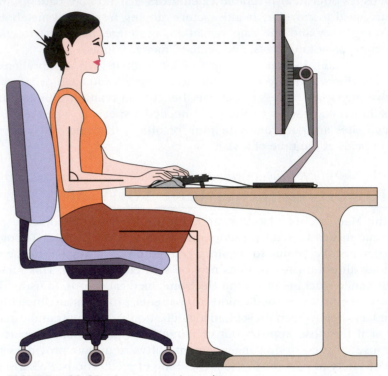

FIGURE ■ 10-15   An ergonomic workspace.

Case Study Questions

Refer to the case study presented at the beginning of this chapter to answer the following questions:

1. How might Nick make certain that each of his new employees receives the proper training on the computers and software used in the medical office?
2. What should Nick do if the employee with extensive computer experience says she does not want to attend training classes?

Chapter Review

Summary

- The basic components of a computer system consist of a hard drive, monitor, and keyboard. Various other items may be added to this basic system, depending on the needs of the user.

- Basic computer functions are important for the medical office manager to understand. Staff who will use the computers in the medical office must be trained on how to use these functions.

- To keep computers in good working order, proper maintenance must be performed.

- A variety of computer software exists on the market today for use in the medical office. This software is used for tasks such as medical billing and coding and financial management of the clinic.

- Security of the computers in a medical office is mandated by HIPAA legislation. To that end, the medical office manager must ensure that all staff members have unique passwords for computer access.

- Electronic medical records have multiple advantages over paper records. With the requirements for heightened security for patient information, as well as patient safety, Medicare offers an incentive program for medical providers who use their electronic medical record in a meaningful way.

- Several companies offer software designed for use in coding diagnoses or procedure codes for patient visits. This makes the coding process more efficient.

- Medical offices today use the Internet to gather information for their patients. It is important for the medical office manager to alert staff to using only reputable sites for the gathering of information and to consult the physicians before distributing any such information to patients.

- Prescription management software is commonly used with the electronic medical record. Physicians using this type of software are alerted to any contraindications in medications or possible medication prescribing errors. If the provider is not alerted to any problems with the prescription, it can be sent to the pharmacy immediately, while the patient is in the examination room. This means that the prescription will be ready for the patient when he arrives at the pharmacy.

- The use of ergonomic equipment in the medical office helps to ensure that those working in the office retain good posture and limit the number of work-related injuries.

Multiple Choice

Choose the letter that best answers each question or completes each statement.

1. A person who illegally enters a computer network is called:
   a. an alien.
   b. an outlaw.
   c. a hacker.
   d. a programmer.

2. Coding software is designed to do which of the following?
   a. Offer the provider a suggested diagnosis code.
   b. Alert the provider to fraud and abuse.
   c. Contact the health department for certain diagnoses.
   d. Ensure the office receives a higher level of reimbursement than the service performed.

3. Computer viruses perform:
   a. mischievous functions.
   b. destructive functions.
   c. funny jokes on the computer user.
   d. helpful tasks.

4. Which of the following presidents most recently issued a mandate about the use of electronic medical records?
   a. George W. Bush
   b. Bill Clinton
   c. Barack Obama
   d. Jimmy Carter

5. Medicare, via the meaningful use criteria, will offer incentives of up to _____ to providers for proof of proper use of electronic medical records.
   a. $44,000
   b. $66,000
   c. $88,000
   d. $144,000

6. Health-related calculators are used for tracking which of the following?
   a. Basal metabolic rate
   b. Account balance
   c. Appointments with the physician this year
   d. IRS tax-deductible benefits

7. HIPAA law dictates which of the following with regard to electronic patient information?
   a. A backup plan and disaster recovery plan must be in place.
   b. Physicians must swear an oath to patient privacy.
   c. Medical office managers must properly train all staff regarding patient privacy.
   d. Privacy curtains must be provided to all patients in healthcare.

8. Medical management software may perform which of the following functions?
   a. Appointment scheduling
   b. Patient charting
   c. Electronic medical record management
   d. All of the above

9. Which of the following would be used to facilitate the reduction of wrist injuries in the medical office?
   a. High-backed office chair
   b. Ergonomic keyboard
   c. Flat-screen monitor
   d. Scanner

10. Which of the following items might be scanned into an electronic medical record?
    a. A patient's records from an outside medical office
    b. A photo of the patient before a plastic surgery procedure
    c. A health evaluation form filled out for the patient
    d. All of the above

True/False

Determine if each of the following statements is true or false.

_____ 1. Prescription management software is commonly used with the electronic medical record.

_____ 2. Security of the computers in the medical office is mandated by ADA legislation.

_____ 3. Physicians using prescription management software are alerted to any contraindications in medications.

_____ 4. The American Medical Association has a reputable website for gathering medical information.

_____ 5. Ergonomics is the use of equipment to reduce injuries to workers.

_____ 6. Many physicians subscribe to online journals that charge for access but offer the latest information on research, medications, and techniques.

_____ 7. Medical management software may be used to process patient credit card payments.

_____ 8. A number of software companies market programs that allow the medical provider to efficiently assign diagnosis or procedure codes to their patients.

_____ 9. As of 2011, Medicaid, at the direction of President Barack Obama, has enacted the Electronic Health Record Incentive Program.

_____ 10. Medical offices often need source material for patient brochures or presentations; the Internet is an unacceptable resource for this material.

Matching

Match each of the following terms with its definition.

a. ergonomic

b. Electronic Health Record Incentive Program

c. central processing unit (CPU)

d. medical management software

e. health-related calculators

f. narcotics

g. hacker

h. Internet search engines

i. computer virus

j. malware

1. The microchip inside the computer that processes the software programs

2. A program designed to perform mischievous functions

3. Something designed to promoted good posture and limit physical injuries

4. Persons who illegally enter into a computer network

5. Internet sites that provide calculators for determining pregnancy due dates, body mass index, and other numbers

6. Search areas on the Internet used for locating needed information

7. Software designed to destroy portions of a computer; more malicious than a computer virus

8. Computer software used in the medical office to assist in tasks such as billing, coding, or payroll

9. Controlled substances

10. This program provides financial incentives to healthcare providers for demonstrating meaningful use of an electronic health record

Chapter Resources

Centricity Electronic Medical Record software: http://www3.gehealthcare.com/en/Products/Categories/Healthcare_IT/Electronic_Medical_Records/Centricity_EMR

EPIC electronic medical record software: http://www.epic.com

Medicare Electronic Health Record Incentive Program: http://www.cms.gov/ehrincentiveprograms

U.S. Department of Health and Human Services – health information privacy: http://www.hhs.gov/ocr/privacy

PEARSON myhealthprofessionskit

Additional interactive resources for this chapter can be found at **www.myhealthprofessionskit.com.** Choose "Medical Assisting" from the discipline menu and then click on the book cover for *Medical Office Management*.

CHAPTER 11

Office Policies and Procedures

CHAPTER OUTLINE

- Creating Patient Education Pamphlets
- Creating a Personnel Manual
- Creating Policies and Procedures for the Medical Office

LEARNING OBJECTIVES

Upon completion of this chapter, you should be able to:

- Spell and define the key terms in this chapter.
- Create a patient education pamphlet.
- List the steps for creating a personnel manual.
- Create a policy and procedure manual for the medical office.
- Describe the different types of procedures (clinical, administrative, infection control, and quality improvement and risk management) in the medical office.

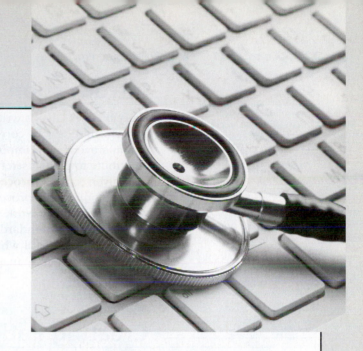

brochure   organizational chart   procedure
chain of command   personnel manual
mission statement   policy

Case Study

Take note of the following scenario and answer the case study questions that appear at the end of this chapter.

Steve Croffut has recently obtained his first job as a medical office manager. On Steve's first day, he asks one of the physicians if there is a manual that outlines office procedures. The physician tells Steve that the previous office manager never took the time to compose a procedures manual. She asks Steve if he would be willing to take on such a task.

Introduction

Every business needs written policies and procedures to ensure that employees know how to perform their jobs correctly, and healthcare is no exception. Policies and procedures are perhaps even more important in the medical field than in other fields because they may contribute to patient safety and risk reduction. A **policy** is a statement of guidelines or rules on a given topic. A **procedure** describes the steps used to perform a given task or project.

The policy and procedure manual in the medical office allows management to set up standards for how work is to be performed and to monitor the employees' performance based on those standards. New employees will find a policy and procedure manual to be extremely helpful while training for their new job. By using the manual for training, the medical office manager knows all new employees understand the expectations for performance.

policy
statement of guidelines or rules on a given topic

procedure
steps used to perform a given task or project

Creating Patient Education Pamphlets

Every member of the healthcare team is responsible for educating patients. Much of the information physicians ask that patients receive may be in written form. Many medical offices buy educational **brochures** to give to patients. These documents are available on a multitude of topics, including back pain, child immunizations, and menopause (Figure ■ 11-1). Educational brochures and pamphlets do not take the place of face-to-face education of the patient; they are a supplement to the education given in verbal form. These brochures allow the patient to review material after the visit or to give information to a spouse after the medical visit.

brochure
document containing information about a topic

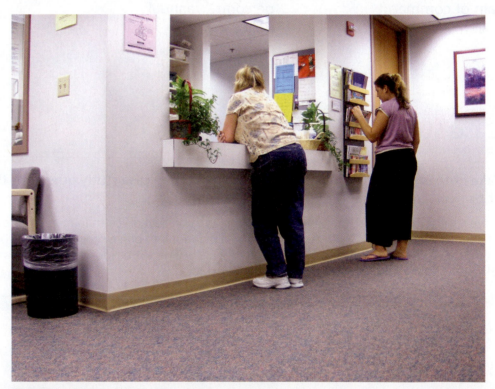

FIGURE ■ 11-1 Having educational materials available to the patients in the reception area is very common.
Source: Leticia Wilson/Fotolia.com.

Critical Thinking 11.1 ?

Why would giving educational brochures to patients be helpful to the physician treating those patients?

Typically, medical offices will have a supply of brochures or pamphlets that pertain to the type of care or type of patient seen in that practice. For example, a pediatrics practice might have educational pamphlets with information on preventing accidental injuries. An OB/GYN practice might have educational brochures with information about pregnancy or other women's health conditions. Depending on the cultural makeup of an office's patients, brochures may be printed in various languages.

Brochures may be purchased from vendors, or physicians may want to create their own brochures. Brochures can provide patients with more details about how a certain physician treats a certain condition or list a particular physician's recommendations regarding medications or care. These types of brochures can be created with the help of in-house staff or a professional printing company. Regardless of how the office chooses to create patient education pamphlets, those pamphlets must be professional. Any educational material given to the patient should be printed using layman's terms; the material should be easily understood by any person with an education level no higher than the 10th grade. All printed material must be accurate and free of typographical errors.

Critical Thinking 11.2 ?

Why do you think brochures should be printed using layman's terms only? Do you think there is any problem with giving a patient an educational pamphlet that is far above that patient's level of medical understanding? Why or why not?

Creating a Personnel Manual

A **personnel manual**, also called an employee handbook, lists the rules and regulations that apply to all staff in the medical office (Figure ■ 11-2). This manual also thoroughly explains the office's benefits for health, life, and disability insurance, among others. Many offices give all new employees copies of their personnel manuals upon hire. Other offices keep single copies in central locations. In many healthcare facilities, personnel manuals are kept electronically on the organization's intranet. This allows employees to search the manual for a desired policy, and for policies to be updated as needed without having to reprint manuals for employees.

personnel manual
a compilation of employment policies for an office; also called an employee handbook

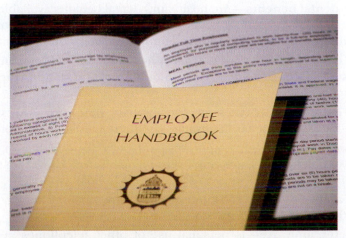

FIGURE ■ 11-2 The employee handbook should be updated on a regular basis and made available to each new employee.
Source: Tony Freeman/PhotoEdit, Inc.

Critical Thinking 11.3 ?

Why might a new employee find the office personnel manual helpful? What are some policies you think a new employee would want to review first?

To create a personnel manual, the office manager and/or physician should start by listing the topics they would like to see included. The personnel manual should have a section for all events or occurrences that might conceivably happen in the office. One way to start this process is to create a list of all policies or procedures for which a new employee will need training. Each of these items should be included in the personnel manual. For ideas, a medical office manager might consult the personnel manuals of other medical offices. It is important to keep federal and state laws in mind for all content included in the manual to ensure all policies are within legal boundaries. The following items are commonly found in personnel manuals:

- **Evaluation process**—How often will employee evaluations occur? What information are employees required to provide before evaluations? Are pay raises associated with evaluations?

- **Absentee policies**—Whom should employees call in the event they must miss work? Are employees responsible for finding replacements when they must miss work? Are doctors' notes required in the event of illness?

- **Confidentiality policy**—What are the penalties for violating patient confidentiality? What constitutes a violation of patient confidentiality? How does the office require certain situations be handled, such as calling out the patient's name in the reception room?

- **Continuing education requirements**—Does the office require written verification of attendance or completion of continuing education? Does the office require more hours of continuing education than the employee needs for recertification/relicensure? Does the office require certain types of continuing education, such as clinical or administrative? Are all members of the staff required to have basic life support training?

- **Grievance procedures**—How should employees handle situations in which they disagree with their supervisors?

- **Orientation process**—What are employees responsible for during orientation? Who do employees answer to during orientation? How long does orientation last?

- **Parking**—Are employees required to park in certain areas? Are employees required to pay for their own parking? Are there incentives for employees who carpool or take public transportation?

- **Pay**—What is the starting rate of pay? At what point are pay increases possible?

- **Health and dental benefits**—Are health and dental benefits available? At what point are employees eligible for these plans? Are employees able to add coverage for their spouses/children? Where can employees find information on benefits?

- **Staff meetings**—How often are staff meetings held? Are staff meetings compulsory? Where are staff meetings held? What type of information should employees bring to staff meetings?

- **Paid time off**—Are employees eligible for paid time off? How should time off requests be handled? How far in advance should requests for time off be submitted?

- **Holiday compensation**—Are employees paid extra for working on holidays? If the office is closed on holidays, are employees compensated? How does the office manager determine which employees to schedule for holiday work?

- **Sexual harassment**—What constitutes sexual harassment? How should employees handle incidences of sexual harassment?

- **Personal telephone use**—Is personal use of office telephones permitted? Under what circumstances? What are the penalties for excessive personal telephone use?

- **Personal computer use**—Is personal use of the office computers permitted? Under what circumstances? What are the penalties for excessive personal computer use?

- **Vacation days**—Are employees eligible for paid or unpaid vacation days? At what intervals? How do employees request vacation days?

- **Severe weather or power outage**—What is the policy should severe weather prevent employees from traveling to the office? What is the policy should the office lose power?

- **Emergency fire procedures**—How are fire emergencies handled? Who is responsible for clearing patients from the office?

- **Emergency procedures for patient accidental injury**—How are patient injuries handled in the office? Under what circumstances are emergency personnel called to the office?

- **Jury duty**—How should employees notify the office of jury duty? Does the office pay employees during jury duty?

- **Maternity leave**—Employers with 50 or more employees must give employees up to 12 weeks off after the birth or adoption of a child under the Family Medical Leave Act. Will the employer offer any of that time paid? Is the employee able to use accrued vacation time for maternity leave? Are male employees able to take time off after the birth or adoption of a child?

Critical Thinking 11.4 ?

Imagine you are starting a personnel manual for a medical office. Reviewing the policies described in the previous section, which of these do you think should be worked on first? Why did you choose those?

Creating Policies and Procedures for the Medical Office

The medical office's policy and procedure manual may contain both policies and procedures, or policies and procedures may be separated. Policies are written instructions outlining what an organization's rule is regarding a certain topic, such as benefits, vacation accrual, and time off. Procedures are written steps for how one is expected to carry out an individual policy. Whatever the approach, each policy and procedure manual should contain the following items in separate sections:

- Mission statement
- Organizational chart
- Personnel policies
- Clinical procedures
- Administrative procedures.

A table of contents should clearly direct readers to desired pages. Per Occupational Safety and Health Administration (OSHA) and HIPAA regulations, infection control and quality improvement and risk management procedures must be kept in separate notebooks and reviewed and updated regularly.

One of the most important reasons for having a medical office policy and procedure manual is to clarify rules and regulations and the physicians' expectations for procedures. Strict adherence to policies as they are outlined achieves uniformity in the office and provides a fair method of treating staff equally.

To ensure ongoing compliance and relevance, all medical office policies should be reviewed and updated regularly. Many large medical offices separate their policy manuals into clinical and administrative sections. Some offices further divide their manuals according to position or department. Table ■ 11-1 identifies ancillary policies that may be found in medical office policy and procedure manuals.

Critical Thinking 11.5 ?

Why do you think a policy and procedure manual should be reviewed and updated regularly? What do you think could happen in a medical office if the policies and procedures are allowed to become out of date?

TABLE ■ 11-1   Ancillary Policies That May Be Found in Medical Office Policy and Procedure Manuals

Policy or Procedure	Purpose
Emergency Closure Policy	Outlines the steps to take in the event the office closes due to an emergency.
Opening Office Policy	Outlines the steps to take to open the office at the beginning of the day.
Building Lockup Policy	Describes the steps to take to lock the building at the end of the day.
Publications and Distribution Policy	Outlines the policy with regard to allowing publications or pamphlets to be distributed to patients and staff.
Smoking Policy	Describes the availability of smoking areas near the office.
Personal Relationships Between Office Staff Members	Outlines the policy for personal relationships between coworkers.
Personal Relationships Between Staff and Patients	Outlines the policy for personal relationships between office staff and patients.
Termination Policy	Describes the policy for terminating employment.
Disciplinary Policy	Describes the policy for disciplining of employees. Includes an outline of the offenses justifying discipline.
Grievance Policy	Describes the process staff must follow to file grievances.
Continuing Education	Outlines the requirements for continuing education.
Malpractice Insurance	Describes the requirements for holding malpractice insurance.
Reimbursement for Seminars	Outlines the policy for reimbursing staff who attend medical-related seminars.
Computers for Personal Use Policy	Describes the policy for personal use of office computers.
Petty Cash Funds	Describes the policy for using petty cash, including the type of expenses that qualify as petty cash and the amount to be kept as petty cash.
Parking Policy	Outlines where employees may park, as well as reimbursement for parking expenses.
Dress Code Policy	Describes the dress code for each office position.
Disclosure of Patient Information Policy	Describes the procedure for disclosing patient information, including the forms required and the HIPAA regulations.
Job Descriptions	Provides a job description for each office position.
HIPAA Privacy Officer Duties	Outlines the duties of the HIPAA privacy officer in the medical office.
Calling Patients from the Reception Room	Describes the procedure for calling patients from the reception room.
Missed Patient Appointments	Describes the steps to take when patients miss their appointments. Includes proper charting technique.
Termination of the Physician/Patient Relationship	Outlines the steps to be followed to legally terminate a physician/patient relationship.
E-Mail Policy	Describes the conditions under which the medical office may e-mail information to patients or other facilities.
Obtaining Consent for a Procedure	Describes the consent forms used in the medical office and outlines the process of witnessing patient signatures.
Prescription Refill Requests	Outlines the policy for taking telephone calls for prescription refills, including documentation in the patient's medical record.
Jury Duty Policy	Describes the policy for employees called for jury duty.
Sick Leave Policy	Describes the policy for employees who take sick leave.
Personal Telephone Calls	Describes the policy for employees making and receiving personal telephone calls.

MISSION STATEMENT

The policy and procedure manual for a medical office should begin with an office **mission statement** that is concise and communicated to all staff. For example, a mission statement might read "To care for all patients in a compassionate and dignified manner, with a focus on patient safety and satisfaction." Many medical offices frame and hang their mission statements for patients to see.

The mission statement should be short so that it is easily remembered by members of the healthcare team. In many organizations, the mission statement is created by soliciting feedback from all employees. This allows an organization to create a mission statement that has input from everyone in the organization.

In many practices, annual employee performance evaluations include feedback on how the employee performs in relation to the organization's mission statement. For example, in a practice with the mission statement listed above, employees might be evaluated on how well they do toward treating patients in a compassionate and dignified manner, and how they do at avoiding patient injury and increasing patient satisfaction.

mission statement
statement that describes a medical office's reason for existing

Critical Thinking 11.6 ?

Why do you think some organizations solicit feedback from all employees in creating a mission statement? How might that organization benefit from this practice? How might the employees benefit?

ORGANIZATIONAL CHARTS

In addition to the mission statement, all policy and procedure manuals should break down the offices' organizational structures in an **organizational chart** (Figure ■ 11-3). Organizational charts are maps to office hierarchies, from physicians to entry-level staff. Members of the healthcare team should be able to use these charts to identify their supervisors, as well as their supervisor's supervisor, all the way to the top of the **chain of command**. In addition to reporting structure, an organizational chart might explain how employees can contact varied healthcare staff. Because organization charts change as people move in and out of positions, these charts should be updated on a regular basis.

organizational chart
visual breakdown of the chain of command in a business

chain of command
a series of positions in which each position has authority over the position below

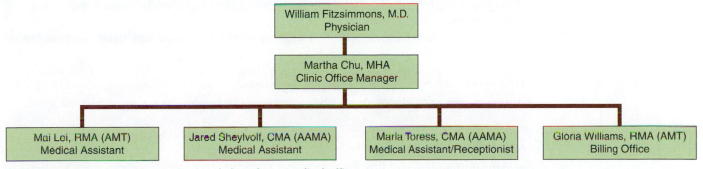

FIGURE ■ 11-3 Sample organizational chart for a medical office.

Critical Thinking 11.7 ?

How does having access to the clinic's organizational chart potentially help an employee?

CLINICAL PROCEDURES

Any clinical procedure that requires staff to interact with a patient should be documented for employee reference. Procedures should clearly list appropriate steps, as well as information on patient education, documentation, and infection control. The type of clinical procedures found in a policy and procedure manual vary according to the type of medical practice and the physician's specialty (Figure ■ 11-4). Clinical procedures should be documented to include such specific topics as:

- Use of the automated external defibrillator
- Procedures, instruments, and positions for various physical examinations
- Draping procedures for physical examinations
- Taking and documenting height, weight, vision, hearing, and chief complaint from the patient
- Procedure for emergencies in the medical office
- Dressing, bandaging, and splinting
- Taking and documenting subjective and objective findings
- Administering injectable medications.

Policy: Administering Injectable Medications
Purpose: To provide injectable medications to the patient per physician orders.

1. Verify the Five Rights of Medication.
   - Verify patient identity by asking the patient his full name and birthdate.
   - Verify the route the medication is to be delivered by checking physician orders.
   - Verify that the correct dose of medication has been drawn by checking the physician orders.
   - Verify that the time of the medication administration is correct by checking the physician orders.
   - Verify that the medication is correct by checking physician orders and the label on the medication.
2. Administer the medication according to physician orders.
3. Discard the syringe in the sharp's container.
4. Document the medication administered, including dose and route, in the patient's medical record.

FIGURE ■ 11-4 Sample clinical procedure.

Critical Thinking 11.8 ?

How might the clinical procedures in a pediatric practice differ from the procedures in a cardiology practice? What might be included in the pediatric procedure manual that is not needed in the cardiology manual?

ADMINISTRATIVE PROCEDURES

Administrative procedures should be documented to include such specific topics as:

- Office opening and closing
- Inventory and supply ordering
- Appointment scheduling
- Patient accounting and bookkeeping
- Insurance processing
- Insurance benefit verification
- Patients' records release
- Medical records management
- Operation of administrative office machinery.

Like clinical procedures, administrative procedures vary according to the type of medical practice, but the vast majority of administrative policies remain constant from office to office (Figure ■ 11-5).

Policy: Releasing Medical Records to a Patient
Purpose: To release medical records to the patient following legal guidelines.

1. Verify the patient's identity by requesting photo identification.
2. Obtain the patient's signature on the release-of-records form.
3. Ensure the patient has dated the release form.
4. Check to see if the patient has made any alterations to the release form, such as restricting the records release to a limited date.
5. Check to see if the patient has checked the boxes allowing release of information regarding HIV/AIDS, reproductive health, mental health, or drug and alcohol rehabilitation.
6. Pull the patient's medical record.
7. Photocopy the appropriate parts of the medical record according to any limitations noted by the patient on the release form.
8. Send copies of the records to the patient.
9. Note in the patient's file when the records were released.
10. File the original signed release form.

FIGURE ■ 11-5 Sample administrative procedure.

Critical Thinking 11.9 ?

Do you think the administrative procedures in a pediatric practice would differ much from those in a cardiology practice? If so, in what way?

INFECTION CONTROL PROCEDURES

Infection control procedures should be written for all of a medical office's applicable procedures, including:

- Biohazardous waste disposal
- Employee needlestick injuries
- Employee exposure to infectious materials
- Employee education for infection control
- OSHA-required documentation
- Local, state, and federal reporting requirements for infectious agents.

As mandated by OSHA, infection control procedures must be part of the office's exposure control plan, which must be kept separate from other procedure manuals in the office and must be made available to an OSHA inspector when needed. In many practices, new employees must sign a form after training on infection control policies. This practice ensures that employees fully understand how to avoid spread of infection for that particular procedure.

Critical Thinking 11.10 ?

Do you think it would be beneficial to a new employee to have him sign the infection control policies after training on each one? Why or why not? Do you think it would be beneficial to the employer to have the employee sign after training? Why or why not?

QUALITY IMPROVEMENT AND RISK MANAGEMENT PROCEDURES

Risk management procedures are those designed to reduce patient or staff injury in the medical office. These policies range from information on washing children's toys in the reception room to handling life-threatening patient events in the office. Often these policies arise as a result of an event that has happened in the office. For example, if a patient who is unsteady on her feet falls while walking from the reception room to the exam room, a risk management policy may be written to address a safer way to escort a patient who is unsteady (Figure ■ 11-6).

Policy: Escorting patients while in the medical office
Purpose: To keep patients from falling while in the medical office.

- When greeting the patient, visually determine if the patient is able to walk unassisted. If the patient is in a wheelchair, or using a device (walker or cane), or appears unsteady in their gait, offer to assist.
- Assist any patient who needs help by gently taking the patient's arm.
- Walk at the same pace as the patient and do not allow the patient to be out of your site as you escort them.

FIGURE ■ 11-6 Risk management policy for escorting patients.

Quality improvement policies are those that address potential problems in the office, such as those relating to patient satisfaction. For example, a medical office may create a quality improvement policy in order to reduce the patient wait time on the telephone (Figure ■ 11-7).

Policy: Patient Wait Time on the Telephone
Purpose: To keep patients from waiting on the telephone longer than 1 minute before call is taken.

- When patients call into the office, the call is sent to a queue for the next available receptionist
- Patent wait time is to be no longer than 1 minute in the call queue
- If a receptionist sees that there are more calls in the queue than the reception team can answer within 1 minute, she should alert the medical assistants to assist with answering the calls

---

FIGURE ■ 11-7 Quality improvement policy for reducing patient wait time on the telephone.

While quality improvement and risk management procedures and policies vary according to office needs, the vast majority apply to all office types. HIPAA legislation mandates that quality improvement and risk management policies be kept in a separate notebook that is clearly marked and updated regularly.

Critical Thinking 11.11 ?

What other ideas can you think of that would qualify as a risk management or quality improvement policy? How would this policy help with care of patients in the medical office?

Case Study Questions

Refer to the case study presented at the beginning of this chapter to answer the following questions:

1. How would you suggest Steve begin to create a policy and procedure manual for his medical office?
2. Who should Steve speak to regarding the needed policies?
3. Where might Steve look for information on what should be included?
4. What type of policies would you suggest Steve begin with first?

Chapter Review

Summary

- Patient education pamphlets or brochures are an excellent way to reinforce information provided by the physician or medical office staff. Brochures may be purchased from vendors, or they may be created by the office for a more personal touch.

- To create a personnel manual, the medical office manager should work in concert with the practice physicians to determine the type of policies needed, as well as the content. Included in the manual are the mission statement, organizational chart, clinical and administrative procedures, infection control procedures, and quality improvement and risk management procedures.

  - A mission statement is the practice's statement of purpose; it is the stated reason why the practice exists.

  - An organizational chart visually demonstrates the hierarchy in the organization. This chart should be updated as needed as people move in and out of their positions.

  - Clinical procedures are any that cause staff to interact with the patient on a clinical level. Examples include the process for taking vital signs or assisting in a physical examination.

  - Administrative procedures are those that pertain to the administrative functions of the medical office. These include the insurance billing process and the scheduling of patient appointments.

  - Infection control procedures include those that keep infection from spreading from one person to another. An example is a procedure on how to sterilize equipment after use.

  - Quality improvement and risk management procedures pertain to patient care and safety in the medical office. These policies may result from an event that occurs in the office, such as a patient fall.

Multiple Choice

Choose the letter that best answers each question or completes each statement.

1. Quality improvement procedures and policies pertain to which of the following?
   a. Addressing a problem with patient satisfaction
   b. Listing the steps to sterilizing equipment after use
   c. Understanding how to answer the telephone
   d. Performing vital signs at the beginning of the patient's visit

2. A mission statement should be:
   a. lengthy and include the names of all physicians in the practice.
   b. concise and easy to remember.
   c. a list of the fees for services in the clinic.
   d. created by copying the statement from another clinic in town.

3. Which of the following is the purpose of an organizational chart?
   a. To alert patients to who they should call with a complaint about quality of care
   b. To provide employees with a list of administrators' salaries
   c. To give employees the telephone numbers of all managers and supervisors in the clinic
   d. None of the above

4. Which of the following is an example of a clinical procedure?
   a. Prevention of patient falls
   b. Employee needlestick injury
   c. Steps for sterilizing equipment
   d. Medical records management

5. Which of the following is an example of an administrative procedure?
   a. Prevention of patient falls
   b. Employee needlestick injury
   c. Steps for sterilizing equipment
   d. Medical records management

6. Which of the following is an example of a risk management policy?
   a. Prevention of patient falls
   b. Employee needlestick injury
   c. Steps for sterilizing equipment
   d. Medical records management

7. Which of the following is an example of an infection control policy?
   a. Prevention of patient falls
   b. Employee needlestick injury
   c. Steps for sterilizing equipment
   d. Medical records management

8. What is one reason for giving an educational brochure to a patient?
   a. The patient will be able to review the material further after the visit.
   b. The patient will be able to provide material for his or her spouse to read after the visit.
   c. The patient will be able to better understand his or her condition.
   d. All of the above

9. How often should an employee handbook be updated?
   a. Monthly
   b. Yearly
   c. As needed
   d. Never

10. A procedure that outlines biohazardous waste disposal would be found in which of the following policy manuals?
    a. Infection Control
    b. Risk Management
    c. Clinical
    d. Administrative

True/False

Determine if each of the following statements is true or false.

_____ 1. OSHA requires every medical office to keep an exposure control plan.

_____ 2. A personnel manual is also known as an employee handbook.

_____ 3. The most important reason for having a medical office policy and procedure manual is so the manager can properly discipline employees.

_____ 4. The organizational chart should list the name of every employee within the organization.

_____ 5. Policies should be clear so that misinterpretation is kept to a minimum.

_____ 6. Policies should be created by the office manager solely, with no input from others.

_____ 7. Offices may copy policies used in other organizations.

_____ 8. The physician is the person who should write all office policies and procedures in the medical office.

_____ 9. New employees should be given access to, or a copy of, the personnel manual upon hire.

_____ 10. Educational brochures should include medical terms, rather than be written in layman's terms.

Matching

Match each of the following procedural descriptions to the correct type of procedure (clinical, administrative, infection control, or risk management).

a. Clinical procedure

b. Administrative procedure

c. Infection control procedure

d. Risk management procedure

1. Outlines the steps to take in the event the office closes due to an emergency
2. Describes the steps taken to sterilize medical equipment after use
3. Lists the steps to take to schedule a patient appointment
4. Outlines the steps required if an employee is exposed to infectious materials
5. Describes the desired process for escorting patients so patients do not fall in the medical office
6. Lists the steps for copying patient medical information
7. Outlines the steps for taking accurate patient vital signs
8. Lists the steps for verifying patient insurance coverage information
9. Describes the steps to take for disposing of biohazardous waste
10. Lists the steps for closing the office at the end of the day

Chapter Resources

Lean Enterprise Institute: http://www.lean.org/whatslean

Occupational Safety and Health Administration: http://www.osha.gov

U.S. Department of Health and Human Services – policies regarding HIPAA: http://www.hhs.gov/ocr/hipaa

PEARSON myhealthprofessionskit™

Additional interactive resources for this chapter can be found at **www.myhealthprofessionskit. com.** Choose "Medical Assisting" from the discipline menu and then click on the book cover for *Medical Office Management.*

CHAPTER 12

Accounting and Payroll in the Medical Office

CHAPTER OUTLINE

- Introduction to Managerial Accounting
- Developing Budgets in the Medical Office
- Petty Cash
- Processing Payroll
- History of Payroll Taxes
- Payroll Laws
- Workers' Compensation
- Creating a Record for a New Employee
- Updating the Employee Record
- Employee Records Must Be Kept Confidential
- Use of the W-4 Form
- Keeping a Record of the Number of Hours Employees Work

- Calculating Payroll
- Computing Payroll Deductions
- IRS Circular E
- Other Deductions
- Using Computer Software to Calculate Employee Payroll
- The W-2 Form
- Garnishment of Wages
- Accounts Payable
- The Checkbook Register
- Preparing a Deposit Slip
- Online Banking
- Reconciling the Bank Statement

LEARNING OBJECTIVES

Upon completion of this chapter, you should be able to:

- Spell and define the key terms in this chapter.
- Describe the function of managerial accounting.
- Understand how a budget is developed in the medical office.
- Describe the purpose of keeping a petty cash fund.
- Understand the process of payroll in the medical office.
- Understand the history of payroll taxes in the United States.
- List laws that govern the payroll function.
- Describe how workers' compensation laws apply to the medical practice.
- Create a record for a new employee.
- Update an employee record.
- Understand that employee records are to be kept confidential.
- Understand how to use and when to update a W-4 form.

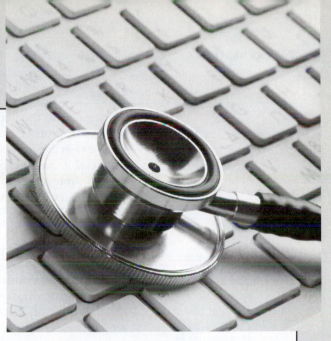

- Keep a record of employee work hours.
- Describe how to calculate payroll and understand the differences between payroll for hourly employees versus payroll for salaried employees.
- Describe how to compute payroll deductions.
- Understand how to use the IRS Circular E publication.
- List other deductions that may apply to the employee payroll.
- Describe the use of computer software to calculate payroll.
- Describe the purpose of the W-2 form.
- Understand how employee wages are garnished.
- Define the accounts payable.
- Understand the purpose and components of the checkbook register.
- Prepare a deposit slip.
- Describe the function of online banking.
- Reconcile a bank statement.

KEY TERMS

auditors
budget
charitable contributions
Circular E
deductions
endorsement stamp
Fair Labor Standards Act (FLSA)
Federal Insurance
Contributions Act (FICA)
Federal Unemployment Tax
Act (FUTA)
financial accounting

fixed costs
gross pay
managerial accounting
net pay
outsource
overtime
payroll
payroll taxes
personnel file
petty cash
products
quarterly payroll reports

security envelope
services
Social Security Act
time clock
unemployment insurance
variable costs
W-2 form
W-4 form
wages
withholding allowances
workers' compensation

Case Study

Take note of the following scenario and answer the case study questions that appear at the end of this chapter.

Barb Rolette is the medical office manager in an internal medicine practice. The physicians in the practice would like to find out if adding a flu shot clinic will be profitable this upcoming flu season. Barb needs to find out if the cost of staffing the clinic and the cost of supplies weighed against the profits from the flu clinic will be profitable to the clinic.

Introduction

Managing the financial aspects of the medical office is one of the most important tasks of the medical office manager. Without sound financial principles and policies in place, no business will succeed, and healthcare is no exception. By paying close attention to all financial areas, the medical office manager allows the physicians to concentrate on the care of their patients. The medical office manager will often be placed in charge of setting up a budget for the medical practice and handling the payroll function.

Introduction to Managerial Accounting

managerial accounting
the function of collecting and applying financial information within an organization in order to make sound business decisions

financial accounting
the process of providing information to stockholders or creditors

Managerial accounting is the function of collecting and applying financial information within an organization in order to make sound business decisions. Another common term for this type of accounting is *cost accounting*. This differs from **financial accounting**, which is the process of providing information to stockholders or creditors.

COSTS OF PRODUCTS AND SERVICES

The medical office manager maintains information on the costs the office incurs for products and services. Examples would be the costs associated with a service contract for equipment and the cost per unit for supplies purchased for use in the medical office. With this information, the medical office manager will be positioned to make the best decisions regarding the type of services the office may want or need to pursue, as well as the best companies to purchase supplies from for office use.

In addition, by understanding the costs associated with the services offered by the medical office, the medical office manager can determine how profitable it is for the physicians to render those services.

> **Critical Thinking 12.1 ?**
>
> Imagine a physician performs a mole removal procedure in the office. If the cost of supplies needed for that procedure is $100 and the reimbursement for the procedure is $1,000, the mole removal procedure seems profitable. But what if the procedure takes over an hour to perform, and the same physician could render four standard office visits during that hour and be reimbursed $1,200 (with no costs for supplies)? Would you suggest the physician perform more mole removals or concentrate on standard office visits?

PRODUCTS AND SERVICES SOLD

products
supplies that the physician prescribes to the patient, such as a splint or crutches

services
things that are provided to the patient in the form of an activity, such as an examination or a surgical procedure

The medical office manager should keep track of the number of **products** and **services** sold or processed in the medical office. Products are supplies that the physician prescribes to the patient, such as a splint or crutches. The medical office must purchase the supplies from a vendor, then charge the patient for the supply when it is distributed. Services are those things that are provided to the patient in the form of an activity, such as an examination or a surgical procedure. Knowing the amount paid for a product, the manager determines if the amount charged to the patient for that product is fair and if the product generates a profit for the organization. In most cases, the charge for a product (a prefabricated arm splint, for example) is billed to the patient's insurance carrier. Medical office managers should stay abreast of the reimbursement amounts provided by insurance carriers for products or supplies in order to determine if the reimbursement is creating a profit or a loss to the organization.

Keeping track of the services in the department consists of tracking the number of patients each physicians sees on a given day. This information is useful in determining physician salaries or the number of staff that it is profitable to employ for a particular physician.

VARIABLE COSTS

Costs that vary with the number of services or products produced are known as **variable costs**. In the medical office, an example of variable costs are medical supplies. A medical office may purchase a case of medicine vials, for example, at a cost of $500. Each time a clinical staff member gives a shot of this medication to a patient, a fee is charged. The amount of money the medical office makes from the case of medicine vials varies with the number of shots given.

variable costs
costs that vary with the number of services or products produced

FIXED COSTS

Unlike variable costs, **fixed costs** remain the same no matter how many products or services are sold in the medical office. Fixed costs are costs for items such as rent, insurance, and housekeeping staff. The amount the medical office pays for these items remains the same whether the office sees 1 patient per day or 100 patients per day.

fixed costs
costs that remain the same no matter how many services are used or produced

Developing Budgets in the Medical Office

A **budget** is a list of planned expenses and revenue. Similar to a household budget, the budget in a medical office is designed to determine the amount of money the medical office can spend, based on the projected amount of income. In the medical office, the medical office manager is often the person who prepares the budget for the practice for each upcoming year.

To calculate the budget, the manager determines the revenue for the past year. With this data, the manager is then able to determine the projected amount of income for the next year. Once the expected amount of income for the next year has been determined, the medical office manager can create a budget of expenses for the upcoming year. This amount will include the amount needed for fixed expenses, such as rent and utilities, as well as the expenses for supplies and other services. Expenses for staffing are also included in the medical office budget.

budget
a list of planned expenses and revenues

Critical Thinking 12.2 ?

What is the importance of having a budget in the medical office? What do you think could happen if the clinic did not create a budget to follow each year?

Petty Cash

Occasionally small expenses crop up in a medical office that require immediate reimbursement. These expenses are not typically formally invoiced, in part because the office staff may not be aware ahead of time that the expense will happen. For example, if office staff use the last receipt in the receipt book, and a new book is needed before an office supply order can be placed, a staff member must go out and purchase the new book right away. For these types of expenses, a small amount of money should be kept in the office. This money is referred to as **petty cash**. The medical office manager should keep a journal or logbook (Figure ■ 12-1) in the office for the staff to document expenses paid via the petty cash fund. A receipt should always accompany the entry into the logbook.

petty cash
a small amount of money kept in the medical office to pay for unexpected items

Critical Thinking 12.3 ?

Aside from the example given in previous section, what other items do you think might be paid from a petty cash fund?

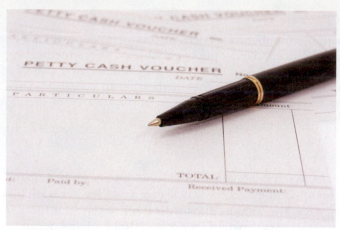

FIGURE ■ 12-1 Receipts must be written for all petty cash expenditures.
Source: Stuartmiles/Dreamstime.com.

payroll
process of calculating the amounts employees receive for their work

gross pay
amount earned before taxes or deductions are subtracted

outsource
to send outside a business to another business for completion

Processing Payroll

Given its role in employees' financial stability, the **payroll** in a medical office is vital. As healthcare has advanced and technology has taken hold, payroll's function has been transformed. Payroll processing today involves far more than paycheck issuance. Various laws and regulations govern just about every phase of payroll, from calculating employees' deductions and the taxes to be withheld from employees' **gross pay** to maintaining and reporting payroll records. The local and national laws impacting payroll practices continue to change, so it is crucial for the medical office manager to track those changes.

Many large offices now use computer software for their payroll functions, but some still calculate payroll manually. Still other offices **outsource** their payroll function to third parties such as accountants. In large and small medical offices alike, the member of the healthcare team who processes payroll (typically the office manager) is assigned a wide range of duties, including:

payroll taxes
monies withheld from wages for federal income, Social Security, and Medicare obligations

deductions
number of allowances to be withheld from an employee's wages

wages
monies paid for work performed

net pay
amount of wages remaining after deductions and taxes have been subtracted

quarterly payroll reports
documents that specify the taxes withheld from wages quarterly

- Staying current with state and federal laws for **payroll taxes**
- Keeping written records of employees' hours and wages
- Computing the taxes and other **deductions** to be taken from employees' paychecks
- Documenting the **wages**, deductions, and **net pay** for each employee
- Preparing and distributing paychecks to employees
- Calculating office payroll taxes and depositing the funds
- Preparing **quarterly payroll reports**.

History of Payroll Taxes

When the Sixteenth Amendment to the Constitution passed in 1913, the U.S. Congress gained the ability to impose a federal income tax on individuals and corporations. Each year when they filed their returns, employees paid the federal government directly. By 1918, the government was collecting just over $1 billion each year as a result. By 1920, that figure had risen to $5.4 billion. When World War II launched and employment increased, taxes climbed to $7.3 billion annually.

In 1935, Congress passed the **Social Security Act** to provide financial security to workers and their families after retirement. Congress followed that legislation with the

Social Security Act
law passed by the U.S. Congress in 1935 to provide workers and their families with financial security after retirement

Fair Labor Standards Act (FLSA) in 1938. This act addressed several worker-related issues, including a federal minimum wage that increases with the inflation rate. As of 2009, the federal minimum wage increased to $7.25, where it stands today. In addition to things like minimum wage, the FLSA requires employers to pay employees **overtime** earnings of 1.5 times the employees' normal hourly wages for any work completed beyond 40 hours in 1 week.

As the years passed, the government tried to remain vigilant to workers' needs, but many employees were finding it difficult to keep up with increasing taxes. Many individual taxpayers found it difficult to pay their full tax bills at the end of each year.

Relief came in 1943, when a law that required withholding of taxes on wages was introduced. Under this law, businesses were responsible for collecting employees' income taxes and sending those taxes to the government. Employers had to keep written records of all the taxes they withheld from employees' pay, as well as records of those employees' addresses, employment dates, and wages. This legislation boosted the number of taxpayers yet further. By 1945, taxes had jumped to $43 billion.

> **Fair Labor Standards Act (FLSA)**
> law passed by the U.S. Congress in 1938 to address employment issues such as the federal minimum wage
>
> **overtime**
> wages paid beyond 40 hours in a workweek, usually at a rate that is 1.5 times the normal rate

Payroll Laws

Throughout the decades, the U.S. government has continued to use legislation to address employment issues. For example, the Social Security Act has evolved over the years into a system that today has two main parts: (1) elderly, survivors, and disability insurance and (2) hospital insurance, known as Medicare. Two other laws address the payment of Social Security and Medicare taxes: (1) the **Federal Insurance Contributions Act (FICA)** and (2) the **Federal Unemployment Tax Act (FUTA).** Still other laws require **unemployment insurance,** a program that benefits employees who have lost their jobs. Employers make quarterly payments to their state and federal governments to support the unemployment program.

When the FICA tax was first collected, it was set at 1 percent. Today, given rising inflation, it rests at 5.65 percent. Of that 5.65 percent FICA tax, employees pay 4.2 percent of their gross income for Social Security and 1.45 percent for Medicare. All employers must pay 7.65 percent of the wage amount, creating a deposit for each employee of 13.3 percent of their gross payrolls. Not all income is subject to FICA tax, however. As of 2011, only the first $106,800 of an individual's wages is subject to FICA tax. The Medicare tax has no wage limit.

The federal agency responsible for enforcing income tax laws is the Internal Revenue Service (IRS). This agency has offices in every major city and employs more than 15,000 **auditors.** Auditors are responsible not only for conducting tax audits but for giving taxpayers federal tax advice. The federal income taxes an employer withholds from an employee's pay must be paid to the IRS each month. FICA taxes, like IRS taxes, must be deposited monthly. Every business must file quarterly payroll reports to the IRS in which they account for all monies withheld as taxes and deposits made to the IRS of those taxes (Figure ▪ 12-2).

Many states have income taxes that are separate from the federal income tax. States laws are similar to federal ones with regard to tax deductions and deposits. From a state perspective, employers must withhold specified amounts and file reports quarterly.

In addition to income taxes, most states have laws that require employers to provide employees coverage should those employees become injured on the job. This coverage, known as workers' compensation (see next section), is used for medical care, lost wages, or death benefits. In many states, the employee pays a portion of the workers' compensation premium, but the employer generally funds the larger share. Employers in high-injury-risk industries, such as construction or mining, pay higher premiums than those in low-risk businesses, such as insurance processing or data entry. However, even employers in low-risk industries will pay higher premiums if too many of their employees are injured on the job.

> **Federal Insurance Contributions Act (FICA)**
> law that addresses Social Security withholding taxes
>
> **Federal Unemployment Tax Act (FUTA)**
> law that addresses federal unemployment tax withholdings
>
> **unemployment insurance**
> program that pays employees who have lost their jobs
>
> **auditors**
> people who review personal or corporate bank or tax records on behalf of an agency like the Internal Revenue Service

Form **941 for 2012:** Employer's QUARTERLY Federal Tax Return

(Rev. January 2012)

Department of the Treasury — Internal Revenue Service

950112

OMB No. 1545-0029

Employer identification number (EIN)

Name (not your trade name)

Trade name (if any)

Address

Number   Street   Suite or room number

City   State   ZIP code

Report for this Quarter of 2012
(Check one.)

☐ 1: January, February, March

☐ 2: April, May, June

☐ 3: July, August, September

☐ 4: October, November, December

Prior-year forms are available at *www.irs.gov/form941.*

Read the separate instructions before you complete Form 941. Type or print within the boxes.

Part 1: Answer these questions for this quarter.

1   Number of employees who received wages, tips, or other compensation for the pay period including: *Mar. 12* (Quarter 1), *June 12* (Quarter 2), *Sept. 12* (Quarter 3), or *Dec. 12* (Quarter 4)   **1**

2   Wages, tips, and other compensation   **2**

3   Income tax withheld from wages, tips, and other compensation   **3**

4   If no wages, tips, and other compensation are subject to social security or Medicare tax   ☐ Check and go to line 6.

	Column 1		Column 2
5a Taxable social security wages .		× .104 =	
5b Taxable social security tips . .		× .104 =	
5c Taxable Medicare wages & tips.		× .029 =	

5d   Add *Column 2* line 5a, *Column 2* line 5b, and *Column 2* line 5c   **5d**

5e   Section 3121(q) Notice and Demand—Tax due on unreported tips (see instructions)   **5e**

6   Total taxes before adjustments (add lines 3, 5d, and 5e)   **6**

7   Current quarter's adjustment for fractions of cents   **7**

8   Current quarter's adjustment for sick pay   **8**

9   Current quarter's adjustments for tips and group-term life insurance   **9**

10   Total taxes after adjustments. Combine lines 6 through 9   **10**

11   Total deposits for this quarter, including overpayment applied from a prior quarter and overpayment applied from Form 941-X or Form 944-X   **11**

12a   COBRA premium assistance payments (see instructions)   **12a**

12b   Number of individuals provided COBRA premium assistance

13   Add lines 11 and 12a   **13**

14   Balance due. If line 10 is more than line 13, enter the difference and see instructions   **14**

15   Overpayment. If line 13 is more than line 10, enter the difference   Check one: ☐ Apply to next return. ☐ Send a refund.

▶ You MUST complete both pages of Form 941 and SIGN it.   Next ▶

For Privacy Act and Paperwork Reduction Act Notice, see the back of the Payment Voucher.   Cat. No. 17001Z   Form **941** (Rev. 1-2012)

FIGURE ■ 12-2 Form 941: Employer's quarterly federal tax return.

Name *(not your trade name)*	Employer identification number (EIN)

Part 2: Tell us about your deposit schedule and tax liability for this quarter.

If you are unsure about whether you are a monthly schedule depositor or a semiweekly schedule depositor, see *Pub. 15 (Circular E)*, section 11.

16 Check one:

☐ **Line 10 on this return is less than $2,500 or line 10 on the return for the prior quarter was less than $2,500, and you did not incur a $100,000 next-day deposit obligation during the current quarter.** If line 10 for the prior quarter was less than $2,500 but line 10 on this return is $100,000 or more, you must provide a record of your federal tax liability. If you are a monthly schedule depositor, complete the deposit schedule below; if you are a semiweekly schedule depositor, attach Schedule B (Form 941). Go to Part 3.

☐ **You were a monthly schedule depositor for the entire quarter.** Enter your tax liability for each month and total liability for the quarter, then go to Part 3.

Tax liability: Month 1 [_____.__]

Month 2 [_____.__]

Month 3 [_____.__]

Total liability for quarter [_____.__] Total must equal line 10.

☐ **You were a semiweekly schedule depositor for any part of this quarter.** Complete *Schedule B (Form 941): Report of Tax Liability for Semiweekly Schedule Depositors,* and attach it to Form 941.

Part 3: Tell us about your business. If a question does NOT apply to your business, leave it blank.

17 If your business has closed or you stopped paying wages . . . . ☐ Check here, and

enter the final date you paid wages [____ / ____ / ____] .

18 If you are a seasonal employer and you do not have to file a return for every quarter of the year . . ☐ Check here.

Part 4: May we speak with your third-party designee?

Do you want to allow an employee, a paid tax preparer, or another person to discuss this return with the IRS? See the instructions for details.

☐ Yes. Designee's name and phone number [_____] [_____]

Select a 5-digit Personal Identification Number (PIN) to use when talking to the IRS. ☐ ☐ ☐ ☐ ☐

☐ No.

Part 5: Sign here. You MUST complete both pages of Form 941 and SIGN it.

Under penalties of perjury, I declare that I have examined this return, including accompanying schedules and statements, and to the best of my knowledge and belief, it is true, correct, and complete. Declaration of preparer (other than taxpayer) is based on all information of which preparer has any knowledge.

X Sign your name here [_____]

Print your name here [_____]

Print your title here [_____]

Date [____ / ____ / ____]

Best daytime phone [_____]

Paid Preparer Use Only

Check if you are self-employed . . . ☐

Preparer's name		PTIN	
Preparer's signature		Date	[____ / ____ / ____]
Firm's name (or yours if self-employed)		EIN	
Address		Phone	
City	State	ZIP code	

Form **941** (Rev. 1-2012)

FIGURE ■ 12-2 (Continued)

Form 941-V,
Payment Voucher

Purpose of Form

Complete Form 941-V, Payment Voucher, if you are making a payment with Form 941, Employer's QUARTERLY Federal Tax Return. We will use the completed voucher to credit your payment more promptly and accurately, and to improve our service to you.

If you have your return prepared by a third party and make a payment with that return, please provide this payment voucher to the return preparer.

Making Payments With Form 941

To avoid a penalty, make your payment with Form 941 **only if:**

• Your net taxes for either the current quarter or the preceding quarter (line 10 on Form 941) are less than $2,500, you did not incur a $100,000 next-day deposit obligation during the current quarter, and you are paying in full with a timely filed return, or

• You are a monthly schedule depositor making a payment in accordance with the Accuracy of Deposits Rule. See section 11 of Pub. 15 (Circular E), Employer's Tax Guide, for details. In this case, the amount of your payment may be $2,500 or more.

Otherwise, you must make deposits by electronic funds transfer. See section 11 of Pub. 15 (Circular E) for deposit instructions. Do not use Form 941-V to make federal tax deposits.

Caution. *Use Form 941-V when making any payment with Form 941. However, if you pay an amount with Form 941 that should have been deposited, you may be subject to a penalty. See* Deposit Penalties *in section 11 of Pub. 15 (Circular E).*

Specific Instructions

Box 1—Employer identification number (EIN). If you do not have an EIN, you may apply for one online. Go to IRS.gov and click on the *Apply for an EIN Online* link. You may also apply for an EIN by calling 1-800-829-4933, or you can fax or mail Form SS-4, Application for Employer Identification Number. If you have not received your EIN by the due date of Form 941, write "Applied For" and the date you applied in this entry space.

Box 2—Amount paid. Enter the amount paid with Form 941.

Box 3—Tax period. Darken the circle identifying the quarter for which the payment is made. Darken only one circle.

Box 4—Name and address. Enter your name and address as shown on Form 941.

• Enclose your check or money order made payable to the "United States Treasury." Be sure to enter your EIN, "Form 941," and the tax period on your check or money order. Do not send cash. Do not staple Form 941-V or your payment to Form 941 (or to each other).

• Detach Form 941-V and send it with your payment and Form 941 to the address in the Instructions for Form 941.

Note. You must also complete the entity information above Part 1 on Form 941.

✂ ------- ▼ **Detach Here and Mail With Your Payment and Form 941.** ▼ ------- ✂

Form **941-V**	**Payment Voucher**	OMB No. 1545-0029
Department of the Treasury Internal Revenue Service	▶ **Do not staple this voucher or your payment to Form 941.**	20**12**

1 Enter your employer identification number (EIN).	2 **Enter the amount of your payment.** ▶	Dollars	Cents

3 Tax Period		4 Enter your business name (individual name if sole proprietor).
○ 1st Quarter	○ 3rd Quarter	Enter your address.
○ 2nd Quarter	○ 4th Quarter	Enter your city, state, and ZIP code.

FIGURE ■ 12-2 (Continued)

Form 941 (Rev. 1-2012)

Privacy Act and Paperwork Reduction Act Notice. We ask for the information on Form 941 to carry out the Internal Revenue laws of the United States. We need it to figure and collect the right amount of tax. Subtitle C, Employment Taxes, of the Internal Revenue Code imposes employment taxes on wages, including income tax withholding. Form 941 is used to determine the amount of taxes that you owe. Section 6011 requires you to provide the requested information if the tax is applicable to you. Section 6109 requires you to provide your identification number. If you fail to provide this information in a timely manner, or provide false or fraudulent information, you may be subject to penalties and interest.

You are not required to provide the information requested on a form that is subject to the Paperwork Reduction Act unless the form displays a valid OMB control number. Books and records relating to a form or its instructions must be retained as long as their contents may become material in the administration of any Internal Revenue law.

Generally, tax returns and return information are confidential, as required by section 6103. However, section 6103 allows or requires the IRS to disclose or give the information shown on your tax return to others as described in the Code. For example, we may disclose your tax information to the Department of

Justice for civil and criminal litigation, and to cities, states, the District of Columbia, and U.S. commonwealths and possessions for use in administering their tax laws. We may also disclose this information to other countries under a tax treaty, to federal and state agencies to enforce federal nontax criminal laws, or to federal law enforcement and intelligence agencies to combat terrorism.

The time needed to complete and file Form 941 will vary depending on individual circumstances. The estimated average time is:

Recordkeeping . . . . 11 hr.

Learning about the law or the form . . . . 47 min.

Preparing, copying, assembling, and sending the form to the IRS . . . . 1 hr.

If you have comments concerning the accuracy of these time estimates or suggestions for making Form 941 simpler, we would be happy to hear from you. You can email us at *taxforms@irs.gov*. Enter "Form 941" on the subject line. Or write to: Internal Revenue Service, Tax Products Coordinating Committee, SE:W:CAR:MP:T:M:S, 1111 Constitution Ave. NW, IR-6526, Washington, DC 20224. **Do not** send Form 941 to this address. Instead, see *Where Should You File?* in the Instructions for Form 941.

FIGURE ■ 12-2 (Continued)

Workers' Compensation

Workers' compensation insurance covers employees injured in the workplace or suffering from a workplace-related illness. Occupational injuries are those that occur during the course of employment, but they do not have to occur on company property or while performing work duties. Accidents that occur off-site, such as while driving on company business, at a remote work site, or during a paid break are covered.

Occupational illnesses are conditions that arise from short- or long-term exposure to a workplace hazard or condition, such as dust, chemical allergens, radiation, repetitive motion, and loud noises. The challenge with occupational illnesses is identifying, diagnosing, and reporting them, because some of these injuries, such as repetitive stress injuries, hearing loss, mental stress–related conditions, and various respiratory disorders, may take years to manifest themselves.

All employers must offer workers' compensation insurance, although laws vary from one state to another. Insurance may be obtained from a state-managed fund, private insurers, or employer self-insurance. Some states do not allow private insurers to offer workers' compensation policies; in such cases, coverage must be obtained from the state or through self-insurance. Federal laws cover workers in Washington, D.C., coal miners, federal employees, and maritime workers.

A workers' compensation claim is initiated by the filing of a *First Report of Illness or Injury*. State laws vary widely on the time frame required for filing and the responsible party. In some states the employer may be required to file this report; in other states the first provider who treats the injured worker is responsible for this filing. Medical office managers need to be familiar with how the filing process works in their state.

workers' compensation insurance coverage for job-related illness or injury provided by employers

Critical Thinking 12.4 ?

The workers' compensation premium for healthcare workers is fairly low, due to the low chance of employees sustaining an injury. What employment areas do you think have higher premiums for this coverage?

Benefits to the injured worker include coverage of the cost of medical care related to the illness or injury, wages for time lost from work due to illness or injury, death benefits for survivors when the accident is the cause of the worker's death, and rehabilitation or retraining benefits that enable the worker to learn a different line of work, if necessary.

A nondisability claim is one in which the worker was injured and treated by a physician, but no time was lost from work. In these claims, no lost wages are paid. Temporary disability claims are ones in which the worker is eventually able to return to his or her previous work or a modified work plan. Permanent disability means that no further improvement is expected and the worker is unable to return to work in any capacity.

Critical Thinking 12.5 ?

What do you think the benefits are to the employee in having coverage for work-related injuries? What are the benefits to the employer in providing this coverage?

Creating a Record for a New Employee

personnel file
set of employment-related documents for an employee; includes the original job application, résumé, credentials, licensing and insurance information, references, federal withholding requests, dates and copies of performance evaluations, and any information about disciplinary actions

For each new employee, the medical office should create a **personnel file** (Figure ■ 12-3) that contains the employee's employment-related documentation, such as the job application, résumé, credentials, licensing and insurance information, and references. To prove their identities at hire, all new employees must provide copies of their driver's license or other photo identification, as well as copies of their Social Security cards. Each employee's personnel file must be kept up to date for the duration of that employee's employment in the clinic. The personnel file will also contain a record of the employee's wage increases, federal withholding requests, and performance evaluations, as well as any information on disciplinary actions.

FIGURE ■ 12-3 A personnel file must be kept for each employee.
Source: Zwolafasola/Dreamstime.com.

Once the employee is no longer employed with that facility, the record should still be kept for a period of time. The amount of time will depend on the employer and the storage available. Employers are often contacted by other organizations looking for job references for former employees. When this happens, the former employer should consult the personnel file. In the event the employee files a legal claim against the employer for discrimination, sexual harassment, wrongful termination, or other workplace-related claim, the employer will need the information in the employee file to defend against the claim.

Updating the Employee Record

A personnel record should reflect all changes to an employee's employment status, such as pay raises, evaluations, disciplinary actions, marital status changes, tax exemptions, and continuing education credits, as those changes occur. Employee records should also include copies of such items as employees' cardiopulmonary resuscitation (CPR) certifications and malpractice insurance documents. In short, personnel records should be accurate, up-to-date pictures of employees.

Critical Thinking 12.6 ?

Imagine an employee is fired due to poor performance, and the employee files a wrongful termination lawsuit against the employer. What information from the personnel file will be helpful to the employer in defending against this claim?

Employee Records Must be Kept Confidential

According to the Health Insurance Portability and Accountability Act (HIPAA), all personal employee information in the medical office, including payroll information, must be kept confidential and in places where only healthcare staff can access it. Nonauthorized parties should not be allowed access under any circumstances. Employees, however, must be allowed to view their personnel files and to request corrections as needed.

Use of the W-4 Form

Every new employee must complete an IRS **W-4 form,** or Employee's Withholding Allowance Certificate, which shows the employer the number of **withholding allowances** the employee is claiming, determined by the employee's marital status and number of dependants (Figure ■ 12-4). This number of allowances determines the amount, if any, to be withheld from the employee's earnings each payroll period.

> **W-4 form**
> U.S. federal form that indicates employees' marital status and federal tax exemptions
>
> **withholding allowances**
> number of exemptions declared on federal tax forms

To ensure timely payroll processing, employees must complete and sign their W-4 forms before their first payroll periods. As employees experience life changes, such as marriage or children, those employees' withholding allowances will change. To keep their payrolls up to date, medical office managers should require employees to notify their personnel departments or payroll staff of any such changes.

UPDATING THE W-4 FORM

When employees wish to change their withholding allowances, they must complete and sign new W-4 forms. W-4 changes should take effect in the next payroll period. When medical offices outsource their payroll functions, W-4 changes may be delayed. When this is the case, offices should notify the affected employees.

Keeping a Record of the Number of Hours Employees Work

To meet FLSA requirements for overtime pay, employers must accurately record the hours their employees work. For all employees, salaried and hourly, employers must also send their states premiums to cover workers' compensation insurance. Such premiums are based on the number of hours all covered employees worked in each quarter. Many medical offices use time clocks for those employees paid on an hourly basis. In these organizations, the record of time punches is all that is needed to account for the employee work hours. Salaried employees, on the other hand, do not typically keep an accounting

Form W-4 (2012)

Purpose. Complete Form W-4 so that your employer can withhold the correct federal income tax from your pay. Consider completing a new Form W-4 each year and when your personal or financial situation changes.

Exemption from withholding. If you are exempt, complete **only** lines 1, 2, 3, 4, and 7 and sign the form to validate it. Your exemption for 2012 expires February 18, 2013. See Pub. 505, Tax Withholding and Estimated Tax.

Note. If another person can claim you as a dependent on his or her tax return, you cannot claim exemption from withholding if your income exceeds $950 and includes more than $300 of unearned income (for example, interest and dividends).

Basic instructions. If you are not exempt, complete the **Personal Allowances Worksheet** below. The worksheets on page 2 further adjust your withholding allowances based on itemized deductions, certain credits, adjustments to income, or two-earners/multiple jobs situations.

Complete all worksheets that apply. However, you may claim fewer (or zero) allowances. For regular wages, withholding must be based on allowances you claimed and may not be a flat amount or percentage of wages.

Head of household. Generally, you can claim head of household filing status on your tax return only if you are unmarried and pay more than 50% of the costs of keeping up a home for yourself and your dependent(s) or other qualifying individuals. See Pub. 501, Exemptions, Standard Deduction, and Filing Information, for information.

Tax credits. You can take projected tax credits into account in figuring your allowable number of withholding allowances. Credits for child or dependent care expenses and the child tax credit may be claimed using the **Personal Allowances Worksheet** below. See Pub. 505 for information on converting your other credits into withholding allowances.

Nonwage income. If you have a large amount of nonwage income, such as interest or dividends, consider making estimated tax payments using Form 1040-ES, Estimated Tax for Individuals. Otherwise, you may owe additional tax. If you have pension or annuity income, see Pub. 505 to find out if you should adjust your withholding on Form W-4 or W-4P.

Two earners or multiple jobs. If you have a working spouse or more than one job, figure the total number of allowances you are entitled to claim on all jobs using worksheets from only one Form W-4. Your withholding usually will be most accurate when all allowances are claimed on the Form W-4 for the highest paying job and zero allowances are claimed on the others. See Pub. 505 for details.

Nonresident alien. If you are a nonresident alien, see Notice 1392, Supplemental Form W-4 Instructions for Nonresident Aliens, before completing this form.

Check your withholding. After your Form W-4 takes effect, use Pub. 505 to see how the amount you are having withheld compares to your projected total tax for 2012. See Pub. 505, especially if your earnings exceed $130,000 (Single) or $180,000 (Married).

Future developments. The IRS has created a page on IRS.gov for information about Form W-4, at www.irs.gov/w4. Information about any future developments affecting Form W-4 (such as legislation enacted after we release it) will be posted on that page.

Personal Allowances Worksheet (Keep for your records.)

A	Enter "1" for **yourself** if no one else can claim you as a dependent	A ____
B	Enter "1" if: { • You are single and have only one job; or • You are married, have only one job, and your spouse does not work; or • Your wages from a second job or your spouse's wages (or the total of both) are $1,500 or less. } . . .	B ____
C	Enter "1" for your **spouse**. But, you may choose to enter "-0-" if you are married and have either a working spouse or more than one job. (Entering "-0-" may help you avoid having too little tax withheld.)	C ____
D	Enter number of **dependents** (other than your spouse or yourself) you will claim on your tax return	D ____
E	Enter "1" if you will file as **head of household** on your tax return (see conditions under **Head of household** above) . .	E ____
F	Enter "1" if you have at least $1,900 of **child or dependent care expenses** for which you plan to claim a credit . . .	F ____
	(**Note.** Do **not** include child support payments. See Pub. 503, Child and Dependent Care Expenses, for details.)	
G	**Child Tax Credit** (including additional child tax credit). See Pub. 972, Child Tax Credit, for more information.	
	• If your total income will be less than $61,000 ($90,000 if married), enter "2" for each eligible child; then **less** "1" if you have three to seven eligible children or **less** "2" if you have eight or more eligible children.	
	• If your total income will be between $61,000 and $84,000 ($90,000 and $119,000 if married), enter "1" for each eligible child . . .	G ____
H	Add lines A through G and enter total here. (**Note.** This may be different from the number of exemptions you claim on your tax return.) ▶	H ____

For accuracy, complete all worksheets that apply.	• If you plan to **itemize** or **claim adjustments to income** and want to reduce your withholding, see the **Deductions and Adjustments Worksheet** on page 2. • If you are **single and have more than one job** or are **married and you and your spouse both work** and the combined earnings from all jobs exceed $40,000 ($10,000 if married), see the **Two-Earners/Multiple Jobs Worksheet** on page 2 to avoid having too little tax withheld. • If **neither** of the above situations applies, **stop here** and enter the number from line H on line 5 of Form W-4 below.

------------------------------ Separate here and give Form W-4 to your employer. Keep the top part for your records. ------------------------------

Form W-4
Department of the Treasury
Internal Revenue Service

Employee's Withholding Allowance Certificate

▶ Whether you are entitled to claim a certain number of allowances or exemption from withholding is subject to review by the IRS. Your employer may be required to send a copy of this form to the IRS.

OMB No. 1545-0074

2012

1 Your first name and middle initial	Last name	2 Your social security number

Home address (number and street or rural route)	3 ☐ Single ☐ Married ☐ Married, but withhold at higher Single rate.
	Note. If married, but legally separated, or spouse is a nonresident alien, check the "Single" box.
City or town, state, and ZIP code	4 If your last name differs from that shown on your social security card, check here. You must call 1-800-772-1213 for a replacement card. ▶ ☐

5	Total number of allowances you are claiming (from line **H** above **or** from the applicable worksheet on page 2)	5 ____
6	Additional amount, if any, you want withheld from each paycheck	6 $ ____
7	I claim exemption from withholding for 2012, and I certify that I meet **both** of the following conditions for exemption.	
	• Last year I had a right to a refund of **all** federal income tax withheld because I had **no** tax liability, **and**	
	• This year I expect a refund of **all** federal income tax withheld because I expect to have **no** tax liability.	
	If you meet both conditions, write "Exempt" here . . . . ▶ 7 ____	

Under penalties of perjury, I declare that I have examined this certificate and, to the best of my knowledge and belief, it is true, correct, and complete.

Employee's signature
(This form is not valid unless you sign it.) ▶ _____ Date ▶ _____

8 Employer's name and address (Employer: Complete lines 8 and 10 only if sending to the IRS.)	9 Office code (optional)	10 Employer identification number (EIN)

For Privacy Act and Paperwork Reduction Act Notice, see page 2.   Cat. No. 10220Q   Form **W-4** (2012)

FIGURE 12-4 W-4 form.

Deductions and Adjustments Worksheet

Note. Use this worksheet *only* if you plan to itemize deductions or claim certain credits or adjustments to income.

1	Enter an estimate of your 2012 itemized deductions. These include qualifying home mortgage interest, charitable contributions, state and local taxes, medical expenses in excess of 7.5% of your income, and miscellaneous deductions	**1**	$
2	Enter: { $11,900 if married filing jointly or qualifying widow(er) / $8,700 if head of household / $5,950 if single or married filing separately } . . .	**2**	$
3	**Subtract** line 2 from line 1. If zero or less, enter "-0-"	**3**	$
4	Enter an estimate of your 2012 adjustments to income and any additional standard deduction (see Pub. 505)	**4**	$
5	**Add** lines 3 and 4 and enter the total. (Include any amount for credits from the *Converting Credits to Withholding Allowances for 2012 Form W-4* worksheet in Pub. 505.)	**5**	$
6	Enter an estimate of your 2012 nonwage income (such as dividends or interest)	**6**	$
7	**Subtract** line 6 from line 5. If zero or less, enter "-0-"	**7**	$
8	**Divide** the amount on line 7 by $3,800 and enter the result here. Drop any fraction	**8**	
9	Enter the number from the **Personal Allowances Worksheet,** line H, page 1	**9**	
10	**Add** lines 8 and 9 and enter the total here. If you plan to use the **Two-Earners/Multiple Jobs Worksheet,** also enter this total on line 1 below. Otherwise, **stop here** and enter this total on Form W-4, line 5, page 1	**10**	

Two-Earners/Multiple Jobs Worksheet (See *Two earners or multiple jobs* on page 1.)

Note. Use this worksheet *only* if the instructions under line H on page 1 direct you here.

1	Enter the number from line H, page 1 (or from line 10 above if you used the **Deductions and Adjustments Worksheet**)	**1**	
2	Find the number in **Table 1** below that applies to the **LOWEST** paying job and enter it here. **However,** if you are married filing jointly and wages from the highest paying job are $65,000 or less, do not enter more than "3"	**2**	
3	If line 1 is **more than or equal to** line 2, subtract line 2 from line 1. Enter the result here (if zero, enter "-0-") and on Form W-4, line 5, page 1. **Do not** use the rest of this worksheet	**3**	

Note. If line 1 is **less than** line 2, enter "-0-" on Form W-4, line 5, page 1. Complete lines 4 through 9 below to figure the additional withholding amount necessary to avoid a year-end tax bill.

4	Enter the number from line 2 of this worksheet	**4**	
5	Enter the number from line 1 of this worksheet	**5**	
6	**Subtract** line 5 from line 4	**6**	
7	Find the amount in **Table 2** below that applies to the **HIGHEST** paying job and enter it here	**7**	$
8	**Multiply** line 7 by line 6 and enter the result here. This is the additional annual withholding needed . .	**8**	$
9	Divide line 8 by the number of pay periods remaining in 2012. For example, divide by 26 if you are paid every two weeks and you complete this form in December 2011. Enter the result here and on Form W-4, line 6, page 1. This is the additional amount to be withheld from each paycheck	**9**	$

Table 1

Married Filing Jointly		All Others	
If wages from **LOWEST** paying job are—	Enter on line 2 above	If wages from **LOWEST** paying job are—	Enter on line 2 above
$0 - $5,000	0	$0 - $8,000	0
5,001 - 12,000	1	8,001 - 15,000	1
12,001 - 22,000	2	15,001 - 25,000	2
22,001 - 25,000	3	25,001 - 30,000	3
25,001 - 30,000	4	30,001 - 40,000	4
30,001 - 40,000	5	40,001 - 50,000	5
40,001 - 48,000	6	50,001 - 65,000	6
48,001 - 55,000	7	65,001 - 80,000	7
55,001 - 65,000	8	80,001 - 95,000	8
65,001 - 72,000	9	95,001 - 120,000	9
72,001 - 85,000	10	120,001 and over	10
85,001 - 97,000	11		
97,001 - 110,000	12		
110,001 - 120,000	13		
120,001 - 135,000	14		
135,001 and over	15		

Table 2

Married Filing Jointly		All Others	
If wages from **HIGHEST** paying job are—	Enter on line 7 above	If wages from **HIGHEST** paying job are—	Enter on line 7 above
$0 - $70,000	$570	$0 - $35,000	$570
70,001 - 125,000	950	35,001 - 90,000	950
125,001 - 190,000	1,060	90,001 - 170,000	1,060
190,001 - 340,000	1,250	170,001 - 375,000	1,250
340,001 and over	1,330	375,001 and over	1,330

FIGURE ■ 12-4 (Continued)

of the number of hours actually worked. For those employees, employers will account for the amount of hours the employee is scheduled to work.

Critical Thinking 12.7 ?

Roy Williams is a salaried employee with a medical organization. He is paid to work 40 hours each week. Roy's schedule fluctuates, depending on his workload. There are some weeks where he works under 40 hours in a week and other weeks when he works over 40 hours. How many hours per week will his employer list for him for the purposes of reporting hours worked for workers' compensation?

Calculating Payroll

time clock
piece of equipment that records employees' arrival and departure times for payroll purposes

Employers uses various ways to track employees' work hours. Some employers use **time clocks** that stamp employees' card at the beginnings and ends of shifts (Figure ■ 12-5). Other employers direct employees to track their hours on timesheets they submit when each pay period ends. Some time clocks offer highly advanced functions such as tracking employees' vacation hours or accounting for the overtime paid in a previous time period. Many of these highly functioning systems have a computerized function that allows both employers and employees to log in and look at hours worked. With these functions, employers are able to manage their employee work hours, including keeping a watchful eye on employees who are approaching overtime or those who are chronically tardy to work.

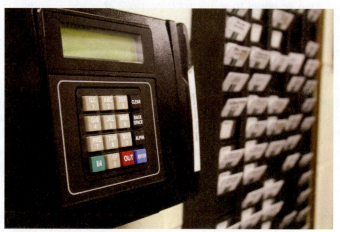

FIGURE ■ 12-5 A time clock.
Source: Cwmgary/Dreamstime.

EMPLOYEES PAID ON AN HOURLY BASIS

The gross earnings of an employee paid hourly are calculated by multiplying the number of regular hours worked by the employee's hourly rate. Any overtime hours are calculated by multiplying the overtime hours worked by 1.5 times the employee's hourly rate. When employees work partial hours, some employers round those hours to the nearest half hour; others round to the nearest quarter hour. Figure ■ 12-6 shows how hourly payroll is calculated.

Jim's regular hourly rate is $15.00, and his regular hours per week are 40. In the past 2-week payroll period, Jim worked 84 hours. To calculate Jim's gross earnings, multiply his regular hours by his hourly wage (80 × $15.00 = $1,200.00). Next, calculate his overtime earnings by calculating his overtime hourly rate (1.5 × $15.00 = $22.50) and then multiply his overtime rate by his overtime hours ($22.50 × 4 = $90.00). Finally, add the amount Jim earned in regular hours with the amount he earned in overtime hours to determine his gross earnings for the payroll period ($1,200.00 + $90.00 = $1,290.00).

FIGURE ■ 12-6 Hourly payroll calculation.

EMPLOYEES PAID ON A SALARIED BASIS

The gross earnings of a salaried employee remain the same each pay period, no matter how many hours are worked, up to 40 hours in 1 week. In general, when salaried employees work more than 40 hours in a week, they must be paid overtime for each hour over 40. Overtime pay is calculated based on an hourly rate, which is calculated by dividing the employee's salaried amount by the number of hours in the pay period. Figure ■ 12-7 explains how salaried payroll is calculated.

Wendy is a salaried employee paid $1,000.00 for each 2-week payroll period. In this pay period, Wendy worked 85 hours. Calculating Wendy's overtime pay entails first determining her normal hourly wage by dividing her $1,000.00 salary by the 80 hours in the 2-week pay period ($1,000.00/80 hours = $12.50 per hour). Next, determine Wendy's overtime rate by multiplying 1.5 by her normal hourly rate (15 × $12.50 = $18.75) and then multiplying that figure by the 5 extra hours she worked during the pay period ($18.75 × 5 hours = $93.75). Finally, add Wendy's base salary to her overtime hours to determine her gross earnings total for the pay period ($1,000.00 + $93.75 = $1093.75).

FIGURE ■ 12-7   Salaried payroll calculation.

Computing Payroll Deductions

Some payroll deductions, like the federal withholding and FICA taxes discussed earlier, are mandated by law. Other deductions, such as benefits for health and life insurance or disability policies, are voluntary. Medical offices should give new employees lists of benefits offered so they can choose to participate if desired. Many organizations pay their employees twice a month, or 26 payroll cycles in a given year. For monthly payroll deductions, such as health insurance, these employers will deduct half of the amount from employees' paychecks for each of the two pay periods each month.

IRS Circular E

When employers calculate payroll manually, medical office managers need an IRS publication called the **Circular E** (Figure ■ 12-8). This publication, revised annually, tells employers how much federal tax to withhold for each employee. Married and single employees appear in separate tables, as do weekly, biweekly, semimonthly, and monthly pay periods. To use the Circular E form properly, medical office managers need employees' completed W-4 forms. Figure ■ 12-9 describes how to use the Circular E tables.

To determine employees' FICA withholding amounts, the medical office manager must first multiply the employees' gross earnings from regular and overtime pay by 6.2 percent for Social Security. Next, the manager must multiply the employees' gross earnings by 1.45 percent for Medicare withholding. When managers work in states with state and local income taxes, they will consult state and local tax tables to determine state and local taxes.

Circular E
yearly booklet published by the IRS that outlines the federal tax

Other Deductions

To determine total deductions from employees' paychecks, amounts for items like workers' compensation insurance, health insurance, retirement plans, and **charitable contributions** must be calculated and added to federal and state or local taxes. Once all deductions have been subtracted, the balance, called the net payroll or "take-home pay," is the amount the employee will receive in a check.

charitable contributions
cash or other donations given to charitable organizations

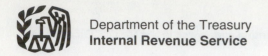

Department of the Treasury
Internal Revenue Service

Publication 15
Cat. No. 10000W

(Circular E), Employer's Tax Guide

For use in **2012**

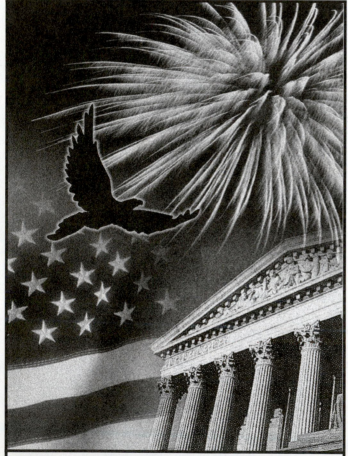

Get forms and other information faster and easier by:

Internet **IRS.gov**

What's New

Future developments. The IRS has created a page on IRS.gov for information about Publication 15 (Circular E), at *www.irs.gov/pub15*. Information about any future developments affecting Publication 15 (Circular E) (such as legislation enacted after we release it) will be posted on that page.

Social security and Medicare tax for 2012. The employee tax rate for social security is 4.2% on wages paid and tips received before March 1, 2012. The employee tax rate for social security increases to 6.2% on wages paid and tips received after February 29, 2012. The employer tax rate for social security remains unchanged at 6.2%. The social security wage base limit is $110,100. The Medicare tax rate is 1.45% each for the employee and employer, unchanged from 2011. There is no wage base limit for Medicare tax.

Employers should implement the 4.2% employee social security tax rate as soon as possible, but not later than

Maria is married and claims four withholding allowances from her payroll. Her gross earnings this biweekly payroll period are $855.00. To determine the federal tax to withhold from Maria's earnings, consult the married persons, biweekly payroll period chart (Figure 12-10). Move down the left column to Maria's wages, and then move across the row to the number for people claiming four exemptions. This amount is the federal tax to withhold from Maria's earnings

MARRIED Persons—WEEKLY Payroll Period
(For Wages Paid through December 2012)

And the wages are—		And the number of withholding allowances claimed is—										
At least	But less than	0	1	2	3	4	5	6	7	8	9	10
		The amount of income tax to be withheld is—										
$800	$810	$81	$70	$59	$48	$37	$28	$21	$14	$6	$0	$0
810	820	82	71	60	49	38	29	22	15	7	0	0
820	830	84	73	62	51	40	30	23	16	8	1	0
830	840	85	74	63	52	41	31	24	17	9	2	0
840	850	87	76	65	54	43	32	25	18	10	3	0
850	860	88	77	66	55	44	33	26	19	11	4	0
860	870	90	79	68	57	46	35	27	20	12	5	0
870	880	91	80	69	58	47	36	28	21	13	6	0
880	890	93	82	71	60	49	38	29	22	14	7	0
890	900	94	83	72	61	50	39	30	23	15	8	1
900	910	96	85	74	63	52	41	31	24	16	9	2
910	920	97	86	75	64	53	42	32	25	17	10	3
920	930	99	88	77	66	55	44	33	26	18	11	4
930	940	100	89	78	67	56	45	34	27	19	12	5
940	950	102	91	80	69	58	47	36	28	20	13	6
950	960	103	92	81	70	59	48	37	29	21	14	7
960	970	105	94	83	72	61	50	39	30	22	15	8
970	980	106	95	84	73	62	51	40	31	23	16	9
980	990	108	97	86	75	64	53	42	32	24	17	10
990	1,000	109	98	87	76	65	54	43	33	25	18	11
1,000	1,010	111	100	89	78	67	56	45	34	26	19	12
1,010	1,020	112	101	90	79	68	57	46	35	27	20	13
1,020	1,030	114	103	92	81	70	59	48	37	28	21	14
1,030	1,040	115	104	93	82	71	60	49	38	29	22	15
1,040	1,050	117	106	95	84	73	62	51	40	30	23	16
1,050	1,060	118	107	96	85	74	63	52	41	31	24	17
1,060	1,070	120	109	98	87	76	65	54	43	32	25	18
1,070	1,080	121	110	99	88	77	66	55	44	33	26	19
1,080	1,090	123	112	101	90	79	68	57	46	35	27	20
1,090	1,100	124	113	102	91	80	69	58	47	36	28	21
1,100	1,110	126	115	104	93	82	71	60	49	38	29	22
1,110	1,120	127	116	105	94	83	72	61	50	39	30	23
1,120	1,130	129	118	107	96	85	74	63	52	41	31	24
1,130	1,140	130	119	108	97	86	75	64	53	42	32	25
1,140	1,150	132	121	110	99	88	77	66	55	44	33	26
1,150	1,160	133	122	111	100	89	78	67	56	45	35	27
1,160	1,170	135	124	113	102	91	80	69	58	47	36	28
1,170	1,180	136	125	114	103	92	81	70	59	48	38	29
1,180	1,190	138	127	116	105	94	83	72	61	50	39	30
1,190	1,200	139	128	117	106	95	84	73	62	51	41	31
1,200	1,210	141	130	119	108	97	86	75	64	53	42	32
1,210	1,220	142	131	120	109	98	87	76	65	54	44	33
1,220	1,230	144	133	122	111	100	89	78	67	56	45	34
1,230	1,240	145	134	123	112	101	90	79	68	57	47	36
1,240	1,250	147	136	125	114	103	92	81	70	59	48	37
1,250	1,260	148	137	126	115	104	93	82	71	60	50	39
1,260	1,270	150	139	128	117	106	95	84	73	62	51	40
1,270	1,280	151	140	129	118	107	96	85	74	63	53	42
1,280	1,290	153	142	131	120	109	98	87	76	65	54	43
1,290	1,300	154	143	132	121	110	99	88	77	66	56	45
1,300	1,310	156	145	134	123	112	101	90	79	68	57	46
1,310	1,320	157	146	135	124	113	102	91	80	69	59	48
1,320	1,330	159	148	137	126	115	104	93	82	71	60	49
1,330	1,340	160	149	138	127	116	105	94	83	72	62	51
1,340	1,350	162	151	140	129	118	107	96	85	74	63	52
1,350	1,360	163	152	141	130	119	108	97	86	75	65	54
1,360	1,370	165	154	143	132	121	110	99	88	77	66	55
1,370	1,380	166	155	144	133	122	111	100	89	78	68	57
1,380	1,390	168	157	146	135	124	113	102	91	80	69	58
1,390	1,400	169	158	147	136	125	114	103	92	81	71	60

$1,400 and over   Use Table 1(b) for a **MARRIED person** on page 36. Also see the instructions on page 35.

FIGURE ■ 12-9 Example of Circular E use.

Using Computer Software to Calculate Payroll

Using a computer software to calculate a payroll is far simpler than calculating it manually. Although payroll software requires employers to set up a file for each new employee, it streamlines the process of entering employees' hours and calculating withholding amounts. Many such software packages also print payroll checks, quarterly payroll tax reports, and W-2 forms.

The W-2 Form

W-2 form
U.S. federal form that annually documents the wages employees drew during the previous year

W-2 forms (Figure ■ 12-10) outline employees' payroll information for the previous year. Because employees need these forms to file their personal taxes, federal law requires employers to send these forms to employees with January 31 postmarks.

22222	Void ☐	**a** Employee's social security number	For Official Use Only ▶ OMB No. 1545-0008	
b Employer identification number (EIN)			**1** Wages, tips, other compensation	**2** Federal income tax withheld
c Employer's name, address, and ZIP code			**3** Social security wages	**4** Social security tax withheld
			5 Medicare wages and tips	**6** Medicare tax withheld
			7 Social security tips	**8** Allocated tips
d Control number			**9**	**10** Dependent care benefits
e Employee's first name and initial	Last name	Suff.	**11** Nonqualified plans	**12a** See instructions for box 12
			13 Statutory employee ☐ Retirement plan ☐ Third-party sick pay ☐	**12b**
			14 Other	**12c**
				12d
f Employee's address and ZIP code				

15 State Employer's state ID number	**16** State wages, tips, etc.	**17** State income tax	**18** Local wages, tips, etc.	**19** Local income tax	**20** Locality name

Form **W-2** Wage and Tax Statement   **2012**

Copy A For Social Security Administration — Send this entire page with Form W-3 to the Social Security Administration; photocopies are **not** acceptable.

Department of the Treasury—Internal Revenue Service
For Privacy Act and Paperwork Reduction Act Notice, see the separate instructions.
Cat. No. 10134D

Do Not Cut, Fold, or Staple Forms on This Page

FIGURE ■ 12-10   W-2 form.

Garnishment of Wages

Employees' wages may be garnished, or taken, for many reasons. Wages may be garnished to repay loans, honor child or spousal support, or pay monetary judgments against employees. Medical office managers who handle payroll must keep accurate records of all garnishment requests, which arise from court orders. These court orders specify the amounts to be taken from employees' gross wages, as well as the parties who are to receive those amounts. Occasionally, a percentage of an employee's gross wages, rather than a set dollar amount, is garnished. Separate checks for the garnished amounts must be sent to whomever is specified on the court orders. Whenever medical office managers mail checks to agencies, insurance carriers, or patients, they should use **security envelopes**, which are nontransparent, to mask the contents. When wages are garnished, corresponding deductions appear on employees' payroll sheets. The employees receive the balance of their wages, less the garnished amount, any other deductions, and taxes.

> **security envelope**
> an envelope that does not allow for the contents to be viewed without opening the envelope

Accounts Payable

The accounts payable function in the medical office is like the financial function most people have in their homes: Bills come in and must be paid. In the medical office, bills may include those for office rent, utilities, insurance, and supplies. Some accounts are paid in single installments, whereas others are paid monthly or on other, similarly regular schedules. The medical office manager in charge of the accounts payable function must determine the accuracy of bills before making payment and keep accurate records of all checks going out.

Several suppliers offer discounts for bills paid by set dates, which are typically 10, 15, or 30 days after the supplies are shipped. Other suppliers offer discounts when supplies are paid by credit card, rather than by invoice. To take advantage of such discounts, medical office managers should research suppliers' and vendors' policies, especially before making a large purchase for the medical office.

The Checkbook Register

Whether medical offices keep their checkbook registers electronically or in handwritten form, those registers must be accurate and clear as to payment purpose and receiver. Clarity, like the availability of the information, is especially important when the IRS conducts audits. To ensure clarity, checkbook registers should have columns with labels such as "Utilities," "Payroll," and "Supplies." Categorized expenditures help the medical office manager track payments. Figure ■ 12-11 lists some common expenditure categories found in the medical office.

- Rent—rental fee for office space
- Utilities—cost for electric, telephone, Internet, and gas services
- Payroll—wages paid to employees
- Taxes—monies paid to city, state, or federal agencies
- Office supplies—costs of items such as pens, paper, and envelopes
- Clinical supplies—cost of items for clinical activities such as gowns, syringes, and lab supplies
- Maintenance—costs for repairs or cleaning staff and equipment maintenance and upkeep
- Continuing education—tuition payments for physicians and staff to attend professional classes
- Insurance—cost of liability insurance for the office
- Travel—expenses for office-related travel such as travel to a seminar
- Marketing—price of office advertising

FIGURE ■ 12-11   Expenditure categories found in the medical office.

Preparing a Deposit Slip

At the end of each business day, medical offices should make a deposit of their daily receipts (Figure ■ 12-12). Such deposits include cash and personal checks collected from patients, usually for copays, and insurance and patient payments received in the mail. Patients may sometimes pay for their care via traveler's checks, which are purchased while traveling as a safe alternative to cash. These are deposited with the daily receipts. Computerized offices can print their days' collections via the medical office software. Such reports, which detail the day's receipts, should cross-check against the money to be deposited. In offices using a manual system for accounting, such as a pegboard, staff must total the payment columns and match that to the amount to be deposited.

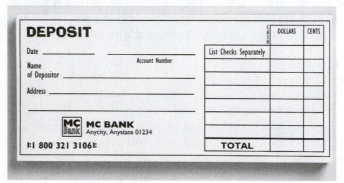

FIGURE ■ 12-12 Sample deposit slip.

The receptionists are often responsible for totaling the receipts they have personally collected at the end of each day. This collection is then given to the medical office manager for deposit to the bank. The medical office manager must ensure that the amounts the computers, pegboards, or receptionists indicate as their daily collections match the deposit amount. When these figures fail to match, managers must then search for and correct the errors. Only when the figures match may the deposit slip be prepared.

ENDORSEMENT STAMPS

endorsement stamp
a method of endorsing a check so that the office's name and account number and the bank's name are listed on the back

Medical offices use **endorsement stamps** to endorse the backs of all checks received (Figure ■ 12-13). Such a stamp lists the office's name and bank account number and the bank's name. The phrase "For Deposit Only" should also appear on these stamps. Checks stamped in this manner are difficult to cash by unauthorized parties. The "For Deposit Only" stamp is known as a *restrictive endorsement*. In offices with more than one receptionist checking in patients and collecting payments at the front desk, each station should have an endorsement stamp so that checks received can be immediately stamped upon receipt.

Any documents that contain patient information, including personal checks, are considered confidential. As a result, documents like these must be kept out of the view of other patients or staff who do not have the authority to access confidential patient information.

Online Banking

Most banks now allow users to access their bank accounts and complete banking functions, such as bill paying, via the Internet. These services are convenient, because they are available 24 hours a day, 7 days a week, 365 days a year. Medical offices may receive such payments from patients' banks via the mail. Medical office managers should post these payments after noting the patient account or identification numbers, just as they would post a conventional hardcopy check.

The medical office may use online banking for payment of its own accounts payable. With this system, payments are entered via the office's online bank and a statement of account may be printed for verification. Payment of accounts in this manner saves both time and the cost of postage. By using this system for payment of accounts, the medical office manager can

ENDORSE CHECK HERE

X

For Deposit Only
Sound View Medical Center
US Bank
03726457809

DO NOT WRITE, STAMP, OR SIGN BELOW THIS LINE

FIGURE ■ 12-13 Sample endorsed check.

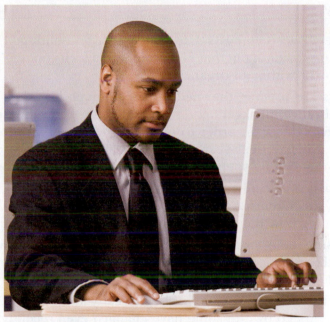

FIGURE ■ 12-14 The medical office manager uses online banking for payment of the office's accounts payable.
Source: AVAVA/Fotolia.com.

choose the date he wishes a particular vendor or supplier to be paid via online payment (Figure ■ 12-14). The date chosen may coincide with a discount offered by the vendor.

Reconciling the Bank Statement

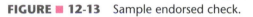

Medical office managers are often responsible for reconciling the medical office's bank statements. Online banking is also a convenient option for this task because it allows the manager to view the office's banking activities in real time. Office managers do not need to wait for statements to arrive or call banks with payment or deposit questions when they are using online banking.

The reconciliation of a medical office's bank statement resembles the reconciliation of a personal bank statement. Once the office's bank statement arrives from the bank, the medical office manager must check off the office's checkbook register the checks and deposits listed as processed on the statement. Next, the manager should add the end-of-month balance on the statement to any outstanding deposits in the office's checkbook register. From that number, any outstanding checks or automatic payments should be deducted. The resulting number should match the amount in the office's checkbook register.

Case Study Questions

Refer to the case study presented at the beginning of this chapter to answer the following questions:

1. How should Barb begin her investigation into the profitability of the proposed flu shot clinic?
2. What information will Barb need to gather?

Chapter Review

Summary

- Managerial accounting is also called cost accounting. This function differs from financial accounting in that it is designed to focus on one organization, or even one department within an organization.

- Budgets are used in the medical office much like they are used in households. Medical office managers review the amount of revenue produced by the practice the previous year in order to make a determination as to the amount of revenue expected in the next year. After that, the manager will determine the amount of money that can be spent in the medical office for all expenses incurred.

- Petty cash is a small amount of money kept in the medical office to pay for unexpected, small items. A journal or log must be kept, along with receipts, in order to account for how the money was spent.

- Processing the payroll is a task that often falls to the medical office manager. Other times, this function is outsourced to another company, or it may be handled by a separate department in the medical organization.

- Payroll taxes have a history that begins early in the 20th century. Laws have changed as the years go by and some have changed even recently.

- Payroll functions are governed by both state and federal laws, so the medical office manager should be familiar with these laws.

- Workers' compensation laws dictate that all employers must purchase coverage for employees in the event the employee becomes injured in the course of employment. This coverage allows injured workers to seek medical care, to be paid for time lost from work, and to be retrained if they can no longer perform their former job.

- Every employee in an organization must have a personnel file. This file contains documents, such as a copy of the Social Security card, that are used as proof of citizenship, as well as the original job application, résumé, credentials, licensing and insurance information, references, federal withholding requests, dates and copies of performance evaluations, and any information about disciplinary actions.

- Employee records must be updated as needed, especially for items that expire, such as certifications.

- All information in the employee record must be kept confidential, including the employee's rate of pay. This confidentiality is outlined in HIPAA legislation.

- The W-4 form outlines the employees' deductions for payroll tax purposes. Employees may update this form as often as they like, though the changes may not take effect immediately.

- Employers must keep an accounting of the number of hours employees work. This is directly related to the premiums employers will pay for workers' compensation insurance coverage.

- Employees who are paid on an hourly basis are paid a certain wage for each hour worked. Employees paid on a salaried basis are paid a set amount each pay period, no matter how many hours they have worked. For all employees, a rate of 1.5 times the hourly wage must be paid if the employee works beyond 40 hours in a week.

- Payroll deductions are taken out of each paycheck an employee receives. Mandatory payroll deductions include payroll taxes, such as Medicare, Social Security, and federal withholding taxes.

- The IRS Circular E form lists the amount of federal withholding tax the employer must withhold from an employee's paycheck. This amount is based on the amount of the wage, the marital status of the employee, and the number of exemptions the employee has claimed.

- Many medical offices use computer software to assist in the payroll function. This software allows employers to manage the payroll function in a quicker, more efficient manner.

- The W-2 form is created once each year and sent to every employee on or before January 31. This form includes the employee's total amounts paid in wages, as well as all deductions, for the preceding year. Employees need this form to file their state and federal income tax returns.

- Employees who have had court orders issued against them for outstanding monies owed to another may have their wages garnished. When this happens, the medical office manager will receive a copy of the court order indicating the amount to withhold from the employee's check and where to send that amount each pay period. Employers are governed by law in cases of garnished wages and must comply when a court order is received.

- The accounts payable are those monies that are owed to others. The medical office interacts with a variety of businesses as it pays for services and supplies. It also has regular, ongoing accounts payable for items such as rent and utilities.

- The checkbook register is usually managed by the medical office manager. Similar to a personal checkbook register, the medical office register must be balanced as deposits and payments are registered.

- Preparation of deposit slips is done at the end of each business day. Receptionists are often responsible for itemizing and totaling their receipts from the day. Then the office manager adds in receipts received via the mail and completes a daily deposit slip.

- Online banking is a function used by many medical offices. This service allows the medical office manager to pay for items online, saving time and the cost of postage.

- The medical office bank statement must be balanced monthly in order to determine if all expenses and deposits have been properly accounted for.

Multiple Choice

Choose the letter that best answers each question or completes each statement.

1. The IRS Circular E is used to:
   a. determine the correct hourly wage for an employee.
   b. give the employee an accounting of wages and withholdings from the previous year.
   c. locate the amount of federal withholding tax to withhold from an employee's paycheck.
   d. determine the number of exemptions the employee is claiming.

2. The W-4 form is used to:
   a. determine the correct hourly wage for an employee.
   b. give the employee an accounting of wages and withholdings from the previous year.
   c. locate the amount of federal withholding tax to withhold from an employee's paycheck.
   d. determine the number of exemptions the employee is claiming.

3. The W-2 form is used to:
   a. determine the correct hourly wage for an employee.
   b. give the employee an accounting of wages and with-holdings from the previous year.
   c. locate the amount of federal withholding tax to with-hold from an employee's paycheck.
   d. determine the number of exemptions the employee is claiming.

4. Martin Holden receives a paycheck for the same amount of money every 2 weeks. There is no variation in the amount he receives. What type of employee is Martin?
   a. An employee paid on an hourly basis
   b. An employee being paid for overtime
   c. An employee who is off work due to a workers' compensation claim
   d. An employee paid on a salaried basis

5. Penny Chi has been sued for outstanding child support. A court order demanding that her employer hold back $250 out of every pay period has been received by Penny's employer. What is this situation called?
   a. Garnishment of wages
   b. Withholding taxes
   c. Prepayment penalty
   d. None of the above

6. To be in compliance with _____, employers must keep an accounting of employee hours worked.
   a. HIPAA
   b. OSHA
   c. FLSA
   d. FDA

7. A _____ cost is one that remains the same no matter how many services are used or produced.
   a. withholding
   b. tax
   c. fixed
   d. variable

8. The federal income tax program began in:
   a. 1903.
   b. 1913.
   c. 1923.
   d. 1933.

9. As of 2009, the federal minimum wage was:
   a. $5.25.
   b. $6.25.
   c. $7.25.
   d. $8.25.

10. Which of the following is a reason an employer needs to keep a copy of an employee's disciplinary actions in the employee's file?
   a. To defend against a claim of wrongful termination
   b. To provide to the employee upon discharge
   c. To provide to the IRS for filing with the employee's federal income tax
   d. To defend against a claim involving a HIPAA violation

True/False

Determine if each of the following statements is true or false.

_____ 1. All employers must offer workers' compensation insurance.

_____ 2. Employees do not have the right to view their own personnel file.

_____ 3. Salaried employees are never paid overtime wages.

_____ 4. The amount paid for overtime wages is decided by each individual employer.

_____ 5. Workers' compensation claims may be filed for injuries caused by repetitive stress in the workplace.

_____ 6. IRS auditors are responsible for giving taxpayers federal tax advice.

_____ 7. Variable costs are costs that vary with the number of services used or produced.

_____ 8. Salaried employees are those who punch a time clock to record their hours worked.

_____ 9. Managerial accounting is another term for financial accounting.

_____ 10. Medical office managers are often given the task of preparing the payroll in the medical office.

Matching

Match each of the following terms with its definition.

a. Circular E

b. deductions

c. Fair Labor Standards Act (FLSA)

d. charitable contributions

e. budget

f. Federal Insurance Contributions Act (FICA)

g. products

h. petty cash

i. Federal Unemployment Tax Act (FUTA)

j. quarterly payroll reports

1. A list of planned expenses and revenues

2. Documents that specify the taxes withheld from wages quarterly

3. Yearly booklet published by the IRS that outlines the federal tax

4. Cash or other donations given to charitable organizations

5. Law that addresses Social Security withholding taxes

6. Number of allowances to be withheld from wages

7. Law passed by U.S. Congress in 1938 to address employment issues such as the federal minimum wage

8. A small amount of money kept in the medical office to pay for unexpected items

9. Law that addresses federal unemployment tax withholdings

10. Supplies that the physician prescribes to the patient, such as a splint or crutches

Chapter Resources

Internal Revenue Service: www.irs.gov

Johnson, H. T., & Kaplan, R. S. (1987). *Relevance lost: The rise and fall of management accounting.* Boston, MA: Harvard Business School Press.

Social Security Administration: www.ssa.gov

PEARSON myhealthprofessionskit

Additional interactive resources for this chapter can be found at **www.myhealthprofessionskit. com.** Choose "Medical Assisting" from the discipline menu and then click on the book cover for *Medical Office Management.*

CHAPTER 13

Billing and Collections

CHAPTER OUTLINE

LEARNING OBJECTIVES

Upon completion of this chapter, you should be able to:

- Spell and define the key terms in this chapter.
- Understand how a fee schedule is created.
- Understand how to analyze a participating provider agreement.
- Describe credit and collection policies to patients prior to rendering services.
- Understand how preprinted brochures are used in the medical office.
- Describe how the medical office works to collect from patients.
- Understand how patient identification is verified.
- List the tasks involved in managing the accounts receivable.
- Describe the use of collection policies when working with managed care.
- List the types of payments received in the medical office.
- Understand how professional courtesies are used in the medical office.
- Describe the steps in creating patient billing statements.

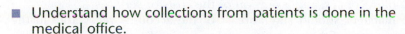

- Understand how collections from patients is done in the medical office.
- List the steps necessary for dismissing a patient from care due to nonpayment of a medical bill.
- Understand the legalities of charging interest on medical accounts.
- Describe how to handle the situation when the patient's check is returned by the bank.
- List the steps for collecting from the patient who does not pay his or her bill.
- Understand how collection agencies are used.
- Define uncollectible accounts.
- Describe the steps to take in collecting payment from a patient's estate.
- Understand the types of bankruptcy and how they apply to medical bills.
- Process overpayments on accounts.
- File a claim in small claims court.

KEY TERMS

accounts receivable (AR)
aging report
certified letter
collection agency
community property laws
Fair Debt Collection Practices Act
fee schedule

geographical practice cost index (GPCI)
hardship agreement
insurance fraud
national conversion factor
national standard
Omnibus Budget Reconciliation Act (OBRA)

patient billing statement
professional courtesy
relative value unit (RVU)
tickler file
uncollectible account
write off

Case Study

Take note of the following scenario and answer the case study questions that appear at the end of this chapter.

Molly Garrison was recently hired as the medical office manager for Wayside Family Practice. As she is going through overdue patient accounts, Molly sees that there are several outstanding accounts that have not had any payments made on them in months.

Introduction

In today's healthcare setting, the vast majority of patients do not pay for their care in full at the time of service. Many patients have health insurance carriers who will pay a portion of their bills, but the patients are responsible for the rest. Most patients will be expected to pay deductibles, copays, and a portion of the costs of services.

The medical office manager should stay abreast of the accounts receivable in the medical office. The management of the amounts owed to the medical office is vital to the practice maintaining a steady cash flow for services rendered.

Fee Schedules

Omnibus Budget Reconciliation Act (OBRA)
legislation passed by Congress in 1993 to calculate healthcare service fees by formula

fee schedule
list of services and their fees

national standard
point of reference for developing charges for healthcare services used throughout the United States

In 1993, U.S. Congress passed the **Omnibus Budget Reconciliation Act (OBRA)** in part to require that physician reimbursement for Medicare services be based on a **fee schedule** (Figure ■ 13-1). Fee schedules set maximum amounts for services using the resource-based relative value scale (RBRVS), which is designed to reduce Medicare costs and establish a **national standard** for physician payment. This national standard is itself based on the Current Procedural Terminology (CPT) codes used for patient visits.

AUDIOLOGY SERVICES		
Screening audio air only	92551	$ 38.00
Pure tone air	92552	$ 37.00
Pure tone air and bone	92553	$ 50.00
Comprehensive audio	92557	$101.00
Loudness balance test	92562	$ 38.00
Tone decay	92563	$ 41.00
Tympanography	92567	$ 40.00
Acoustic reflex	92568	$ 42.00
Reflex decay	92569	$ 43.00
Visual reinforced audio	92579	$ 78.00
Brain stem audiogram	92585	$327.00

FIGURE ■ **13-1** Sample fee schedule.

Medicare service fees are calculated based on the five following factors:

- Service intensity
- Time needed for the service
- Skills needed to perform the service
- Practice's overhead
- Practice's malpractice premiums.

geographical practice cost index (GPCI)
Medicare system of adjusting fees based on the county in which the healthcare provider practices

relative value unit (RVU)
numeric value assigned by Medicare to formulate fee schedules for healthcare providers

Physicians' fees are adjusted according to a **geographical practice cost index (GPCI)**, which factors in the differing healthcare costs across the United States. Together, these factors determine a healthcare provider's **relative value unit (RVU)**. The RVU was devised by the Centers for Medicare and Medicaid Services (CMS) as a way for physicians to create a fee schedule for the services they render. RVUs take into account three factors: how much work by the physician is involved in performing the service, the type of expertise the physician needs to have to perform the service, and the cost of the physician's malpractice insurance policy.

Each year, Medicare assigns a **national conversion factor** that is added to the RVU. The national conversion factor is a number released by Medicare each year that determines fee schedules for all healthcare services. The national conversion factor is multiplied by the physician's RVU for any given service or procedure to determine the allowed fee for that service. For example, imagine CPT code 99205 has an RVU of 4.78 for a healthcare provider practicing in the Los Angeles area, and the national conversion factor is 37.5623. This would make the Medicare-allowed charge for this service $179.55 (4.78 × 37.5623 = $179.55). Because most health insurance plans base their fee schedules on the Medicare fee schedule, the Medicare allowed charge is typically considered the maximum charge any insurance plan will allow for any given service or procedure.

> **national conversion factor**
> number released by Medicare each year that determines fee schedules for all healthcare services

Participating Provider Agreements

Most patients with private health insurance are covered by managed care plans. As a condition of participation, managed care plans credential healthcare providers and require those providers to apply. When providers agree to participate in managed care plans, they agree to accept predetermined fee schedules. Some managed care plans also dictate the type of medications providers can prescribe and the types of specialist referrals those providers are allowed to make.

Participating provider agreements range from several pages long to small-book size. Though it may be time consuming, physicians and their medical office managers should read their agreements in full. Once providers have signed with plans, they are obligated to see patients with that coverage for the agreed-on fees, which may be lower than providers are willing to accept; hence, the need to understand the managed care agreement in full.

The best way to review participating provider agreements is with a highlighter. Medical office managers should highlight all areas of interest or concern, especially any details about fee schedules or provider care restrictions, and then review the highlighted areas with the physicians. Objections to any item may be grounds for declining plan participation.

Critical Thinking 13.1 ?

What kind of problems do you think might arise if the physician signs a managed care contract without reading all of the language? If you were working with a physician who told you she did not see any reason for reading the contract before signing, how might you explain the importance of reviewing the contract?

Credit and Collections

The best way to ensure patients pay their bills properly is to discuss the medical office's credit and collection policies before services are rendered. Medical office managers should discuss all fees and outline all payment policies. When patients arrange to make regular payments on their balances, for example, managers should provide written contracts that stipulate the payment amounts and due dates (Figure ■ 13-2). Such contracts avoid confusion and reduce or eliminate patient questions. Patients who clearly understand fees for physician services are better equipped to make healthcare choices and to understand their bills. When a patient does not understand the fees they incur in the medical facility, this confusion can lead to nonpayment of a bill.

Critical Thinking 13.2 ?

Why do you think it is important to have a written contract that outlines a patient's agreement regarding payments? How might this benefit the patient? How might it benefit the medical office?

May 21, 2013

I, [patient's name], agree to pay Monroe Family Practice $100 every 2 weeks until my $800 balance is paid in full. I understand that finance charges will not accrue while I am making these payments and that if I stop making payments before my balance is paid in full finance charges will begin to accrue on the remaining balance.

Patient Signature   Date

_____

Witness Signature   Date

_____

FIGURE ■ 13-2   Sample payment contract.

Using Preprinted Brochures

To further help ensure that payment terms are clear, many medical offices include important financial information in their office brochures and send these brochures, along with registration paperwork and fee and credit policies, before patients arrive for their first visits. Table ■ 13-1 identifies some items that should be included in introductory brochures. Ensuring that patients are well informed helps avoid collection problems. Copayments, for example, should be paid at visit check in.

TABLE ■ 13-1   Payment Policies in an Office Brochure

- Requirement for payment at the time of service, if any
- Allowable time frame for payment (e.g., "within 30 days")
- Guidelines for insurance claim submission on patients' behalf
- Time the medical office will carry an outstanding balance
- Credit limit extended to patients
- Percentage of finance charges that will accrue on a balance and when charges start accruing (e.g., after 30 days, after 60 days)
- Point at which accounts are turned over to collection agencies
- Process for assigning benefits to the provider

Collecting from Patients

Medical offices should request certain pieces of information on their patient registration forms to make tracking patients, and therefore debt collection, easier. For example, offices should request patients' employers' names and telephone numbers, as well as the names and numbers of emergency contacts who do not live with the patients. Emergency contact information helps provide options when patients' accounts become past due and medical office managers cannot reach patients at home.

Each state has a statute of limitations that sets the maximum time in which healthcare providers can collect patient debts. Because Medicare and many managed care insurance companies prohibit providers from billing patients until insurance companies have issued explanations of benefits outlining the amounts patients owe, it is crucial to bill insurance providers soon after the service is provided so that the patient portion can be billed in a timely manner. Table ■ 13-2 outlines the number of years from the patient's last date of service or last billing statement that a healthcare provider may send a bill to a patient.

TABLE ■ 13-2 Statutes of Limitations on Healthcare Debts

State	Number of Years	State	Number of Years
AL	6	MT	8
AK	6	NE	5
AZ	6	NV	6
AR	5	NH	3
CA	4	NJ	6
CO	6	NM	6
CT	6	NY	6
DE	3	NC	3
D.C.	3	ND	6
FL	5	OH	15
GA	6	OK	5
HI	6	OR	6
ID	5	PA	6
IL	10	RI	15
IN	10	SC	10
IA	10	SD	6
KS	5	TN	6
KY	15	TX	4
LA	10	UT	6
ME	6	VT	6
MD	3	VA	5
MA	6	WA	6
MI	6	WV	10
MN	6	WI	6
MS	3	WY	10
MO	10		

SELECTING A CREDIT LIMIT TO EXTEND TO PATIENTS

In terms of credit, medical offices should predetermine the amounts they are willing to extend to patients, document those amounts in policies, and apply the policies equitably. The amount of credit the medical office wishes to extend will vary from one office to the next. The important thing to keep in mind is that the amount must be the same for all patients; the medical provider or manager may not deem one patient worthy of a higher credit amount than others. This would be a violation of the Fair Debt Collection Practices Act.

Critical Thinking 13.4 ?

What factors do you think a physician and medical office manager may want to consider before determining an amount to extend for credit? What problems might they incur if they set that number too low? What problems might occur if they set that number too high?

Verifying Patient Identification

In 2008, The Federal Trade Commission (FTC) passed the Red Flags rule (see Chapter 8). The purpose of this legislation is to reduce fraud and identity theft. The Red Flags rule applies to any business or entity that extends credit. Healthcare offices that allow patients to be seen for care, without requiring payment in full for services at the time of service, are extending credit and must therefore abide by the Red Flags rule. In essence, this legislation requires the medical office to have a written program in place to verify patient identity, before extending credit. The easiest way to accomplish this is to require patients to show photo identification when they check in at the medical office.

When new patients visit the medical office, receptionists must copy those patients' driver's licenses and insurance cards, front and back (Figure ■ 13-3). Such documentation confirms patients' identities and can help the medical office manager track patients for collection purposes.

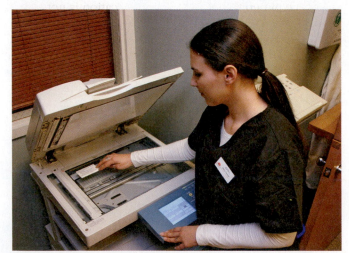

FIGURE ■ 13-3 The receptionist should make a copy of both sides of the patient's insurance card.
Source: Dylan Malone/Pearson Education.

Critical Thinking 13.5 ?

What problems might the medical office experience if a patient is using another person's identity?

Managing the Accounts Receivable

Any successful medical office must manage its **accounts receivable (AR)**, which is the money owed the office from all sources, including patients, insurance companies, workers' compensation, Medicare, and Medicaid. AR management, which entails documenting how much money is owed the office, by whom, and for how long, is a weighty task and so must be done regularly and thoroughly.

accounts receivable (AR)
money owed the medical practice

With the decline of manual billing systems in the medical office, computerized systems have become the norm. Although computerized systems vary, most allow the medical office manager to:

- Post charges and payments to patient accounts
- Print insurance billing forms and patient billing forms
- Create **aging reports** (documentation of the money owed the medical office and how long the account has been outstanding) that detail the amounts owed by patients.

aging report
documentation of the money owed the medical office and how long accounts have been outstanding

Most medical billing programs offer a wide variety of reports. Such reports can list information like all patients with birthdays in any given month or all female patients over age 40 who have not had mammograms in the past year.

Billing systems with basic features like reports are affordable for most medical offices. Higher-level features increase the price of a system. Some systems, for example, offer integrated electronic appointment books. Others send insurance claims electronically and receive insurance payments electronically. Some systems even allow remote access, which means healthcare team members can access their billing system when out of the office.

To ensure that the office receives the software package it needs, the office manager should research a number of options. Online, the website www.2020software.com lists the most popular medical billing programs on the market and allows users to order demo CDs of programs at no charge.

The aging reports mentioned earlier are important to AR management for a number of reasons. When physicians wish to take business loans, for example, banks will request documentation on AR accounts. Some malpractice insurance companies examine physicians' AR before extending policies. Physicians with high or old AR are considered greater risks to insure.

The most effective way to collect money on past due accounts is to speak with patients while they are in the office. When face-to-face communication is not possible, the next most effective method is calling patients, but from private office locations to safeguard patient confidentiality. Medical office managers making such calls must pay strict attention to the law regarding collections and document all calls and conversations, as well as any patient messages, in patients' financial records. Table ■ 13-3 outlines procedures for telephone

TABLE ■ 13-3 Dos and Don'ts for Collection Telephone Calls

Do	Don't
Call the patient from a private location in the medical office.	Call the patient from a location where other patients can hear.
Call the patient between 8 a.m. and 9 p.m.	Call the patient if the patient asks not to be called.
Verify the patient's identity.	Speak with anyone except the patient or the patient's parent or guardian about the patient's bill.
Be respectful, polite, and professional.	Call repeatedly if the patient fails to answer or return messages.
Tell the patient the reason for the call.	Become angry if the emotion arises.
Keep the conversation short and to the point.	Make promises that cannot be kept, such as reducing the bill.
Document any promises the patient makes.	Converse about topics other than the subject of the call.
Follow up on any of the patient's promises.	Neglect to document all parts of the conversation with the patient.

Source: Malone, Christine, *Administrative Medical Assisting: Foundations and Practices, 1st Ed.,* © 2010. Reprinted and electronically reproduced by permission of Pearson Education, Inc., Upper Saddle River, NJ.

collection calls. When calling patients regarding past due bills, the medical office manager should offer the option of payment via credit card while the patient is on the telephone.

Collection Policies and Working with Managed Care

Some medical offices collect entire visit fees from patients the first time they are seen in the office for care, but this practice is not common. Some managed care plans strictly govern how much money, if any, providers may collect from patients at the time care is rendered. When offices participate with Medicare, for example, providers are not allowed to charge patients for covered services at the time of service. Instead, those providers must bill Medicare and then bill the patients for the portions Medicare states those patients owe.

When speaking with patients about fees or payments, it is important to remember that people tend to associate payment with value. When medical office managers act embarrassed about fees, or fail to ask for payment, they give the impression that the physician's services lack value.

insurance fraud
illegal act by a healthcare provider involving an insurance company

hardship agreement
agreement a patient signs to indicate an inability to pay full healthcare costs due to financial hardship

FORGIVING DEDUCTIBLES OR COPAYMENTS

It is illegal, and is in fact considered **insurance fraud**, for healthcare providers to forgive patients' deductibles or copayments. When patients cannot pay their bills and physicians agree to treat them for lesser or no fees, those patients must sign and date **hardship agreement** letters for their file (Figure ■ 13-4). Hardship letters become part of patients' permanent medical records. Having a hardship letter on file allows providers to treat patients for reduced fees.

I am receiving treatment with Dr. Josephine Smith. Due to my financial hardship, Dr. Smith is giving me a discount for her services. I understand that the fee I am receiving is not Dr. Smith's conventional charges for these services.

Patient Signature   Date

_____ _____

FIGURE ■ 13-4 Sample hardship agreement.

Types of Payments

Patients typically make three types of payment in the medical office: (1) cash, (2) check, and (3) debit or credit card. With cash payments, receptionists should write receipts to document the transaction both for the patient and the office. Receipts also help discourage stealing. With a paper trail, medical office managers can easily track all office cash.

When a patient offers a personal check as payment, receptionists must verify that the spelled-out amount of the check matches the check's numeral amount. Receptionists must also ensure that checks are dated and signed. When a receptionist takes a check from a party other than a patient, the receptionist should request the check writer's photo identification to verify the writer's identity. When checks are suspicious or for large amounts, receptionists should call the issuing banks to ensure funds are available. When checks are marked "Payment in Full," receptionists must verify that the checks are in the amounts patients owe. If they are not, patients may later argue that no additional payment is required.

Some offices use check-verification systems that, although costly, guarantee checks. Some of these systems simply check to see if patients have written bad checks. Others are more sophisticated, holding patients' bank funds until checks clear. As such systems become more sophisticated, however, their costs increase.

For the third payment type, debit or credit cards, providers pay bank fees in the amount of 1 to 3 percent of charges, depending on the providers' credit card use.

Offering a Professional Courtesy

Physicians who treat other physicians for free or at greatly reduced fees extend what is called **professional courtesy**. Such courtesy is also extended to family or friends of the physician, to the family of other physicians, or even to such professional associates as the physician's attorney or accountant. Even if the physician is treating the patient at no charge, a complete patient medical record must be kept in the medical office for that patient.

In cases of professional courtesy, accurate patient charts are vital to avoid the appearance of fraud or impropriety. Medical office managers should have any patients in these situations sign professional courtesy agreements, such as "I understand Dr. Jones is giving me a professional courtesy discount for services rendered."

Medicare prohibits physicians from billing for the treatment they provide their relatives or household members. Immediate relatives include the physician's spouse, parent, children, siblings, grandparents, grandchildren, stepparents, stepsisters, stepbrothers, and stepchildren. Household members include anyone living in the same home as the physician, like a nanny, maid, butler, chauffer, medical caregiver, or assistant. Boarders, people who rent rooms from physicians, are not considered household members.

professional courtesy
a discount offered to friends, colleagues, and family members of the physician

Patient Billing Statements

patient billing statement

monthly statement sent to patients who have outstanding balances

Medical offices should set aside a day each month to send **patient billing statements** to patients with balances due (Figure ■ 13-5), preferably after the first of the month when rent and mortgages are typically due. Patient billing statements that arrive mid- to late month are more likely to be paid in a timely fashion.

Heritage Park Women's Clinic
14 Heritage Way
Heritage Park, IN 12345

STATEMENT

CLOSING DATE	PREVIOUS BALANCE	BALANCE DUE
10/2/13	0	20.00

NOTE: ALL PAYMENTS AND CHARGES POSTED AFTER THE ABOVE CLOSING DATE WILL APPEAR ON THE NEXT STATEMENT.

AMOUNT PAID $ _____

BANKCARD PAYMENT AUTHORIZATION	☐ VISA	☐ M/C
VISA M/C ACCOUNT NUMBER		
CARDHOLDER SIGNATURE		EXP. DATE

Lillian Vidali
2715-16th Drive SW
Heritage Park, IN 12345

PLEASE DETACH AND **RETURN** THIS STUB WITH YOUR PAYMENT TO INSURE PROPER CREDIT

RETAIN THIS PORTION FOR YOUR RECORDS.

DATE OF SERVICE	DOCTOR / CPT CODE	DESCRIPTION	CHARGES	CREDITS
9/7/13	Wilson/99211	Office Visit	62.00	
9/20/13	Wilson	Insurance payment 9/7/13		42.00

PAST DUE				CURRENT		BALANCE DUE
0	0	0	0	20.00	▶	20.00
OVER 120 DAYS	OVER 90 DAYS	OVER 60 DAYS	OVER 30 DAYS	0 - 30 DAYS		

COMMENTS: Payment due by 11/10/13

FIGURE ■ **13-5** Sample patient billing statement.

Nearly every medical office sends monthly billing statements to patients with outstanding balances. These billing statements must be Health Insurance Portability and Accountability Act (HIPAA) compliant and sent on or near the same day each month.

In order to be HIPAA compliant, the statement must be sent in a security envelope (one that does not allow for the contents to be viewed without opening the envelope).

Although patient billing statements are one means of securing patients' payment, collecting any payment due at the time of an office visit is far more cost effective. Monthly billing statements have been shown to cost about $8 per month per bill. To provide an incentive to pay, healthcare providers can offer discounts, called *cash discounts*, to patients who pay their bills in full. However, to avoid being considered a form of fraud, such discounts should not exceed 5 percent of total fees. Billing statements should offer patients the option of supplying credit card information for payment of their bill. Many medical offices today include a payment feature on the clinic website, allowing patients to pay their bill online via credit card or direct transfer from their bank account.

Collecting from the Patient in the Office

Asking patients to pay while they are in the office is the most effective way to collect payment. When patients with past due accounts are due in for appointments, medical office managers should ask the receptionist to see those patients before those patients receive treatment. In private areas out of other patients' hearing range, the managers can then remind the patients of their balances due. When patients cannot provide payment in full, the managers should make other arrangements (Figure ■ 13-6). Those arrangements should always include a commitment from the patient to the amount of payment and a date by which the patient will make that payment. After the conversation, the medical office manager should ask the patient to sign a contract that outlines the agreement made.

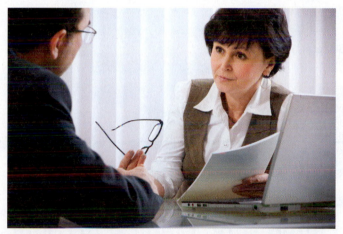

FIGURE ■ 13-6   When patients cannot provide payment in full, the manager should make other arrangements with the patient.
Source: Alexraths/Dreamstime.com.

Dismissing a Patient from Care due to Nonpayment of a Bill

When patients are chronically late with payments or refuse to pay at all, providers can dismiss those patients from care via **certified letter**. Figure ■ 13-7 provides an example of a dismissal letter to a patient. Providers must give patients at least 30 days to receive care, but after that period providers are no longer bound to provide treatment. Physicians who do not honor this commitment may be sued for patient abandonment. Patients should be dismissed only after physicians' have given their consent and signed receipts verifying that patients received their certified letters have been filed in those patients' permanent medical records.

certified letter
postal service letter that the recipient must sign for

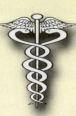

Marian Williams, MD
Markson Family Practice
2323 Front Street
Yonkers, NY 12345

Joseph Paterniti
41 Bronxville Ave
Yonkers, NY 12345

January 31, 2013

Dear Mr. Paterniti:

Our office has tried several times to contact you regarding
your outstanding balance with us. Because we have failed to
reach you, I must dismiss you as a patient. Please find a new
physician and notify this office within 30 days if you would
like your medical records transferred. If you need care within
the next 30 days, you may still patronize this office. After 30
days, you will be disallowed from making another appointment with us.

Sincerely,

Marian Williams, MD

FIGURE ■ 13-7   Sample dismissal letter.

Charging Interest on Medical Accounts

Medical providers who wish to charge interest on past due balances must be sure to
check the laws in their states. Any changes in financial policy, including the decision to
charge interest on accounts, requires providers to post written notices in prominent office
locations at least 30 days before the financial changes occur.

It is important to note that those bills patients receive that are accruing interest will
typically be paid before those bills that are not accruing interest. To be paid in a timely
manner, it is advisable for the medical office to charge interest on outstanding accounts.

When a Patient's Check is Returned by the Bank

When patients write nonsufficient funds (NSF) checks that "bounce," most banks charge
the medical office a fee. An NSF check is one that is written for more money than is in
the checking account. If an office receives an NSF check, it can legally charge patients a

fee in return. Most banks redeposit NSF checks only once, so when checks cannot be redeposited, medical office managers must contact the patients to inform them of their checks' return and communicate the fee charged by the office. In such conversations, managers should determine the dates by which patients will send replacement payments. At the end of the interactions, managers should make any relevant notations in the patients' billing ledgers.

When a Patient Does Not Pay a Bill

When patients fail to pay their monthly billing statements by the due date, medical office managers should try to contact the patients regarding payment. Unless patients have instructed otherwise, it is legal to contact patients at their places of employment. Once managers reach patients, they should communicate the outstanding balances and ask when to expect payment on the balances. When patients agree to dates and amounts, managers should make notations in a **tickler file**. Serving as a reminder, a tickler file facilitates follow-up should payment fail to arrive when expected. Tickler files can be manual, such as index cards in a small box, or computerized. Many medical software programs have such reminder mechanisms.

> **tickler file**
> tool for tracking future events, such as patient appointments

In addition to making notes in tickler files, managers should follow up with patients in writing. Letters should outline conversation details, including the amount owed on the account, the agreed-on payment amount and due date, and any follow-up actions in the event of nonpayment.

HIPAA regulations prevent members of the healthcare team from leaving messages with live parties or on voice mail when those messages may violate patient confidentiality. It is inappropriate, for example, to mention that a message is about a past due balance. An appropriate message is "This is Steve from Dr. Sutcliffe's office. I need to leave a message for Jorge Rodriguez to call me at (425) 555-9899." Document all phone calls in the patient's financial ledger.

SENDING COLLECTION LETTERS TO PATIENTS

When patients continue to be delinquent in their accounts, medical office managers can send those patients letters stating the amounts owed and any requested payment terms. Figure ■ 13-8 gives an example. Some offices have their clinic directors or healthcare providers try to contact the patients. Whatever procedure an office follows, the medical office manager must be sure to consistently and carefully apply the same guidelines to all patients.

Use of Collection Agencies

When offices choose **collection agencies** to collect past due accounts, those companies must be reputable. Other medical offices are good sources for agency references. Collections companies should actively pursue accounts, not harass or offend patients. Such agencies must also abide by federal guidelines for debt collection (Figure ■ 13-9). The **Fair Debt Collection Practices Act** was enacted to eliminate abusive, deceptive, and unfair collection practices. This law applies to all consumer debt for personal, family, or household purposes.

> **collection agency**
> company that pursues overdue accounts for a fee
>
> **Fair Debt Collection Practices Act**
> law that dictates how debts may be collected

Once accounts go to collection agencies, offices typically write off the balances owed. Collection agencies typically charge percentage fees for their services. As patients' amounts owed increase, so, too, do collection agencies' fees. The standard rate is 33 percent of the amount owing. Therefore, if a patient owes $99 when the office sends the account to collections, the provider is paid $66 when the collection agency collects payment on the account ($99 − $33 = $66). Some collection agencies charge flat dollar amounts to collect accounts, which is most cost effective for large accounts. To maximize their collections efforts, medical offices can use multiple collection agencies.

Russ Bowman, RMA (AMT)
Markson Family Practice
2323 Front Street
Yonkers, NY 12345

Joseph Paterniti
41 Bronxville Ave
Yonkers, NY 12345

January 31, 2013

Dear Mr. Paterniti:

It has come to my attention that your account is now past due. We received the last payment on your account on [date of last payment]. To render your account current, we must receive your payment by [date 10 days from the letter's date].

If you cannot meet this deadline, please contact this office immediately to make other arrangements. If we do not receive your payment or fail to hear from you by the date listed previously, we will refer your account to a third-party collection agency.

Sincerely,

Russ Bowman, RMA (AMT)

FIGURE ■ 13-8 Sample collection letter.

Medical offices must:

- Threaten to take only action that is legal or intended to come to fruition. For example, offices that threaten to sue patients for nonpayment must file lawsuits or face harassment accusations.

- Accurately represent themselves and the amounts patients owe.

- Make collection phone cells outside the hours of 9 p.m. and 8 a.m. unless directed by patients.

- Stop calling about accounts upon patients' request. Continued calling would be considered harassment.

FIGURE ■ 13-9 Highlights of the federal Fair Debt Collection Practices Act guidelines.

Critical Thinking 13.8 ?

Can you name some benefits to the medical office of using a collection agency, rather than continuing to pursue the collection with the patients themselves? Can you think of any drawbacks to using a collection agency?

Uncollectible Accounts

Some offices choose to **write off** accounts deemed **uncollectible** to maintain patient relations. Patients may have legitimate reasons for nonpayment, such as the death of a spouse or the loss of a job. When medical offices choose to write off patients' owed balances, which is legal, the medical office manager must send the patients letters to that effect (Figure ■ 13-10). Copies of the letters should reside in the patients' files.

write off
to remove a balance from a patient account

uncollectible account
account that will likely never be paid

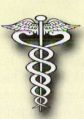

Adam Nichols, CMA (AAMA)
Markson Family Practice
2323 Front Street
Yonkers, NY 12345

Joseph Paterniti
41 Bronxville Ave
Yonkers, NY 12345

January 31, 2013

Dear Mr. Paterniti:

Our medical office has been unable to collect the $55 outstanding on your account. At this time, we are forgiving that balance and bringing your account balance to zero.

If you should again seek care in this office, you will be required to pay any patient portion of your bill at the time of service.

Sincerely,

Adam Nichols, CMA (AAMA)

FIGURE ■ 13-10 Sample letter forgiving a patient balance.

Collecting from Estates

Sometimes patients die with balances owed to a medical office. Providers may choose to forgive the balances if the deceased was unmarried, for example, or lacked assets. When providers choose to pursue the amounts, however, medical office managers should send statements to the deceased's estates in the following format:

Estate of [patient's name]

c/o [name of patient's spouse or next of kin]

Patient's last known address

In return, the person handling the deceased's estate should contact the medical office to arrange for payment. If the office receives no response, the medical office manager can contact the County Recorder's Office in the Probate Department of the Superior Court in the county where the deceased resided. This office should provide the name of the estate's executor. If the office receives no response from the estate's executor, the medical office manager should gather the proper forms from the County Clerk's office to file a claim against the estate for the amount owed. In general, medical offices have from 2 to 36 months to act. While a claim remains outstanding, the manager should continue sending the estate's executor monthly billing statements.

When Patients File Bankruptcy

Patients who are unable to pay their medical bill may file bankruptcy. A Harvard study performed in 2005 found that inability to pay medical bills is the leading cause of bankruptcy filings, affecting nearly 2 million Americans each year. Depending on the type of bankruptcy the patient files, the medical office may or may not be repaid any of the amount outstanding on the patient's account. Since bankruptcy is designed to protect debtors from further collection activity, the medical office may no longer contact the patient for payment of his account once the patient has filed a bankruptcy claim. Patients may file bankruptcy in one of the five following types:

1. **Chapter 7**—All nonexempt patient assets are sold and the proceeds distributed to creditors. Secured creditors, like mortgage or car loans, are paid first; unsecured creditors, like medical providers, are paid last. This type of bankruptcy is considered complete in that most or all patient debt dissolves. If the patient's assets are less than their debts, the medical office may not receive any of the amount outstanding and may have to write off the patient's balance.

2. **Chapter 9**—Used for town reorganizations. This does not apply to medical bills.

3. **Chapter 11**—Used for business reorganizations. This does not apply to medical bills.

4. **Chapter 12**—Used by farmers who cannot meet their financial obligations. This does not apply to medical bills.

5. **Chapter 13**—Protects debtors from creditors while the debtors arrange to repay all or some of their debts over 3- to 5-year periods. When those periods end, the balances on most debts dissolve. With this type of bankruptcy, the medical office may receive a portion of the amount outstanding on the patient account over the 3- to 5-year period of time.

Overpayments on Accounts

Account overpayments can occur for a number of reasons, including when patients pay on their accounts and their insurance policies pay unexpectedly high amounts or when patients have multiple policies that together pay more than owed. When overpayments occur, careful review is needed to identify the party who should receive the refund. The refund may be due to the patient, or it may be due to the insurance carrier. The medical office manager should determine the correct amount to return and the correct person or company owed the refund.

When posting the amount of the refund to the patient's account, the medical office manager should note the reason for the refund, as well as the person and address to whom the refund was sent. A letter from the medical office manager should accompany the refund so that the recipient is aware of the purpose for the refund check.

Small Claims Court

Small claims court is yet another option for collecting on past due accounts. To pursue a small claims suit, the patient's balance owing must fit the "small claim" criteria in the state where the provider's office is located.

Depending on the laws in the states where medical office managers work, those managers may be able to file claims online or through the mail. Some states require claims to be filed in person at the local county courthouse. All methods incur a cost at the time of filing. Notice of the suit must be served on the patient by someone outside the medical office. Often, offices hire companies specializing in this task.

When small claims cases enter court, someone from the medical office must appear to testify. The office representative will need a copy of the patient's account ledger and any documentation proving the healthcare provider treated the patient. Any signed documentation indicating the patient agreed to pay any outstanding bill is also important to bring. Typically, in small claims court, the healthcare provider's office need only prove that the patient was treated and that the patient knew of the charges for the service. Providers often win judgment in these cases, and patients are ordered to pay their bills.

When patients fail to pay their ordered amounts, physicians may opt to garnish those patients' wages. In states with **community property laws**, patients' spouses are also responsible for the bills. As a result, spouses' wages can also be garnished. To act appropriately, medical office managers must check the laws in their states.

community property laws
legislation that deems one spouse financially responsible for the other spouse's debts

Case Study Questions

Refer to the case study presented at the beginning of this chapter to answer the following questions:

1. How would you suggest Molly begin the task of collecting the overdue accounts she has discovered?
2. What steps would you suggest Molly follow?
3. How would you suggest Molly document the work she is doing, as well as any conversations she has with patients?

Chapter Review

Summary

- Fee schedules are created based on formulas released by Medicare. These formulas are based on a variety of factors, from office location to physician specialty.

- Participating provider agreements are contracts between physicians and managed care insurance companies. Physicians and office managers will want to carefully read the contacts before agreeing to sign them.

- Credit and collections in the medical office require attention on a regular basis. Without proper collection policies in place, the medical office may find it is not collecting on patient debts.

- Many medical offices use preprinted brochures to explain payment and collection policies to patients. These are especially helpful in practices where patients will have a large out-of-pocket expense.

- Collecting from patients can be done in person, over the telephone, or by sending the patient a billing statement. To avoid collection problems with patients, medical offices should have clear policies on when payment is due and those policies should be explained to patients before any expense is incurred.

- Medical offices need to verify patient identification as part of the Red Flags rule. This legislation is aimed at reducing fraud in healthcare when patients use another's identity.

- Management of the accounts receivable includes maintaining open conversations with patients about amounts owed for medical care.

- Managed care plans have rules set out in their contracts regarding how medical offices are allowed to collect fees from patients. These rules should be carefully considered prior to signing managed care contracts. The rules must be followed or the office risks cancellation of its managed care contract.

- The types of payments seen in the medical office include cash, personal checks, and credit cards.

- A professional courtesy is a discount offered to friends, colleagues, and family of the physician.

- Patient billing statements should be sent out on the same day each month. Because most patients have bills that are due at the first of the month, it is advisable for medical offices to send their statements out later in the month.

- When a patient who owes money to the medical office is in the office for care, the medical office manager should take the patient to a private office to discuss payment of her bill.

- Patients who do not pay their bills may be dismissed from care in the medical office. Offices must give the patients adequate notice in the form of a certified letter.

- Medical offices may charge interest on accounts owed by patients. Those offices that choose not to charge interest may find their accounts are not given as high a priority as other, interest-accruing accounts that the patient may have to pay.

- When a patient does not have adequate funds in his bank to cover the amount of a check, that check is returned to the medical office. In these cases, the medical office manager should contact the patient to discuss payment of the bill.

- Patients who do not pay their medical office bills should be contacted on a regular basis. Collection laws must be followed.

- Medical offices may choose to turn past due patient accounts over to a collection agency. These agencies must follow collection laws regarding how they contact patients for payment. With some collection agencies, the medical office pays a percentage of the amount owed when the patient makes payment. With other agencies, there is a flat fee associated with payment.

- At times the medical office manager or physician may determine a patient account is uncollectible and should be written off. These are typically cases where the patient is unemployed, or the amount owed is too small to consider worthy of further collection activity. When this happens, the medical office manager should send a letter to the patient notifying her of the release of the amount owed.

- When patients die while still owing for care in the medical office, the medical office manager may pursue the patient's estate for payment of the amount due.

- When patients file bankruptcy, medical office managers need to respond to the claim in order to pursue payment.

- Sometimes patients incur an overpayment on their account. This may happen when the patient makes a payment and then the insurance carrier pays as well. In these cases, the medical office manager should investigate the claim to determine who is due the refund.

- Medical offices may choose to file a case in small claims court for past due accounts. In these cases, the medical office manager should research and follow the laws in the state where the claim is to be filed.

Multiple Choice

Choose the letter that best answers each question or completes each statement.

1. Your patient has a $50 balance owing from care received last month. What is the best option for collecting that amount from the patient?
   a. Ask the patient for payment when he comes in for care next week.
   b. File a claim in small claims court.
   c. Send the patient account to a collection agency.
   d. Ask the patient to sign a hardship letter.

2. Your patient passed away while still owing $150 for medical services. Which of the following is the option you would choose as the medical office manager?
   a. Write the amount off as uncollectible.
   b. Contact the patient's estate to arrange payment of the account.
   c. Send the claim to a collection agency.
   d. File a claim in small claims court against the estate.

3. Mrs. Tiki has been a patient of Dr. Yi's for over 20 years. Her husband has been out of work for the past 2 years and Mrs. Tiki has been unable to make payment on the $75 owing on her account. What would you suggest Dr. Yi do with this account?
   a. Send the account to a collection agency.
   b. File a claim in small claims court.
   c. Forgive the debt and send Mrs. Tiki a letter to let her know.
   d. Call Mrs. Tiki and ask her to make payment in full by the end of the month.

4. Which of the following pertains to the Red Flags rule?
   a. Avoiding identity theft
   b. Collecting patient accounts
   c. Filing claims in small claims court
   d. Making a note of patient allergies in the medical record

5. Why would the medical office manager care about the statute of limitations on healthcare debt?
   a. To determine how much credit to extend to patients
   b. To determine the time of day a collection telephone call can be made
   c. To determine the number of years the medical office can pursue a patient's debt
   d. To determine if a patient should have credit extended to them

6. Which of the following describes the accounts receivable in the medical office?
   a. It is the amount of money the medical office owes to others for services or supplies.
   b. It is the amount of money the medical office pays in salary and wages each pay period.
   c. It is the amount of money the physicians pay themselves for salaries.
   d. It is the amount of money owed to the medical office for services rendered.

7. Which of the following is true about collection policies and managed care?
   a. Managed care policies dictate the amount of money that can be collected from patients.
   b. Managed care policies dictate how much credit the medical office can extend to patients.
   c. Managed care policies stipulate the date by which the patient account should be sent to a collection agency.
   d. Managed care policies state that spouses cannot be held responsible for their partner's medical bills.

8. Which of the following is **not** part of Medicare service fee calculations?
   a. Service intensity
   b. Time needed for the service
   c. Skills needed to perform the service
   d. Age of the patient

9. Which of the following is the best way to avoid collection problems in the medical office?
   a. Discuss fees and payment policies with patients prior to rendering services.
   b. Post a list of fees in the reception area for patients to view.
   c. Hand out a list of fees to patients at every visit.
   d. Require all patients to pay in full for their care at the time of service.

10. Which of the following is illegal under the Fair Debt Collection Practices Act?
   a. Calling patients at their place of employment
   b. Calling the patient's spouse about a past due bill in a community property state
   c. Failing to identify yourself when you place a call to the patient
   d. Sending the patient account to a collection agency

True/False

Determine if each of the following statements is true or false.

_____ 1. It is insurance fraud to forgive patient deductibles without a hardship agreement.

_____ 2. It is not important to carefully choose a collection agency for the medical office; they will all perform at the same level.

_____ 3. The Red Flags rule does not apply to healthcare clinics.

_____ 4. The best way to collect payment from patients is to do so while the patient is in the medical office.

_____ 5. Medical offices are not legally allowed to take patients to small claims court for past due bills.

_____ 6. All managed care contracts are the same.

_____ 7. When accepting credit card payments in the medical office, providers pay bank fees in the amount of 1 to 3 percent of charges.

_____ 8. Aging reports detail the amount of money owed to the medical office.

_____ 9. Accounts receivable include only those amounts owed by patients personally.

_____ 10. Some clinics have the healthcare providers attempt to contact patients who have past due accounts.

Matching

Match the following terms with their definition.

a. aging report

b. certified letter

c. collection agency

d. community property laws

e. Fair Debt Collection Practices Act

f. fee schedule

g. relative value unit (RVU)

h. tickler file

i. uncollectible account

j. accounts receivable (AR)

1. Money owed the medical practice

2. Postal service letter that the recipient must sign

3. Documentation of the money owed the medical office and how long accounts have been outstanding

4. Legislation that deems one spouse financially responsible for the other spouse's debts

5. Law that dictates how debts may be collected

6. Company that pursues overdue accounts for a fee

7. Account that will likely never be paid

8. List of services and their fees

9. Numeric value assigned by Medicare to formulate fee schedules for healthcare providers

10. Tool for tracking future events, such as patient appointments

Chapter Resources

Federal Trade Commission, Fair Debt Collection Practices Act: www.ftc.gov/bcp/edu/pubs/consumer/credit/cre18.shtm

Federal Trade Commission, Red Flags rule: www.ftc.gov/bcp/edu/microsites/redflagsrule/index.shtml

PEARSON
myhealthprofessionskit™

Additional interactive resources for this chapter can be found at **www.myhealthprofessionskit.com.** Choose "Medical Assisting" from the discipline menu and then click on the book cover for *Medical Office Management.*

CHAPTER 14

Health Insurance

CHAPTER OUTLINE

LEARNING OBJECTIVES

Upon completion of this chapter, you should be able to:

- Spell and define the key terms in this chapter.
- Discuss the history of health insurance in the United States, and issues of healthcare today, including the Health Care Reform of 2010.
- Define health insurance terminology.
- List and describe the various types of health insurance plans.
- Define COBRA coverage and describe how it works.
- Understand how individual health insurance plans function.
- Describe the use of flexible spending, healthcare savings accounts, and consumer-directed healthcare plans.
- Describe various elective procedures that may not be covered by health insurance.
- Describe how prescription drug coverage is applied.
- Explain Medicare coverage, including Parts A, B, C, and D.
- Describe how the Medicaid program covers medical care.
- Describe the use of TRICARE and CHAMPVA.
- Explain the function of insurance for accidental injuries and the use of disability insurance.

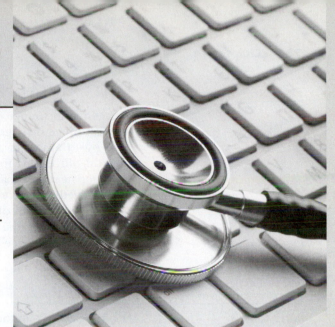

- Understand how insurance claims are processed.
- Describe and complete the health insurance claim form.
- Reconcile payments and rejections from insurance carriers.

KEY TERMS

accept assignment
advance beneficiary notice
(ABN)
allowed amount
balance billing
beneficiary
birthday rule
capitated plan
catastrophic
certificate of coverage
CHAMPVA
Children's Health Insurance
Program (CHIP)
COBRA
coinsurance
consumer-directed healthcare
plan
copayment
deductible

dependent
e-billing
elective procedure
exclusions
exclusive provider
organization (EPO)
experimental
fee-for-service plan
flexible spending account
(FSA)
form locators
formulary
gatekeeper
group health insurance
health insurance
health maintenance
organization (HMO)
Healthcare and Education
Reconciliation Act of 2010

holistic healthcare
hospice
indemnity plan
individual health insurance
insured
liability insurance
lifetime maximum benefits
maintenance medications
managed care
Medicaid
Medicare
member
national provider identifier
(NPI)
nonparticipating provider
participating provider
Patient Protection and
Affordable Care Act
payer number

point-of-service option
policyholder
preauthorization
precertification
preexisting condition
preferred provider
organization (PPO)
premium
preventive care
respite care
self-insure
skilled nursing facility
sliding fee scale
stop loss
subscriber
superbill
TRICARE
waiting period
waiver

Case Study

Take note of the following scenario and answer the case study questions that appear at the end of this chapter.

Roland Rubowski works as the medical office manager in a cardiology practice. Many of the patients seen in his clinic are covered by Medicare as well as a supplemental insurance plan. Roland has just hired three new medical assistants and needs to train them on the basics of Medicare coverage, so that the medical assistants will be able to properly communicate coverage information to their patients.

Introduction

Processing insurance claims accurately is vital to the success of any medical practice. The medical office manager must have a strong grasp on how managed care plans work and how owed amounts are determined for specific procedures. Patients will look to the medical office staff for information about their insurance plans, and the medical office manager needs to make sure staff are trained to answer these questions. The size and type of medical office are determining factors in the size of the billing office. In smaller offices, the function of insurance billing may rest solely with the medical office manager. In larger facilities, this function may be performed by a separate billing department. The function of insurance billing may also be outsourced to an outside billing agency.

History of Health Insurance

Health insurance in the United States began in the mid-1800s, when it was used to replace the income of people injured in accidents or ill from certain diseases. Massachusetts Health Insurance of Boston offered the first group policy providing comprehensive benefits in 1847. Insurance companies issued the first individual disability and illness policies around 1890. Hospital insurance coverage began in 1929, when a group of public school teachers in Texas formed a contract with a local hospital to guarantee up to 21 days of hospital care for a premium of $6 per year. This plan became quite popular, and other groups of employers joined the plan, which eventually became known as the Blue Cross plan.

During World War II, when wages were frozen, employers began offering their employees **group health insurance** as a benefit. Group health insurance plans cover entire groups of individuals, usually through employers or other large associations or defined groups. These early plans were designed to protect employees from the high costs of hospitalization and eventually evolved into the healthcare plans common today.

Employee benefit plans became popular in the 1940s and 1950s. The unions that represented large groups of workers bargained for better benefit packages, including tax-free, employer-sponsored health insurance.

During the 1950s and 1960s, government programs began to cover healthcare costs. Social Security coverage included disability benefits for the first time in 1954 and the government created the Medicare and Medicaid programs in 1965. By the end of 2008, about 45% of Americans received health insurance benefits from their employer.

The 1980s and 1990s saw a rapid rise in the cost of healthcare. During this time the majority of employer-sponsored group insurance plans moved to less expensive managed care plans. This move was facilitated by the federal HMO Act of 1973, which created policies and allowed use of federal funds to promote health maintenance organizations (HMOs), and the Tax Equity and Fiscal Responsibility Act (TEFRA) in 1982, which made it easier and more attractive for HMOs to contract with the Medicare program. By the mid-1990s, most Americans who had health insurance were enrolled in managed care plans.

Although most insurance plans began as safety mechanisms in the event of **catastrophic** health events, most plans today cover **preventive care**. Catastrophic health events are defined as chronic illnesses or serious injuries that require expensive, specialized, or long-term care. An example is a person diagnosed with cancer or a person who needs several surgeries after a serious accident. Preventive care is any care a patient receives to stay well. Examples include well-child checks and yearly mammograms or physicals. Insurance company administrators realize that covering preventive care encourages patients to seek such care, thereby avoiding or reducing the need for more expensive or long-term care for many conditions.

group health insurance
a commercial insurance policy with rates based on a group of people; usually offered by an employer

catastrophic
large and usually unforeseen

preventive care
healthcare designed to keep a person healthy

Critical Thinking 14.1 ?

Why do you think patients who seek preventive care might be able to avoid expensive or long-term care for certain health conditions? What healthcare conditions can you think of that would likely be less serious if discovered during a preventive healthcare visit, instead of waiting for symptoms to arise?

Health Insurance Today

Today, Americans obtain health insurance from a variety of sources. Medical office managers need to be knowledgeable about the rules and requirements of each source. About half of insured Americans have health insurance through a private or commercial insurance company. Usually, this is through a group policy sponsored by an employer. Some employers **self-insure** by paying directly for employees' medical expenses. Individuals who do not have employer-sponsored health insurance may purchase an **individual health insurance** policy. **Liability insurance**, such as automobile and homeowner insurance, provides for medical expenses related to certain types of accidents.

Many Americans who do not have private insurance receive health insurance benefits from the state or federal government. Government programs such as **Medicare**, a federal program for people over age 65 and people with end-stage kidney disease or long-term disabilities; **Medicaid**, a federal/state program primarily for those with low incomes; **TRICARE**, for active-duty and retired service personnel and their families; and **CHAMPVA** for spouses and children of veterans. Workers' compensation provides coverage for employees who experience job-related injuries or illnesses.

Despite the many options available for health insurance, approximately 50 million Americans did not have any health insurance coverage as of 2010. Often this is because individuals do not have or do not qualify for employer-based coverage, do not qualify for federal programs, and cannot afford individual policies. For these patients, some medical offices establish a **sliding fee scale** where fees are charged based on a patient's financial ability to pay. Some cities and counties have free or low-cost clinics established and run by volunteers or not-for-profit agencies. These clinics will often provide access to low-income patients to seek primary care services, though not all have access to specialty services, such as cardiology or orthopedics.

In addition to determining the source of patients' insurance, medical office managers need to determine what type of coverage the patients have. Insurance may cover hospital services, physician services, preventive care, catastrophic care, long-term care, and ancillary services such as prescription drugs, vision, dental, and chiropractic. With each type of coverage and each source of coverage, medical office managers need to identify how patients' insurance plans relate to the specific services being provided in each situation. Research, attention to detail, careful communication, and patient advocacy are skills that successful medical office managers use in the insurance area. In addition to the medical office manager mastering this knowledge, he or she will also need to train appropriate staff about insurance plans (Figure ■ 14-1).

Critical Thinking 14.2 ?

What types of problems might result if a medical office manager is not thoroughly knowledgeable about how patients' health insurance coverage applies to the patients' care?

Healthcare Reform of 2010

Two major pieces of healthcare legislation were passed in 2010: the **Patient Protection and Affordable Care Act**, and the **Healthcare and Education Reconciliation Act of 2010**. These acts, scheduled to phase in over 4 years, were designed to provide health insurance coverage for more Americans. Part of the legislation includes language that targets reform of the insurance industry. The elimination of lifetime and annual caps on the amount of coverage an individual is allowed and the mandate that insurance carriers cannot deny coverage to individuals with chronic healthcare conditions meant that more Americans would be able to receive care for long-term and expensive care and that they would not experience gaps in coverage for health conditions when the patient changes employers.

self-insure
insurance program in which an employer sets aside funds to pay for employee health expenses

individual health insurance
a commercial insurance policy with rates based on individual health criteria

liability insurance
type of insurance that covers injuries that occur on, in, or because of the insured's property

Medicare
federal program that covers medical expenses for those ages 65 and over, those with end-stage kidney disease, and those with long-term disabilities

Medicaid
a joint federal and state program that helps with medical costs for eligible people with low incomes and limited resources

TRICARE
health insurance for active-duty military personnel, retired service personnel, and their eligible dependents

CHAMPVA
Civilian Health and Medical Program of the Department of Veterans Affairs; health insurance for spouses and children of veterans

sliding fee scale
a provider's fee schedule that charges varying fees for a service based on a patient's financial ability to pay

Patient Protection and Affordable Care Act
healthcare legislation passed in 2010

Healthcare and Education Reconciliation Act of 2010
healthcare legislation produced to amend the Patient Protection and Affordable Care Act

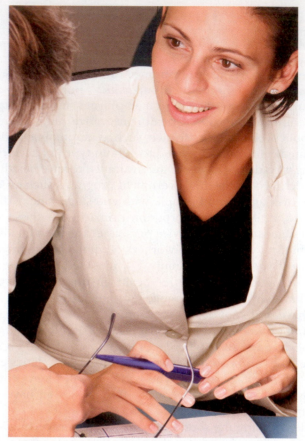

FIGURE ■ **14-1**   All members of the medical office team must understand patients' insurance coverage.
Source: Endostock/Dreamstime.com.

These healthcare reform acts included the expansion of the Medicaid program, which allows individuals and families who previously earned too much to qualify for Medicaid—yet too little to purchase individual plans—to obtain health insurance coverage. Sliding fee scales were enacted, with the government subsidizing premiums for health insurance coverage based on the income of the family or individual. Incentives to businesses for providing coverage to their employees were included in order to encourage more employer-provided health insurance coverage.

As of 2014, the law prohibits insurance carriers from refusing coverage for individuals who have chronic healthcare conditions. That same year is set as the date by which all individuals are required to purchase government-approved health insurance plans. These plans are designed to offer competitive prices for premiums and a fine will be waged against any individual who does not purchase an approved plan by 2014. Government studies show that this mandate reduces the number of uninsured Americans from 19 percent in 2010 to 8 percent in 2014. Of the remaining 8 percent, approximately 5 percent are expected to be illegal immigrants. In 2008, approximately $43 billion was spent in providing unreimbursed healthcare to the uninsured. Those costs are passed on through the healthcare system by raising the cost of care. By requiring all Americans to purchase health insurance coverage, the goal is to reduce the rising cost of healthcare in the United States.

Critical Thinking 14.3 ?

Do you think more Americans will seek preventive care if they have coverage? Some policy makers believe that forcing individuals to purchase health insurance coverage will result in patients seeking care unnecessarily. This train of thought surrounds the belief that if individuals have to pay for a policy, they will think they need to seek care in order to get their money's worth. What do you think of this line of thought?

Health Insurance Terminology

Just as medical office managers need to understand medical terminology in order to provide the best care for patients, knowledge of insurance terminology is critical to helping patients utilize their health insurance. In many situations, multiple terms are used to essentially mean the same thing. In other situations, terms that seem similar to the layperson have different and specific meanings in the world of health insurance. Patients are often unfamiliar with their insurance benefits and may not understand the terms they hear. Medical office managers who understand insurance terms can advocate for patients and communicate in ways that patients understand. This is another area where the medical office manager should provide training for staff so that the entire team is using the terminology correctly.

Critical Thinking 14.4 **?**

What problems could result if a member of the medical office staff does not properly understand certain medical insurance terms? If that person were talking to a patient about his health insurance coverage, do you believe the patient would feel confident in the competence of the staff with regard to insurance?

MEMBERS AND THEIR FAMILIES

Health insurance, also referred to as medical insurance, is a contract between an insurance carrier and the person who owns the policy. The person who owns the policy is known as the **member**, **subscriber**, **insured**, or **policyholder**. For those who receive insurance through their employers, the member is the employee. For those who buy individual policies, the member is the person who purchased the plan. For those covered by government policies, the term **beneficiary** is often used and refers to the individual who qualifies for the program.

Many commercial policies allow policyholders to include family members on the plan. Family members are also called **dependents** and may include a spouse, children, unmarried domestic partner, and stepchildren. Inclusion of family members is not automatic and it is possible for some, but not all, members of the family to be covered. The policyholder must obtain forms from the employer or the insurance company to specifically designate coverage for dependents. The medical office manager should ask the patient, and possibly contact the insurance carrier, to determine who is eligible for benefits. It is also important to know exactly how each dependent is legally related to the member.

PREMIUMS

To obtain a commercial health insurance policy, the policyholder pays a **premium** to the insurance carrier. The premium is typically paid in monthly installments for the next month's coverage. In group coverage, the employer often pays the majority of the premium and employees may pay the remainder of the premium as a deduction from their paychecks. If dependent coverage is selected, the premium is usually higher. Some government plans require policyholders to pay a premium as well.

ALLOWED AMOUNTS

Providers that contract as preferred providers with insurance companies agree to a set fee schedule for reimbursement. Insurance companies are not required to pay providers' usual charges. Most insurance companies calculate reimbursement prices based on the average price among providers of the same specialty in the same geographic area. The amount the insurance company approves is called the **allowed amount**. When a provider's actual charge is more than the allowed amount, the provider has to write off the

---

health insurance
insurance purchased to cover medical expenses

member
the person who owns the insurance policy; also referred to as subscriber and insured

policyholder
the person who owns an insurance policy

beneficiary
person who is eligible to receive benefits and services under an insurance policy

dependent
a family member or other individual who qualifies for coverage on the insured's policy

premium
dollar amount paid to an insurance company to have coverage in force

allowed amount
the dollar amount for a service that an insurance company considers acceptable and uses to determine benefit payments

balance billing
billing a patient for the dollar difference between the provider's charge and the amount approved by the insurance agency

deductible
monetary amount patients must pay to a provider for healthcare services before their health insurance benefits begin to pay

difference between the actual charge and the insurance company allowed charge. Billing the patient for that difference, a practice called **balance billing**, is in violation of the preferred provider contract.

DEDUCTIBLES

Very few health insurance plans cover 100 percent of the care patients receive, so patients are responsible for several different kinds of out-of-pocket expenses. Before the insurance plan pays any benefits, patients may have a **deductible** to meet. The deductible is a monetary amount patients must pay to the provider for healthcare services before health insurance benefits begin to pay. Deductible amounts can be as low as $100 or as high as $10,000. Plans with low deductibles tend to have higher premiums than plans with high deductibles. Some government plans also have deductibles. When calculating benefits and amount owed, the deductible must be subtracted from the allowed charge (Figure ■ 14-2).

Scenario #1: Frida Roberts has health insurance through her employer's plan. She has a yearly deductible of $100, then she is covered at 100%. Frida sees Dr. Sheridan for an office call. The cost of the office call is $128. How much does Frida owe for her visit?

$128 charge for medical services

$100 for Frida's deductible

Frida must pay her $100 deductible and the insurance company will pay the $28 balance.

Scenario #1: Mallory Discman has an individual health insurance plan. She has a $1000 yearly deductible and then is covered at 80%. Mallory sees Dr. Price for an office call. The cost of the office call is $217. How much does Mallory owe out of pocket for this visit?

$217 charge for medical services

$1000 for Mallory's yearly deductible

Mallory's insurance company will pay $0 because she has not met her $1000 yearly deductible. Mallory must pay the full $217 charge.

FIGURE ■ **14-2** Calculating a patient's insurance deductible.

In some policies, the deductible does not apply to all services. A preventive care visit may not be subject to a deductible, whereas a sick call typically will be. This is to encourage patients to seek preventive care. Deductibles vary according to the type of physician or facility as well. For example, most plans have a higher deductible for care in the emergency department. This is to encourage patients to be seen by their primary care provider, rather than incur the higher costs associated with the emergency department.

When patients include family members on their policy, there is typically an individual deductible and a family deductible. The individual deductible is the maximum deductible that any given family member must pay; the family deductible is the maximum deductible for all family members combined. For example, imagine Joyce Shawger is the policyholder and carries coverage for her husband Tim and their two children on the policy. The individual deductible is $100 and the family deductible is $300. Once three of the family members have individually satisfied their $100 deductible, the family deductible has been met.

copayment
set dollar fee per visit or service that patients are responsible for according to their insurance plan contracts

coinsurance
percentage of medical charges patients are responsible for according to their insurance plan contracts

COPAYMENTS AND COINSURANCE

After the deductible has been met, most patients will have an out-of-pocket expense for a portion of their care. This cost sharing of the expense of medical care takes the form of a **copayment** or **coinsurance**. Copayments are set dollar amounts that patients must pay at the time of service, no matter what service is rendered. Copayments can range from $5 to $50 per visit, depending on the policy. Coinsurance is a set percentage of charges that patients pay. An 80/20 coinsurance plan is one in which the insurance covers 80 percent of the allowed charge and the patient pays the remaining 20 percent. Figure ■ 14-3 shows how copayments and coinsurance amounts are calculated.

Scenario #1: Dr. Brown charges $75 for an office call. Monique Walters is insured with Premera Blue Cross Insurance and has a 20% coinsurance obligation. Dr. Brown is a preferred provider with Premera Blue Cross and has a contractual agreement to accept $64.25 as payment in full for his office call. Mary owes 20% of the $64.25 fee ($12.85).

Scenario #2: Dr. Cubby charges $70 for an office call. Jennifer Smith is insured with Regence Blue Shield Insurance and has a $20 copayment obligation. Dr. Cubby is a preferred provider with Regence Blue Shield and has a contractual agreement to accept $67.25 as payment in full for her office call. Jennifer owes $20 of the $67.25 fee.

FIGURE ■ **14-3** Calculating copayments and deductibles.

Similar to deductibles, certain types of care do not incur a copayment or coinsurance. Preventive care, for example, is typically covered at 100 percent of the allowed amount with no copayment or coinsurance. Specialty care may require a higher copayment or coinsurance than primary care. Each insurance company sets its rules for individual policies. The medical office manager should determine the amount of payment due from the patient and have a conversation with the patient to discuss those fees. These conversations should ideally take place prior to expensive care being rendered, and the conversation should be documented in the patient's medical record.

STOP LOSS AND LIFETIME MAXIMUMS

Many insurance policies have stop loss and lifetime maximum benefit clauses. A **stop loss** is the maximum amount the patient must pay out of pocket for copayments and coinsurance yearly. After this amount is reached, the insurance policy pays 100 percent of the allowed amount for any additional covered medical care. The stop loss amount starts over at the beginning of the next year. The stop loss amount may not apply to all care the patient pays for. Services for behavioral health or prescription drug medications are often excluded from the stop loss calculation.

Lifetime maximum benefits are the maximum benefits an insurance company pays for patients over the course of a lifetime. A common lifetime maximum is $1 million, but it could be as low as $100,000 in a very inexpensive policy. Sometimes patients will select a low-cost policy and not be aware of provisions such as the lifetime maximum. While $1 million or even $100,000 may seem like a lot of money to pay for healthcare expenses, these expenses can accumulate quickly with a serious illness or injury. As mentioned earlier in the chapter, the Patient Protection and Affordable Care Act of 2010 mandates that lifetime maximums be eliminated as of 2014.

WAITING PERIODS, EXCLUSIONS, AND PREEXISTING CONDITIONS

In addition to out-of-pocket expenses, many health insurance plans have waiting periods and exclusions that limit what the insurance plan needs to pay in benefits. A **waiting period** is a set period of time that must pass before a member's **preexisting condition** is covered. A preexisting condition is any condition a patient was diagnosed with or treated for, including prescription medications, before beginning coverage with a new insurance plan.

Although waiting periods for preexisting conditions vary from one insurance plan to the next, a preexisting condition is covered without a waiting period when the patient has been insured the 24 months before joining the new plan. Therefore, if patients remain insured for 24 months or more, they can change jobs and retain preexisting condition coverage without added waiting periods even when they have chronic conditions. Patients

stop loss
the maximum amount the patient must pay out of pocket for copayments and coinsurance

lifetime maximum benefits
monetary amount allowed by an insurance carrier for a member's covered expenses over the member's lifetime

waiting period
period after a new health insurance plan begins during which certain services are not covered

preexisting condition
condition for which a patient received treatment in a certain period before beginning coverage with a new insurance plan

should obtain a **certificate of coverage** from the previous insurance plan. This letter documents the nature and length of coverage with the plan. Patients submit this letter to the new plan to establish proof of continuous coverage. If patients have had more than one insurance plan during the previous 24 months, certificates of coverage from each plan should be submitted.

Even when patients have not been insured the 24 months before joining a new insurance plan, Health Insurance Portability and Accountability Act (HIPAA) legislation restricts insurance companies from requiring patients wait any longer than 12 months from the date the new insurance begins before preexisting conditions are covered. As mentioned earlier in the chapter, the Patient Protection and Affordable Care Act of 2010 mandates that preexisting condition exclusions be eliminated as of 2014.

Exclusions are those items that an insurance carrier denies coverage for. These items may be those considered **experimental**, or not yet approved by the Food and Drug Administration. Other items that may be excluded are those that may not require a physician's prescription or orders. An example would be vitamins or a neck brace. These items may be purchased over the counter at a pharmacy and therefore may not be covered by the insurance carrier. Eye exams and hearing tests are often excluded items in health insurance policies (Figure ■ 14-4). Other items that may not be covered are those considered **holistic healthcare**, such as acupuncture, massage, or chiropractic. In some policies, certain items are limited to a specific dollar amount or specific number of visits, rather than excluded entirely. Generally, the fewer the exclusions in a health insurance policy, the more expensive the policy premiums.

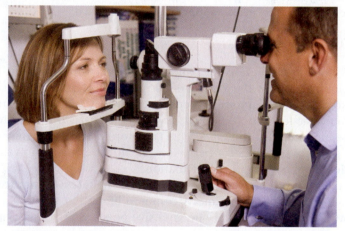

FIGURE ■ 14-4   Eye exams are often excluded in health insurance policies.
Source: Monkeybusiness/Dreamstime.com.

Critical Thinking 14.5 ?

Given the information provided so far in this chapter, do you think it is important for the medical office manager to remain up-to-date about the changes in the medical industry? How do you think the medical office manager should go about staying educated on healthcare policy changes? How often should the manager seek information on changes?

Types of Health Insurance Plans

Since the passage of the HMO Act of 1973 and the Tax Equity and Fiscal Responsibility Act (TEFRA) of 1982, the insurance industry has introduced health insurance plans that provide patients with a variety of ways to access providers and share in the cost of care. These various plans also differ in how insurance companies pay providers for services rendered. The medical office manager should not only need to be aware of how these plans affect the patients' cost burden, but should also carefully review reimbursement contracts between the physicians and the insurance carriers to be certain the practice is not losing money by seeing patients for certain types of care.

FEE-FOR-SERVICE PLANS

In the 1980s, **fee-for-service plans**, also known as **indemnity plans**, were the norm. These plans are far less common today and typically are among the most expensive plans to purchase. Fee-for-service plans allow patients to seek care with any covered healthcare provider, for any covered service. Neither the list of physicians patients may see, nor the fee schedules are preapproved. These plans are private health insurance plans that reimburse healthcare providers on the basis of a fee for each health service provided to the covered person. Fee-for-service plans typically include a yearly deductible, after which the insurance company will pay at a certain coinsurance rate. Most commonly, the coinsurance rate is 80/20 or 70/30 percent, with the insurance company paying the larger share of the costs and the policyholder paying the lower.

These plans are costly because they do not contain managed care or cost control measures. The type of person who generally opts for the fee-for-service plan is an individual with a serious medical condition who needs frequent treatment, and those who can afford the plan and want to have complete freedom of choice to see the provider of their choice whenever they wish (Figure ■ 14-5).

fee-for-service plan
plan in which insurance companies pay providers fees for each service provided to covered patients, also known as an indemnity plan

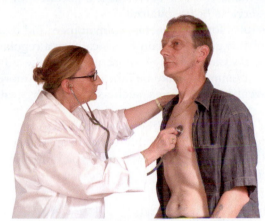

FIGURE ■ **14-5** Individuals who opt for fee-for-service plans usually have a serious medical condition that requires frequent treatment.
Source: Patrick/Dreamstime.com.

Critical Thinking 14.6 ?

Why do you think fee-for-service plans, with their absence of managed care provisions, are so much more costly than other plans?

MANAGED CARE PLANS

Today, most patients are covered by **managed care**. Managed care plans control the costs associated with plan purchase by controlling the amounts they reimburse healthcare providers. Managed care organizations (MCOs) contract with healthcare providers to provide care for a certain group of patients. Those providers, called **participating providers**, sign a contract with the MCO that stipulates discounted reimbursement rates, billing guidelines, and other rules. A provider usually has contracts with several different MCOs. The MCO then contracts with insurance companies to offer lower reimbursement rates through its network of participating providers. The MCO will list the provider's name in a directory given to patients. Patients will have lower out-of-pocket expenses if they use a participating provider.

managed care
a system of healthcare delivery focused on reducing costs by transferring risk to the provider; may limit the type and frequency of care members may receive

participating provider
healthcare provider who has contracted with a particular health insurance carrier

nonparticipating provider
healthcare provider who has not contracted with a particular health insurance carrier

Providers who do not contract with a specific MCO are called **nonparticipating providers**. Some MCOs cover patients who see nonparticipating providers, but typically at a higher out-of-pocket expense for the patient. Other MCOs offer no coverage if the patient sees a nonparticipating provider. It is very important for the medical office manager to let patients know whether the providers are participating with the patient's healthcare plan before charges are incurred. A provider may be participating with some patients' MCOs and nonparticipating with others. Most offices ask about healthcare coverage when patients call to schedule a first appointment. When in doubt, medical office managers should ask patients for their insurance information and then call the insurance company or check for coverage online.

Managed care plans are divided into four basic types: health maintenance organizations, preferred provider organizations, exclusive provider organizations, and point-of-service plans, as discussed next.

Health Maintenance Organizations

health maintenance organization (HMO)
a group of physicians or medical centers that provide comprehensive services to members

gatekeeper
physician responsible for determining when and if a patient needs specific types of healthcare

Health maintenance organizations (HMOs) are managed care plans that cover members only when those members seek care from a list of healthcare providers and suppliers who have contracted with the HMO. When members wish to seek care from providers not on the list, they must pay for the care out of pocket, with no coverage from the HMO. Most HMOs require patients to choose a primary care provider (PCP) who belongs to the network of covered providers. The PCP serves as the **gatekeeper** and is the person who arranges any specialist services or hospitalizations.

HMOs have various rules for copayments, coinsurance, and deductible amounts. The subscriber to an HMO plan is able to obtain healthcare on a regular basis with unlimited medical attention. Thus, HMOs encourage subscribers to take advantage of preventive healthcare services in an attempt to make healthcare coverage more cost efficient. HMOs tend to cover many preventive procedures, such as annual physicals, mammograms, and colonoscopies.

A distinct feature of the HMO is that the subscriber chooses a primary care provider. The PCP must arrange for and coordinate all referrals to specialists or hospitalizations for the patient. Although HMOs are the most restrictive type of health plan, they are also the lowest cost to the patient in premiums.

Preferred Provider Organizations

preferred provider organization (PPO)
organization that contracts with independent providers to perform services for members at discounted rates

The **preferred provider organization (PPO)** contracts with physicians and facilities to perform services for PPO members at specified rates. These rates, or fees, are contractually adjusted so that the PPO member is charged less than nonmembers. The PPO gives subscribers a list of PPO member-providers from which subscribers can receive healthcare at PPO rates. If a patient chooses to receive treatment from a provider who is not in the PPO network, the patient has to pay any difference between the PPO's rate and the outside provider's rate. PPOs generally require preauthorization for major medical expenses.

Each physician in a practice may be a member of more than one PPO, and all the doctors in the practice may not necessarily belong to the same PPO. Some of the main features of PPOs include the following:

- PPOs are similar to HMOs in that they enter into a contractual agreement with healthcare providers, and together form a provider network.

- Unlike an HMO, members of PPOs do not have to use their primary care provider for permission to seek care with another provider, nor do they have to use an in-network provider for their care. PPOs offer members a higher benefit as a financial incentive for seeing an in-network provider.

- PPO members typically do not have to get a referral to see a specialist. However, there is a financial incentive to see a specialist who is contracted with the PPO.

- PPOs are less restrictive than HMOs in the choice of healthcare provider. However, they tend to require greater out-of-pocket payments from their members.

Exclusive Provider Organizations

Exclusive provider organizations (EPOs) are managed care plans that cover members who seek care from healthcare providers in a small network. In these plans, groups of healthcare providers often form their own networks and then contract with employers to provide exclusive care to their employees. EPOs often have hospitals in their networks, and physicians contracted with these networks must perform their hospital services in the contracted hospitals. Members who wish to seek care outside the EPO must pay for that care in full.

exclusive provider organization (EPO)
a managed care contract with a small network of providers under which the employer agrees to not use any other networks in return for favorable pricing

Point-of-Service Options

Because many patients do not wish to accept services from only their HMO providers, some HMO plans add a **point-of-service option**. Patients who choose this option do not have to see only the HMO's physicians. However, if they choose to see physicians outside the network, they must pay increased deductibles and coinsurance. This option makes the HMO more like a PPO, in terms of choices available to the patients. The reason it is called a point-of-service option is because members choose which option—HMO or PPO—they will use each time they seek healthcare. Like an HMO and PPO plan, a POS plan has a contracted network of providers and facilities.

point-of-service option
an insurance offering in which a patient has access to multiple plans, such as an HMO and PPO

CAPITATED PLANS

Capitated plans are managed care plans in which the risks for the high cost of healthcare rest on the shoulders of the contracted physicians or facilities. In these plans, insurance companies contract with providers and agree to pay the provider a set dollar amount each month to provide care for a group of patients. This amount is called the *per-patient per-month payment*. Patients pay a premium to the insurance plan and are assigned to a contracted physician. Patients must seek care only from their assigned physician. When the patient sees his physician for care, a small copayment is typically paid at that visit. The physician receives the per-patient per-month payment every month no matter how many times she sees each individual patient. Aside from the copayment paid by the patient, no extra fees are paid to the physician when she sees these patients.

capitated plan
healthcare plan in which providers are paid a set fee per month for each member patient

Although the financial incentive may seem to be for the physician to limit the number of visits with each patient because she is only receiving a small copayment each time the patient is seen, there is an additional risk the providers must bear. If the physician is unable to provide the care needed by a particular patient and must refer the patient to another provider, some or all of that cost must be paid by the patient's primary care provider, not the insurance carrier. For this reason, it is in the physician's (as well as the patient's) best interest to provide preventive care to these patients in order to keep them healthy and out of the hospital or in need of specialty care services.

Critical Thinking 14.7 ?

What are some of the pros and cons for the patient for each of the insurance plan types discussed in the previous sections?

COBRA Coverage

When employees have been covered under group insurance and leave employment, they may have the opportunity to continue the group coverage at their own expense. The premium is the same as that for other members of the group, but because the employer has typically been paying a large portion of the employee's premium during employment, employees may be surprised at the cost of the premium. The group premium is typically less than a premium for an individual policy, and for patients who have chronic conditions that require ongoing care and medications, going without health insurance coverage may be far more expensive than the premium.

COBRA
Consolidated Omnibus Budget Reconciliation Act; this act gives workers and their families the ability to continue health insurance coverage for a limited period of time after loss of a job

The federal Consolidated Omnibus Reconciliation Act (**COBRA**) requires employers to extend health insurance coverage, at group rates, usually for up to 18 months, to any employee who is laid off, quits, or is fired, except under certain circumstances. Congress passed COBRA health benefit provisions in 1986 to provide certain former employees, retirees, spouses, former spouses, and dependent children the right to temporarily continue health coverage at group rates. To be eligible for COBRA coverage, employees must have been enrolled in their employers' health plans when they worked and those health plans must continue to be in effect for active employees.

COBRA coverage is available to employees who work for employers with 20 or more employees. Both full- and part-time employees are counted to determine whether a plan is subject to COBRA. A qualified beneficiary is typically an individual who was covered by the employer's group health insurance plan on the day before a qualifying event. This beneficiary can be the employee, the employee's spouse, and the retired employee's dependent children or any child born to or placed for adoption with a covered employee during the period of COBRA coverage.

To qualify for COBRA coverage, the qualified beneficiary must have experienced a qualifying event. Qualifying events for employees include:

- The voluntary or involuntary termination of employment for reasons other than gross misconduct
- A reduction in the number of hours of employment resulting in the termination of health insurance coverage.

Qualifying events for spouses include:

- The covered employee becoming entitled to Medicare coverage
- Divorce or legal separation of the covered employee
- Death of the covered employee.

Qualifying events for dependent children include:

- Loss of dependent child status under the plan rules
- Voluntary or involuntary termination of the covered employee's employment for any reason other than gross misconduct
- Reduction in the hours worked by the covered employee resulting in the termination of health insurance coverage
- Covered employee becoming entitled to Medicare
- Divorce or legal separation of the covered employee
- Death of the covered employee.

To be eligible for COBRA coverage, a qualified beneficiary must notify the employer's plan administrator of a qualifying event within 60 days after divorce or legal separation or a child's ceasing to be a dependent under plan rules. Employers must notify the plan administrator of a qualifying event within 30 days after an employee's death, termination, reduced hours of employment, or entitlement to Medicare.

INDIVIDUAL HEALTH INSURANCE POLICIES

Individual health insurance policies are those that individuals purchase directly from an insurance carrier. These plans are typically the most expensive forms of coverage because group rates are unavailable. The benefits of individual plans are often not as good as those for group policies, resulting in higher deductibles and other out-of-pocket expenses. The minimum level of benefit package for individual insurance policies is regulated by each state and, in some states, only a few companies offer individual policies due to restrictive requirements. Employees who have been on a COBRA plan can convert to an individual policy with the same insurance company when the COBRA benefits expire, but the group rates and benefits will no longer apply.

Flexible Spending and Healthcare Savings Accounts

Flexible spending accounts (FSAs) are also called *healthcare savings accounts*. These accounts allow individuals to set aside a portion of their pretaxed wages to pay for certain out-of-pocket healthcare expenses. Money from flexible spending accounts can be used to pay for expenses not covered by health insurance such as:

- Deductibles and copays
- Prescription drugs and medical supplies
- Dental services, dentures, and orthodontics
- Eyeglasses, contacts, solutions, and eye surgery
- Chiropractic services
- Psychiatric care and psychologist's fees
- Smoking cessation programs
- Weight loss programs
- Exercise programs, including gym fees

flexible spending account (FSA) account into which employees place pretax earnings for projected medical expenses

Money set aside in flexible spending accounts in any given year must be spent by a certain date, typically March 15 of the following year, or the money is forfeited. Figure ■ 14-6 explains how a flexible spending account works.

Margaret McIlroy works for an employer that offers to put Margaret's pretax earnings into a flexible spending account for her health care expenses. Margaret has a health insurance plan through her employer that has a $500 deductible and then covers 80% of her care.

Margaret visits her physician for an office call and lab work. The cost of the visit is $165. During the office call, Margaret gets a prescription that costs $55. Margaret's health insurance policy does not include a prescription benefit.

Cost of physician visit and lab work:	$165
Cost of prescription:	55
Total	$220

Margaret has an annual deductible of $500, so her insurance plan will pay $0 for the physician visit. Because she does not have a prescription drug benefit, Margaret's insurance company will pay $0 for the prescription. Margaret pays the full amount to her physician and the full amount for the prescription. She submits her receipts to her employer. The employer reimburses Margaret $220 out of Margaret's flexible spending account.

FIGURE ■ 14-6   Example of how a flexible spending account works.

CONSUMER-DIRECTED HEALTHCARE PLANS

The newest type of insurance plan, which is becoming increasingly popular in response to rising healthcare costs, is the **consumer-directed healthcare plan**. These plans place consumers in charge of how their healthcare dollars are spent, rendering those consumers more likely to ask questions about, or research the need for, their health-related services. Just as with traditional employer-paid plans, employers who support consumer-directed healthcare plans retain a certain amount of money from employees' paychecks to fund healthcare premiums.

consumer-directed healthcare plan health insurance plans that place patients in charge of how their healthcare dollars are spent

Generally, a consumer-driven health plan includes a three-tier structure of payment for healthcare: a tax-exempt health savings account or medical savings account that an individual uses to pay for health expenses up to a certain amount, a high-deductible health insurance policy that pays for expenses over the deductible, and a gap between those two in which the individual pays any healthcare expenses out of their own pocket.

These out-of-pocket expenses may be eligible for reimbursement through a flexible spending account. Accounts are administered by insurance companies, which process claims and issue payments. Employees receive lists of covered services, just as with traditional plans. From the medical provider's point of view, consumer-directed healthcare plans work much the same as traditional health insurance plans. Patients pay any portion not covered by the healthcare plan.

Elective Procedures

elective procedure
procedure that is generally considered not medically necessary

Elective procedures are those that are generally considered not medically necessary. These procedures are those that the patient wishes to undergo, but may not have a medical reason for doing so. The most common examples are aesthetic procedures, such as cosmetic surgery. A patient who wishes to undergo breast augmentation surgery, or to have a surgical procedure to reduce the size of her nose, would be considered a patient undergoing elective procedures. These procedures are often not covered by health insurance policies because many policies exclude procedures that are not considered medically necessary. In these cases, patients will need to self-pay for medical services.

Critical Thinking 14.8 ?

How would the medical office manager's conversation about medical fees differ when speaking with a patient undergoing a noncovered elective procedure and another who is undergoing a covered procedure?

Prescription Drug Coverage

Most insurance plans today have some form of prescription drug coverage. Prescription medications are often very expensive, and name brands are often far more costly than their generic counterparts. Pharmaceutical representatives often visit medical offices with the intent of meeting with physicians (Figure ■ 14-7). These representatives showcase the latest drugs on the market and, as a marketing tactic, they will often leave samples for physicians to dispense to patients. By using these free samples, physicians are able to give medications to patients on a short-term basis. This can be very helpful to patients who face a financial barrier when purchasing expensive prescription medications. Physicians may also use these drug samples for patients as a trial before writing a prescription for the medication.

Some clinics do not permit pharmaceutical representatives to visit with physicians and leave sample medications. These clinics prohibit these visits because they do not want physicians hearing about medications from pharmaceutical representatives who do not have pharmacy or clinical degrees. They may also feel that by leaving free samples of expensive name brand drugs, there is a higher likelihood physicians will prescribe these name brand medications, instead of less expensive, generic brand medicines. Each clinic's management staff should determine if allowing pharmaceutical representatives to meet with physicians is useful to the physicians and the patients they serve.

formulary
tiered list of drugs covered by an insurance company

Medical insurance plans typically have a **formulary**, which is a list of drugs they will cover. Usually the formulary is subdivided into two or more tiers with each tier having a different level of coverage (Figure ■ 14-8). For example, tier 1 may include most generic drugs and perhaps a few brand name drugs that have no generic equivalent. Patients might have a small copayment, perhaps only a few dollars, for tier 1 drugs. Tier 2 may include preferred name brand drugs, ones for which there is no generic equivalent. Patients would have a slightly higher copayment for those drugs. Tier 3 may include brand name drugs that have generic equivalents or similar brand name drugs that cost less. Patients would have the highest out-of-pocket expense for these drugs, perhaps as high as 50 percent coinsurance.

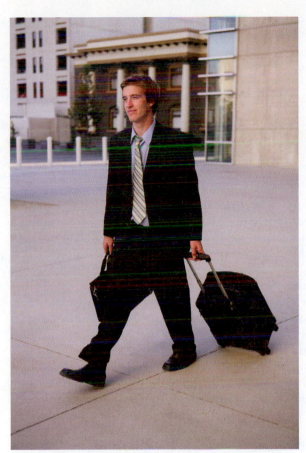

FIGURE ■ 14-7 Pharmaceutical representatives visit medical offices to speak to physicians about the newest drugs on the market.
Source: Nruboc/Dreamstime.com.

Tier 1
Penicillin G Sodium
Penicillin V Potassium
Trimox

Tier 2
Avelox (tablet)
Timentin

Tier 3
Avelox (solution)
Penicillin G Procain
Piperacillin Sodium
Zosyn

FIGURE ■ 14-8 Sample tiered drug formulary for antibiotics.

Some drugs may not be on the formulary at all. Patients need to present evidence of medical necessity in order to receive coverage for nonformulary drugs. Medical office managers can advocate for patients if their plans do not cover a specific drug the provider prescribed. The manager, or her staff, can help identify potentially similar medications from the formulary or from a lower tier of the formulary that the provider could evaluate and consider prescribing for the patient. This could create a financial savings to the patient while maintaining safe and high-quality care for the patient.

Most drug plans are administered separately from the main insurance plan. Patients usually will have a separate deductible and different copayments or coinsurance amounts than their health insurance plan for medical care. This can be confusing to patients who think they have met their medical deductible, only to discover there is an additional drug deductible as well. In addition, prescription deductibles are not part of the costs considered when determining stop loss benefits.

Some drug plans provide a mail-order option for **maintenance medications**, which are medications patients take on a long-term basis to treat a chronic condition such as high blood pressure, arthritis, or a heart condition. The mail-order plan may allow patients to order 3 months of medications for the cost of two copayments. This saves the patient four copayments over the course of a year for each medication ordered in this manner. To fill prescriptions in this manner, the mail-order pharmacy will require the prescription to be written to dispense 90 days of medication at a time, with three refills for the remainder of the year. Medical office managers should be sure their staff are trained on this task so that the prescription can be written in the proper format.

maintenance medications medications patients take on a long-term basis to treat a chronic condition such as high blood pressure, arthritis, or a heart condition

Medicare

Medicare was established in 1965, and is a federal program that provided health insurance for approximately 47.5 million people in 2010. Of that number, 40 million were over the age of 65. The remaining people either had disabilities or were being treated for a chronic kidney disease. As previously discussed, Medicare coverage is available for people who are age 65 or older, those who have been disabled for more than 24 months, and patients with end-stage kidney disease.

As of 2010, Medicare costs accounted for 14 percent of the federal budget in the United States. According to the Kaiser Group, the number of people on Medicare is expected to rise from 46 million to 78 million between 2010 and 2030. Given this projection, it is expected that by the year 2019, the Medicare Part A Hospital Insurance Fund will have insufficient funds to pay for full benefits.

The Medicare program is administered by the Centers for Medicare and Medicaid Services (CMS), formerly known as the Health Care Financing Administration (HCFA). One of CMS's obligations is to keep healthcare providers informed about proper Medicare billing. To accomplish this, CMS keeps up-to-date information on their website, www.cms.gov.

Medicare claims must be submitted within 365 days of the date of service. Claims submitted after that date will be subject to a 10 percent penalty, unless the healthcare provider can prove that late submission was due to factors beyond her control. The final submission deadline for claims to be considered at all is determined by a unique timetable based on the Medicare fiscal year. To simplify, services provided from January 1 to September 30 must be billed by the end of the next calendar year. Services provided between October 1 and December 31 have until the end of two calendar years to be billed. This schedule is longer than most private insurance carriers allow.

The Medicare program has major component parts called Part A (hospitalization coverage), Part B (provider coverage), Part C (Medicare Advantage), and Part D (prescription drug coverage).

NATIONAL PROVIDER IDENTIFIER

national provider identifier (NPI)
a unique, 10-digit number assigned to healthcare providers by the Centers for Medicare and Medicaid Services

A **national provider identifier (NPI)** is a unique, 10-digit number assigned to healthcare providers by the CMS. This number replaces the unique provider identification number (UPIN) formerly assigned by CMS. NPI use was mandated as part of HIPAA administrative simplifications language. As of May 2007, all healthcare providers were required to use NPIs on all patient billing forms.

NPI numbers must be used by all covered entities. A covered entity is any provider who submits claims to Medicare. Specialists who receive referrals from other physicians must place not only their own NPI number on the CMS claim form but also the NPI number and name of the referring physician. Not only does each provider have an NPI, but each facility or medical group that bills for individual providers has a facility or group NPI. Both the rendering provider NPI and group NPI will be entered on the CMS claim form in specific locations.

All members covered by Medicare receive a Medicare identification card that lists the name, identification number of the member, and the plans (Part A, Part B, or both), and effective dates that apply to the member (Figure ■ 14-9).

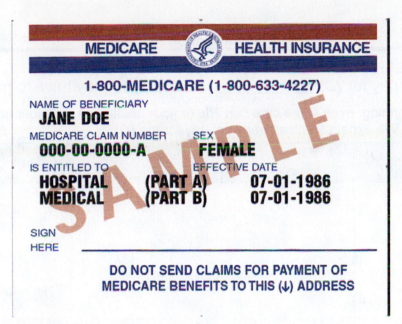

FIGURE ■ 14-9 A Medicare ID card.

MEDICARE PART A

Part A Medicare coverage is hospital insurance that covers most care for patients who have been hospitalized for up to 90 days in a given period of time; patients in a **skilled nursing facility**; patients who receive medical care at home; patients with life-limiting illnesses that require **hospice** care; patients who require psychiatric treatment for a certain period of time; and patients on **respite care**.

Citizens who receive Social Security benefits are automatically enrolled in Medicare Part A, which does not require premiums. Deductibles and coinsurance, however, apply to most services in Part A.

MEDICARE PART B

Medicare Part B coverage applies to services such as physician care, therapy, and laboratory testing. Because Part B is voluntary, members must pay a premium to enroll. This requirement was enacted as of January 1, 2007, and premiums are income based. As of 2011, the standard monthly premium was $115.40, though this premium fluctuates based on the member's income level.

Patients are subject to out-of-pocket expenses under Part B. The annual deduction as of 2011 was $162. This deductible increases every year and patients are also required to pay a 20 percent coinsurance for medical services received.

Physicians may determine whether or not they want to participate in the Medicare program. A participating provider, also known as a PAR, must accept the Medicare fee schedule amounts as payment in full for their services. If the Medicare allowed amount is lower than the billed amount, the participating provider must write off the difference between the fees. PARs must bill Medicare for all services rendered, even those services that they know are not covered by Medicare. PARs are also required to **accept assignment** on all claims, which means they accept the Medicare allowed amount and the payment is sent directly to the provider. Approximately 95 percent of all physicians participate in the Medicare program.

ADVANCE BENEFICIARY NOTICE

One important aspect to be aware of when billing Medicare is a form called the **advance beneficiary notice (ABN)** or **waiver** (Figure ■ 14-10). The ABN must be signed by patients before those patients receive services that may be denied payment by Medicare. If physicians recommend services that may be declined payment by Medicare, the ABN

---

skilled nursing facility
a facility for long-term care or other care facility where the patient must be monitored by nursing staff on a regular basis

hospice
comfort care provided to patients who have 6 or fewer months to live

respite care
care provided in a skilled nursing facility on a short-term basis for patients who are otherwise treated at home

accept assignment
when a physician agrees to accept the amount approved by the insurance company as payment in full for a given service

advance beneficiary notice (ABN)
a form patients sign agreeing to pay for services that may be denied by Medicare; also referred to as a **waiver**

(A) **Notifier(s):**

(B) **Patient Name:**   *(C)* **Identification Number:**

ADVANCE BENEFICIARY NOTICE OF NONCOVERAGE (ABN)

<u>NOTE</u>: If Medicare doesn't pay for *(D)*_____ below, you may have to pay.

Medicare does not pay for everything, even some care that you or your health care provider have good reason to think you need. We expect Medicare may not pay for the *(D)*_____ below.

*(D)*_____	*(E)* Reason Medicare May Not Pay:	*(F)* Estimated Cost:

WHAT YOU NEED TO DO NOW:

- Read this notice, so you can make an informed decision about your care.
- Ask us any questions that you may have after you finish reading.
- Choose an option below about whether to receive the *(D)*_____ listed above.
  Note: If you choose Option 1 or 2, we may help you to use any other insurance that you might have, but Medicare cannot require us to do this.

(G) **OPTIONS:**   **Check only one box. We cannot choose a box for you.**

❑ **OPTION 1.** I want the *(D)*_____ listed above. You may ask to be paid now, but I also want Medicare billed for an official decision on payment, which is sent to me on a Medicare Summary Notice (MSN). I understand that if Medicare doesn't pay, I am responsible for payment, but **I can appeal to Medicare** by following the directions on the MSN. If Medicare does pay, you will refund any payments I made to you, less co-pays or deductibles.

❑ **OPTION 2.** I want the *(D)*_____ listed above, but do not bill Medicare. You may ask to be paid now as I am responsible for payment. **I cannot appeal if Medicare is not billed**.

❑ **OPTION 3.** I don't want the *(D)*_____ listed above. I understand with this choice I am **not** responsible for payment, and **I cannot appeal to see if Medicare would pay**.

(H) **Additional Information:**

This notice gives our opinion, not an official Medicare decision. If you have other questions on this notice or Medicare billing, call **1-800-MEDICARE** (1-800-633-4227/**TTY**: 1-877-486-2048).

Signing below means that you have received and understand this notice. You also receive a copy.

(I) **Signature:**	*(J)* **Date:**

According to the Paperwork Reduction Act of 1995, no persons are required to respond to a collection of information unless it displays a valid OMB control number. The valid OMB control number for this information collection is 0938-0566. The time required to complete this information collection is estimated to average 7 minutes per response, including the time to review instructions, search existing data resources, gather the data needed, and complete and review the information collection. If you have comments concerning the accuracy of the time estimate or suggestions for improving this form, please write to: CMS, 7500 Security Boulevard, Attn: PRA Reports Clearance Officer, Baltimore, Maryland 21244-1850.

Form CMS-R-131 (03/08)   Form Approved OMB No. 0938-0566

FIGURE ■ 14-10 Advance beneficiary notice (ABN).

gives the patient notice of this possible denial, and the opportunity to refuse the non-covered service. If the patient did not understand and sign an ABN form prior to receiving a noncovered service, the provider may not charge the patient for the noncovered service. The medical office manager should clearly explain the ABN and the noncovered services to the patient. A copy of the signed ABN should be given to each patient and the original kept in each patient's file.

MEDICARE PART C

Medicare Part C is managed care and its plans are known as Medicare Advantage plans. Formerly known as Medicare + Choice, these plans are offered by private insurance companies and replace Parts A, B, and D. The benefit to the patient is potentially more comprehensive care at the same or lower cost than Medicare. The disadvantage, as with any managed care plan, is that the choice of providers is limited. As of 2010, 10.1 million individuals were enrolled in a Medicare Advantage plan. This number rose from 5.3 million in 2003.

Patients keep their Medicare identification card and receive an additional card from the Medicare Advantage plan. Because patients may not understand the difference between the two cards, it is a good practice for medical office managers to ask patients if they belong to a Medicare Advantage plan or have another identification card. When billing, the Medicare Advantage plan is billed, not Medicare. When patients have secondary coverage, the medical office manager will bill the secondary plan after the Medicare Advantage plan has made a payment or decision.

Many physicians and clinics today are finding it difficult to make a profit seeing patients who are covered under Medicare Part B instead of a Medicare Advantage plan. Because the reimbursement from Medicare Part B is far lower than that paid by Medicare Advantage plans, many physicians and clinics encourage their Medicare Part B patients to move to a managed care Medicare Advantage plan. As of 2008, the government was paying 113 percent more for beneficiaries enrolled in Medicare Advantage than for beneficiaries enrolled in traditional Medicare.

MEDICARE PART D

Medicare Part D was introduced in January 2006. It is a prescription drug plan. Members may choose to purchase Part D coverage, which covers both name brand and generic prescription drugs at participating pharmacies. The Part D plans are provided by private companies. Not all drugs are covered under every plan, so patients should review various plans and determine which one covers their most common or expensive medications. Medical office managers can assist patients by providing them with complete medication lists. As of 2008, 90 percent of all Medicare beneficiaries had prescription drug coverage.

The Medicare website for patients, www.medicare.gov, has a prescription drug plan finder tool to assist patients to evaluate their options for coverage. Medicare Part D has an annual deductible, copayments or coinsurance, and a maximum benefit level.

Medicare Part D enrollees have several mail-order pharmacy options from which to choose that typically offer low out-of-pocket expenses. Enrollees should view this option cautiously, however. It may be less than ideal for patients on short-term medications, like antibiotics, because delivery may take a week or more.

SECONDARY INSURANCE WITH MEDICARE

Plans that cover the out-of-pocket expenses incurred are known as "Medigap" or Medicare supplemental plans. These plans are regulated by CMS and not all Medigap plans cover the same expenses. The basic benefit is payment of the patient's coinsurance, though some plans also cover yearly deductibles, skilled nursing facility coinsurance, foreign travel, and other specific expenses. Medigap plans are billed after Medicare makes a determination. These supplemental plans are often billed directly by Medicare at the time the decision for payment has been made. Payment from the supplemental coverage is typically made directly to the treating provider.

MEDICARE PATIENTS WHO ARE CURRENTLY EMPLOYED

At times, workers today are staying in the workforce beyond the age of retirement. This means that some patients may have Medicare coverage as well as a commercial health insurance plan through the patient's employer. In these cases, the patient's commercial health insurance plan is the primary insurance plan and Medicare is secondary. In all other cases where the patient has Medigap coverage, Medicare is the primary payer of the covered claims.

PROVIDERS PARTICIPATING IN THE MEDICARE PLAN

Any healthcare provider who wishes to participate with Medicare must file an application with CMS. This application process is similar to that of any other managed care plan. Medical office managers should stay current with the approved Medicare fee schedule, which is updated each year. This fee schedule may be found on the CMS website.

e-billing
electronic transmission of medical claims to insurers

As of 2005, Medicare required all medical offices to file medical claims electronically. This process is known as **e-billing**. Clinics that have no more than 10 full-time employees are allowed to continue to bill Medicare claims on paper.

Medicare prefers to pay providers for claims using electronic funds transfers. This is set up by filling out an Electronic Funds Transfer Authorization Agreement form. This form is returned to Medicare along with a copy of a voided check or deposit slip. After Medicare receives this information, it will begin directly depositing funds into the provider or facility's account within 3 weeks.

Medicare maintains a nationwide directory of participating providers. A search for a provider can be performed by state or specialty. This list contains the provider's name, specialty, education, residency, gender, foreign languages spoken by the physician, hospital affiliation, and practice location.

Medicare provides a variety of in-person as well as online workshops for providers to learn more about topics such as payment notices and reimbursements, the appeals process, using the Medicare website, and updates on changes that apply to physicians or medical facilities.

Critical Thinking 14.10 ?

In order for patients to better understand their Medicare coverage, some medical clinics host no-cost classes for patients who are new to Medicare coverage to attend. How do you think these classes would be beneficial to the patient? How would they be beneficial to the clinic?

Medicaid

Medicaid is a health benefit program for low-income patients. Like Medicare, Medicaid is run by CMS, although each state dictates the amount and type of services Medicaid covers. The federal government provides funds to every state, and every state then adds its own funds to cover qualified enrollees. As of 2009, nearly 48 million people were covered by Medicaid in the United States. With the expansion of the Patient Protection and Affordable Care Act, that number is expected to rise substantially. Every state runs its own Medicaid program, so each state's identification card will differ from that of other states (Figure ■ 14-11).

Medicaid reimbursement to healthcare providers is extremely low in most states, which leads to providers limiting the number of Medicaid patients they will see for care. Any healthcare provider who would like to accept Medicaid-covered patients must apply to become Medicaid accredited in his or her state. As part of this process, which is very similar to any other managed care application process, Medicaid provides physicians with fee schedules of covered expenses.

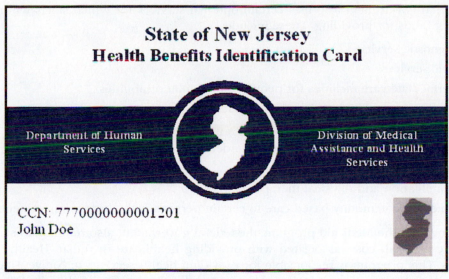

FIGURE ▪ 14-11 Medicaid coupon from New Jersey.

Medicaid programs offer coverage on a month-to-month basis in most states, which means Medicaid may not cover a patient one month just because Medicaid covered the patient in a previous month. It is vital for medical office managers to know the Medicaid rules and regulations in their state as they apply to the various practice types and to ask Medicaid-covered patients for proof of coverage by the plan.

MEDICARE AS PRIMARY, MEDICAID AS SECONDARY

Low-income elderly patients or those with disabilities often have both Medicare and Medicaid coverage. Medicare is always the primary carrier in these cases, and Medicaid is the secondary. Often, Medicare's reimbursement rate is higher than what Medicaid will allow, resulting in no Medicaid payment. The CMS estimates that approximately 6.5 million individuals are receiving benefits from both Medicare and Medicaid.

COVERED MEDICAID SERVICES

Although each state determines who will be covered by Medicaid, what type of services will be covered, and the reimbursement provided for the covered services, the federal government requires certain basic services to be provided in order for the state to qualify for federal funding. These services include:

- Inpatient hospital services
- Outpatient hospital services
- Prenatal care
- Vaccines for children
- Physician services
- Nursing facility services for persons ages 21 or older
- Family planning services and supplies
- Rural health clinic services
- Home healthcare for persons eligible for skilled nursing services
- Laboratory and radiology services
- Pediatric and family nurse practitioner services
- Nurse-midwife services
- Early and periodic screening, diagnostic, and treatment services for children under age 21.

The federal government also lists certain optional services for which states will receive matching funds for providing. These include:

- Diagnostic services
- Clinic services
- Intermediate care facilities for people with mental disabilities
- Prescribed drugs and prosthetic devices
- Optometrist services and eyeglasses
- Nursing facility services for children under age 21
- Transportation services
- Rehabilitation and physical therapy services
- Home and community-based care to certain persons with chronic impairments.

Along with the Medicaid program, the federal government also reimburses states for 100 percent of all costs associated with providing healthcare in Indian Health Service facilities. This program is responsible for providing health services to Native Americans and Alaskan Natives. The federal government also provides financial assistance to the 12 states that provide the highest number of emergency services to undocumented aliens.

Critical Thinking 14.11 ?

Imagine you have a patient who has just moved to your area from out of state. The patient was covered under the Medicaid program in the previous state and tells you he knows the service he needs is covered because it was covered in the previous state. How do you address this with the patient?

STATE CHILDREN'S HEALTH INSURANCE PROGRAM

Children's Health Insurance Program (CHIP)
a program created to cover children who do not have another form of health insurance coverage

The **Children's Health Insurance Program (CHIP),** formerly known as the State Children's Health Insurance Program (SCHIP), was created by the Balanced Budget Act of 1997. This program was created to cover children who did not have another form of health insurance coverage. Similar to basic Medicaid, CHIP was designed to function as a federal/state joint program. Children within families who earned too much income to qualify for Medicaid, but not enough income to purchase other health insurance, are covered by the CHIP program.

Beginning in October 1997, the federal government provided $24 billion in funds over 5 years to help states expand healthcare coverage to the estimated 5 million uninsured children who fall into the category targeted by CHIP. States can choose from three categories in order to comply with the CHIP program:

1. Use the federal CHIP funds to expand Medicaid eligibility to children who did not previously qualify.
2. Design a separate children's health insurance fund that is entirely separate from Medicaid.
3. Combine both the Medicaid and the separate children's health insurance fund.

Every state had an approved CHIP program in place by October 1999. As of 2006, about 6.9 million children were covered under the CHIP program nationwide.

TRICARE

TRICARE, formerly called CHAMPUS, is a federal program that provides healthcare benefits to families of current and retired military personnel. The active-duty service member is called a sponsor and eligible family members are called beneficiaries. To be eligible for TRICARE, sponsors and beneficiaries must be enrolled in the Defense Enrollment Eligibility Reporting System.

TRICARE offers three benefit types:

1. TRICARE Standard, a fee-for-service plan
2. TRICARE Extra, a PPO
3. TRICARE Prime, an HMO.

Active-duty families on TRICARE Standard and TRICARE Extra and most retirees will usually owe copayments and deductibles. Medical office managers should be aware that TRICARE's deductible year begins on October 1, rather than January 1 as is common with most other insurance plans. All TRICARE enrollees are automatically enrolled in TRICARE Standard and TRICARE Extra. TRICARE Prime is an optional plan in which enrollees must specifically enroll. Some patients have TRICARE for Life, a plan that acts as secondary insurance coverage for patients over age 65. For primary insurance, these patients have Medicare. TRICARE requires preauthorization for medical services, and patients must use in-network providers.

TRICARE requires participating providers to submit claims within 60 days of the date care was provided. Non-network providers have up to 1 year from the date the care was provided to submit claims.

CHAMPVA

The Civilian Health and Medical Program of the Department of Veterans Affairs (CHAMPVA) program is a federal program that covers the healthcare expenses of the families of veterans with total, permanent, service-related, covered disabilities and the spouses and dependent children of veterans who died in the line of duty. Patients with CHAMPVA coverage may use any civilian healthcare provider, without preauthorization.

If a patient has other coverage besides CHAMPVA, the other coverage should be billed first. By law, CHAMPVA is always the secondary payer, except to Medicaid, State Victims of Crime Compensation, and supplemental CHAMPVA policies. Once the primary insurance carrier has made payment, a CMS claim form is sent to CHAMPVA along with a copy of the primary carrier's explanation of benefits.

CHAMPVA requires preauthorization in the following areas only:

- Organ and bone marrow transplants
- Hospice care
- Dental care
- Durable medical equipment worth more than $300
- Most mental health or substance abuse services.

Insurance Coverage for Accidental Injuries

When patients are involved in a non–work-related accident, third-party liability insurance may cover medical bills. Most businesses, homeowners, and vehicle owners have liability insurance to cover injuries that occur on their properties or in vehicle accidents (Figure ■ 14-12). For example, when patients are injured in an automobile accident, the automobile owner's liability insurance typically covers the patients' medical expenses.

State laws vary regarding how automobile insurance is handled, but many states have no-fault coverage. Under this type of coverage, the injured person's own auto insurance pays the medical bills, even if someone else was at fault. This is paid under the personal injury protection (PIP) portion of the injured person's policy. The automobile insurance company then works with the at-fault party's insurance company to recover the expenses. If the injured person does not have PIP coverage, or expenses exceed policy limits, then the at-fault party's insurance is billed. If the injured party files a lawsuit against the at-fault party, then medical bills may be sent to the patient's attorney. In these cases, the provider may need to wait until the case is settled to receive payment, which can take

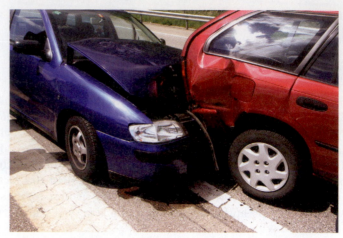

FIGURE ■ 14-12 Injuries due to car accidents are typically paid by car insurance, rather than personal insurance.
Source: Exinocactus/Dreamstime.com.

several years. The medical office manager should ask the practice's own attorney to file a lien against the at-fault party, which establishes the provider's legal right to be paid upon settlement.

If payment from a third-party liability company is delayed by more than a specified number of days, such as 45 or 60 days, some insurers will pay and pursue. This means they will accept claims for services related to injuries, pay them, then pursue the third-party liability insurance company for reimbursement.

When injured patients are already established in the practice, a new medical record and a new financial account should be created specifically for treatment related to an accident. This can be done for both paper as well as electronic medical records. This practice helps clarify what services are accident related and what services are a part of a patient's ongoing healthcare. It also makes it easier to provide copies of accident-relevant records to the insurance carrier. When registering patients involved in an accident, medical office managers should instruct receptionists to gather as much information as possible regarding the accident, the patient's automobile coverage if an auto accident, the at-fault party's name and insurance information, as well as the patient's private health insurance or Medicare coverage. While this information can be confusing to collect and organize, thoroughness up front will make it easier to bill and collect for services later.

Critical Thinking 14.12 ?

Patients who do not have liability insurance for their accident-related claim may use their own health insurance policy to cover their needed care. In a case such as this, do you think the medical office should still choose to keep a separate medical chart for the patient's accident-related care? Why or why not?

Disability Insurance

Disability insurance reimburses a patient for lost wages due to a non-work-related disability that prevents the individual form working. Benefits are based on a percentage of employees' wages, often 66 percent, because benefits are not subject to income tax. Lost wages due to work-related disability are covered by workers' compensation insurance; lost wages due to a disability related to an automobile or other liability accident are covered by liability insurance.

With only a few exceptions, disability insurance does not pay for medical treatment; therefore, medical office managers will not typically bill a disability plan for medical services. However, medical office managers may need to assist patients who are applying for disability coverage or benefits by providing information from the medical record regarding a patient's past health history or current disability. Even though patients have disability insurance, they may not have medical coverage due to their employment status and may not be able to afford or are not eligible for individual health insurance policies.

Processing Claims

The first step in properly reimbursing insurance claims is to obtain accurate information. Many medical offices ask patients for their health insurance information over the telephone, before the patients' first visits. Other offices simply ask patients for their insurance type over the telephone, then ask those patients to bring their insurance card to their first office visit. Medical offices that have a robust website may offer patients the option of registering for appointments online. This service will often include the ability for patients to enter their insurance information, and to verify that the facility is contracted with the patients' insurance carriers.

MEDICAL CLAIMS FOR INJURIES

Any patient who has a medical claim for an injury, whether through workers' compensation or other liability insurance, will have a claim number and a claims manager or department to handle the claim. At the beginning of the patient's care in the medical office, the medical office manager should locate the name and phone number of the claims manager. Having contact information readily available will allow the office to easily contact the claims manager in the event the physician orders tests or procedures that require preauthorization.

PATIENT REGISTRATION

Each new patient in the medical office should complete a registration from (Figure ■ 14-13) that is verified at each visit and updated annually. Before releasing private patient information to insurance carriers, medical office managers must obtain signed authorizations from patients. To do so otherwise is to violate HIPAA regulations for patient confidentiality. Insurance claim forms give patients' names, addresses, birth dates, diagnoses, and types of treatment—all highly protected patient information.

After obtaining pertinent patient information, medical office managers must identify the name and birth date of the insured. When the patient is the spouse or child of the insured, the medical office manager must ask the patient for additional information. The manager should know if the patient is covered by more than one plan. If so, the manager will then have to determine which plan is primary and which is secondary.

Either way, medical office managers must photocopy both sides of patients' insurance identification cards (Figure ■ 14-14) when patients arrive for their first visits. The front of an insurance card typically carries the name and identification number of the insured or member. Each patient is uniquely identified by a member identification number assigned by the insurance company. Patients have a different number for each separate insurance plan they have. HIPAA originally made provision for a unique patient identification number that would be the same for all insurance companies, but concerns about privacy and identity theft have put this on hold indefinitely.

In today's world of identity theft, most insurance plans no longer use Social Security numbers for identification. Instead, member numbers are commonly composed of an alphabetic character, followed by numbers, or a combination of letters and numbers. Each identification number is specific to the policyholder.

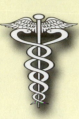

Victory Medical Center
4100 SW Highway 6
Victorville, WA 12345
(509) 555-9832

Patient Name: _____

　　　　　Last Name　　　　　　　　　　　First Name　　　　　　　　　Middle Initial

Address: _____

　　　　　Street　　　　　　　　　　　　City　　　　　　　State　　　Zip

Home Phone: _____ Work Phone:_____

Mobile Phone: _____ Birthdate:_____

Social Security Number: _____ Age:_____

Sex: _____ Marital Status: S M D W Children: _____

How do you prefer to be addressed? _____

Spouse's Name:_____

Primary Care Physician: _____ Phone No:_____

Name of Person Responsible for Bill: _____

Relationship to Patient: _____ Phone No: _____

Address of Person Responsible for Bill: _____

Patient's Employer: _____ Phone No: _____

Occupation: _____

Spouse's Employer: _____ Phone No:_____

Occupation: _____

INSURANCE INFORMATION

Primary Insurance: _____ Policy No: _____

Name of Policyholder: _____ Birthdate: _____

SS#: _____ Relationship to Insured: _____

Secondary Insurance: _____ Policy No: _____

Name of Policyholder: _____ Birthdate: _____

If Injured: Date:_____ Place: _____

Claim Number: _____ Nature or Cause of Injury: _____

Employer at Time of Injury: _____ Phone No: _____

EMERGENCY INFORMATION

In case of emergency, local friend or relative to be notified (not living at same address)

Name:_____ Relationship to Patient: _____

Address: _____ Phone No: _____

I hereby authorize the healthcare professionals in this clinic to diagnose and treat my condition. I clearly understand and agree that all services rendered me are charged directly to me and that I am personally responsible for payment. I agree that I am responsible for all bills incurred at this clinic. I hereby authorize assignment of my insurance rights and benefits directly to the provider for services rendered. I also authorize the healthcare professionals to discuss my care with other health care providers who I am currently treating with.

_____　　　_____

Patient's Signature　　　　　　　　　Date　　　Parent or Guardian Signature　　　　Date

FIGURE ■ 14-13　Sample new patient registration form.

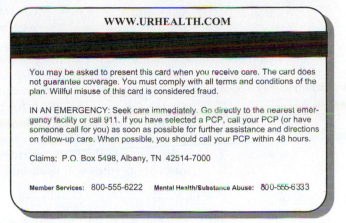

FIGURE ■ 14-14 The front and back of an insurance identification card.

Health insurance cards include telephone numbers for members and providers to contact customer service with questions. These numbers may be used by the medical office manager to verify a patient's insurance benefits. The insurance card will also contain a **payer number**. This is the number that medical offices must include on an electronic claim to identify the insurance company to whom the claim is directed.

payer number
the number that medical offices must include on an electronic claim to identify the insurance company to whom the claim is directed

Critical Thinking 14.13 ?

Many medical offices today offer patients the option of completing registration forms online, before arriving in the office for their first visit. What benefits do you think this allows for the medical office staff? How does this option benefit the patient?

VERIFYING ELIGIBILITY

After obtaining insurance information from patients, medical office managers should verify coverage with the insurance company. There are two common ways to verify patients' insurance eligibility. The first is to call the customer service telephone number listed on the patient's insurance identification card. Once customer service has been reached, the medical office manager should supply the patient's insurance identification number and birth date. Because changes to insurance policies may not be reflected in real time, the customer service representative will tell the office manager that the information given is not a guarantee of benefits and that final determination will be made when a claim is received. The second way to verify insurance benefits is to use computer software to contact the insurance company and verify patients' benefits online. The second way is much faster, but some medical offices do not possess this technology.

COORDINATING INSURANCE BENEFITS

Patients may be covered by more than one insurance plan. Most often this is because spouses each have a group health plan and each has purchased coverage for the other. Also, both spouses may elect to cover their children under both policies. Insurance companies, in cooperation with state insurance commissioners, have established specific rules that determine which coverage is billed first (called the primary carrier) and which is billed second (called the secondary carrier). Patients do not have the option of specifying which insurance should be primary or secondary.

When spouses or partners are covered by each other's policy, the patient's own policy is always primary for them, and the spouse or partner's policy is secondary. Medical office managers should not assume that spouses are covered by each other's policy. It is possible, for example, for the husband's insurance to cover himself and his wife, but the wife's insurance may cover only her. In this case, the husband would have only one insurance, his own. The wife would have two policies; hers would be primary and her husband's would be secondary.

birthday rule
according to this rule, the parent with the birthday earlier in the year is the primary carrier for the children

When both parents carry coverage for their children, most health insurance plans decide which insurance plan is primary and which is secondary based on the **birthday rule** (Figure ■ 14-15). According to this rule, the parent with the birthday earlier in the year is the primary carrier for the children; the parent with the later birthday is the secondary carrier for the children. The birthday rule relies only on the month and day of the parent's birthday. The year is not used. The insurance commissioners of most states have agreed to use the birthday rule. If a state does not use the birthday rule, the coordination of benefits rules will spell out how to determine the primary and secondary carrier.

Betsy and Ed Foreman have a son, Michael. Betsy has an insurance policy through Premera Blue Cross that provides family coverage. Ed has an insurance policy through Aetna U.S. Health Care that also provides family coverage. Betsy's birthday is June 1st and Ed's is August 10th. According to the birthday rule, the primary and secondary coverage for this family would be as follows:

	Primary Coverage	Secondary Coverage
Betsy	Premera Blue Cross	Aetna U.S. Health Care
Ed	Aetna U.S. Health Care	Premera Blue Cross
Michael	Premera Blue Cross	Aetna U.S. Health Care

Because Betsy's birthday falls earlier in the year than Ed's, her policy is primary for her and Michael. Because Ed's birthday falls later, his plan is secondary for Michael. Policyholders are primary on their own policies, so Ed's primary carrier is his own policy through Premera Blue Cross.

FIGURE ■ 14-15   Example of applying the birthday rule.

Medical office managers should ask about coordination of benefits when verifying benefits. Complicated issues can arise with children who are covered by three or more companies. This may happen when a child has two biological parents as well as two stepparents. If three or even all four of the parents have coverage for the child, the child would have coverage with four insurance companies. In these cases, typically the custodial parent's plan is primary, the spouse of the custodial parent's plan is secondary, and the noncustodial parent and stepparent are the third and fourth in line, respectively, for coverage. In these cases, it is always best to call one of the insurance carriers and ask the customer service representative the order in which claims should be submitted to carriers.

Critical Thinking 14.14 ?

Imagine you have a child patient whose parents share the same birth date. How would you determine which insurance carrier is primary and which is secondary?

REFERRALS, AUTHORIZATIONS, AND PRECERTIFICATIONS

preauthorization
the process of obtaining approval from an insurance company for a patient's procedure; also referred to as **precertification**

Before scheduling any nonemergency procedures or costly tests, medical office managers should call insurance carriers to both verify patients' eligibility for those services and to complete any needed **preauthorization**. This process is also referred to as **precertification** and consists of calling the patients' insurance carriers to obtain permission for patients to receive prescribed procedures. Depending on the insurance plan, some managed care plans require referrals from patients' primary care providers for specialized care. In these cases, medical office managers may need to call patients' primary care providers to coordinate the patients' referrals. Any time managers receive preauthorization or precertification numbers for patients, they should include those numbers on the insurance billing form and also make note of them in the patients' files.

When patients require specialist care, managed care plans may require referrals from patients' primary care providers. Medical office managers who work in a primary care setting may be asked to arrange those specialist referrals, which entails verifying that specialists are covered under the patients' managed care plans. To accomplish this task, managers can either call insurance carriers' customer service departments or look online.

Medical office managers in specialist offices must ensure that patients' primary care providers have arranged referrals before those patients visit the specialists' offices. Many HMOs penalize physicians who fail to obtain authorization before rendering service. Many times, insurance carriers will deny claims that were not properly authorized. In managed care, physicians are then restricted from billing the patient for the denied service. In effect, the physician performs the procedure for free. With penalties this severe, it is imperative that medical office managers verify the need for referrals, authorizations, or precertifications before providing service.

DOCUMENTING CALLS TO AND FROM INSURANCE COMPANIES

Because having comprehensive, in-depth knowledge of all insurance plans is unrealistic, medical office managers should know where to find answers and the information needed. Many insurance companies provide coverage information online. Insurance companies' website addresses are usually on the patients' identification cards. These resources are recommended for general information, but not for procedure authorization. When managers have questions about patients' insurance coverage, the insurance customer service department is the best place to call.

Medical office managers should document any calls made to an insurance carrier, including the date and time, number used, party on the phone, and the information obtained. Such data becomes a part of the patient's permanent financial record and can be referenced should there ever be a discrepancy between what the office manager was told by the insurance carrier and how the insurance carrier processed the claim.

Health Insurance Claim Forms

Before the 1990s, health insurance carriers required healthcare providers to use unique forms to bill for patient services. Patients were required to obtain these forms from their employers or insurance carriers. Healthcare providers would attach a **superbill**, also called a *charge slip* or *encounter form* (Figure ■ 14-16), which are preprinted lists of procedures and diagnosis codes commonly used in the office. Providers would circle the services provided, include the applicable diagnoses, attach the superbill to the unique insurance form, and mail the form to the appropriate insurance carrier for reimbursement.

superbill
form used in the medical office for indicating the services rendered to the patient, as well as the diagnosis for the service

CMS-1500 CLAIM FORM

To help standardize the insurance billing industry, the former HCFA (now CMS) created a uniform billing form to be used by physicians and other professional healthcare providers. This form, now called the CMS-1500, is used today by all health insurance carriers, including Medicare, Medicaid, and workers' compensation carriers (Figure ■ 14-17). Dental claims are sent via the American Dental Association (ADA) standard form. The ADA form and the CMS-1500 are the only two insurance claims forms medical offices use to submit paper claims today.

The boxes to be completed on the CMS-1500 form are referred to as **form locators**. The form is divided into two major sections: patient and insured information, and physician or supplier information. The top right portion of the form is the carrier's area and is used to print the insurance company's name and address on the form.

form locators
the boxes on the CMS-1500 insurance claim form

Patient Name _____

Capital City Medical
123 Unknown Boulevard, Capital City, NY 12345-2222

Date of Service
_____

New Patient			Laboratory	
Problem Focused	99201		Amylase	82150
Expanded Problem, Focused	99202		B12	82607
Detailed	99203		CBC & Diff	85025
Comprehensive	99204		Comp Metabolic Panel	80053
Comprehensive/High Complex	99205		Chlamydia Screen	87110
Well Exam Infant (up to 12 mos.)	99381		Cholesterol	82465
Well Exam 1–4 yrs.	99382		Digoxin	80162
Well Exam 5–11 yrs.	99383		Electrolytes	80051
Well Exam 12–17 yrs.	99384		Ferritin	82728
Well Exam 18–39 yrs.	99385		Folate	82746
Well Exam 40–64 yrs.	99386		GC Screen	87070

Arthrocentesis/Aspiration/Injection

Small Joint	20600	
Interm Joint	20605	
Major Joint	20610	

Other Invasive/Noninvasive

Audiometry	92552	
Cast Application		
Location	Long	Short
Catheterization	51701	
Circumcision	54150	
Colposcopy	57452	
Colposcopy w/Biopsy	57454	
Cryosurgery Premalignant Lesion		
Location (s):		
Cryosurgery Warts		

Glucose	82947
Glucose 1 HR	82950
Glycosylated HGB A1C	83036
HCT	85014

Established Patient		
Post-Op Follow Up Visit	99024	
Minimum	99211	
Problem Focused	99212	
Expanded Problem Focused	99213	
Detailed	99214	
Comprehensive/High Complex	99215	
Well Exam Infant (up to 12 mos.)	99391	
Well exam 1–4 yrs.	99392	
Well Exam 5–11 yrs.	99393	
Well Exam 12–17 yrs.	99394	
Well Exam 18–39 yrs.	99395	
Well Exam 40–64 yrs.	99396	

Location (s):		
Curettement Lesion		
Single	11055	
2–4	11056	
>4	11057	
Diaphragm Fitting	57170	
Ear Irrigation	69210	
ECG	93000	
Endometrial Biopsy	58100	
Exc. Lesion Malignant		
Benign		
Location		

HDL	83718
Hep BSAG	87340
Hepatitis panel, acute	80074
HGB	85018
HIV	86703
Iron & TIBC	83550
Kidney Profile	80069
Lead	83655
Liver Profile	80076
Mono Test	86308
Pap Smear	88155
Pregnancy Test	84703

Obstetrics		
Total OB Care	59400	

Injections		
Administration Sub. / IM	90772	
Drug		
Dosage		
Allergy	95115	
Cocci Skin Test	86490	
DPT	90701	
Hemophilus	90646	
Influenza	90658	
MMR	90707	
OPV	90712	
Pneumovax	90732	
TB Skin Test	86580	
TD	90718	
Unlisted Immun	90749	
Tetanus Toxoid	90703	
Vaccine/Toxoid Admin <8 Yr Old w/ Counseling	90465	
Vaccine/Toxoid Administration for Adult	90471	

Exc. Skin Tags (1–15)	11200	
Each Additional 10	11201	
Fracture Treatment		
Loc		
w/Reduc	w/o Reduc	
I & D Abscess Single/Simple	10060	
Multiple or Comp	10061	
I & D Pilonidal Cyst Simple	10080	
Pilonidal Cyst Complex	10081	
IV Therapy—To One Hour	90760	
Each Additional Hour	90761	
Laceration Repair		
Location	Size	Simp/Comp
Laryngoscopy	31505	
Oximetry	94760	
Punch Biopsy		
Rhythm Strip	93040	
Treadmill	93015	
Trigger Point or Tendon Sheath Inj.	20550	
Tympanometry	92567	

Obstetric Panel	80055
Pro Time	85610
PSA	84153
RPR	86592
Sed. Rate	85651
Stool Culture	87045
Stool O & P	87177
Strep Screen	87880
Theophylline	80198
Thyroid Uptake	84479
TSH	84443
Urinalysis	81000
Urine, bacterial culture	87086
Drawing Fee	36415
Specimen Collection	99000
Other:	

Diagnosis/ICD-9: _____

I acknowledge receipt of medical services and authorize the release of any medical information necessary to process this claim for healthcare payment only. I do authorize payment to the provider.

Patient Signature _____

Total Estimated Charges: _____

Payment Amount: _____

Next Appointment: _____

FIGURE ■ 14-16 Sample superbill.

FIGURE ■ 14-17 CMS-1500 claim form.

When completing the form, the medical office manager will use various sources to locate the required information. The patient registration form provides information about the patient's and insured's names, addresses, birth dates, and related data. The insurance card provides information on the insurance policy, identification and group numbers, mailing address for claims, and basic coverage and cost information. The clinic's encounter form provides the date of service, services rendered, and treating provider. The encounter form may contain fees or the medical office manager may need to refer to the clinic's fee schedule for charges. The encounter form or patient registration form may contain the clinic's address, tax identification number, and NPI numbers, or the medical office manager may need to refer to other office records for this information.

Mistakes on the CMS-1500 Claim Form

Even the smallest mistake on the CMS-1500 claim form may cause the claim to be denied or rejected for accurate information. Time spent making sure all data on the CMS-1500 form is correct will keep these rejections and denials from occurring.

Critical Thinking 14.15 ?

What ideas do you have for how mistakes can be avoided on the CMS-1500 claim form?

FILING TIMELINES

Most insurance carriers accept claims for up to 1 year from the date of service, although some have much shorter timelines, such as 90 days. After filing timelines pass, claims are considered past timely filing limits and will likely be rejected. With most managed care plans, claims rejected because the filing timeline passed cannot be billed to the patient. To avoid rejection, it is best to submit claims soon after service is rendered.

ELECTRONIC BILLING

Electronic claims are submitted to the insurance carrier via direct electronic submission. No paper is printed and claims are saved on the computer only. When claims are sent electronically to insurance carriers for processing, an electronic signature is used to verify that the information received is true and correct. With electronic claims, administrative costs are lower due to the elimination of paper and envelopes, as well as postage for mailing paper claims. Fewer claims are rejected with electronic claims because technical errors are detected and corrected before the claim arrives at the payer. Payment of electronic claims is faster with electronic billing because the claim is received instantly by the payer and payment can then be transmitted to the provider's bank. Medicare is required to process electronic claims within 14 days.

Reconciling Payments and Rejections

Insurance claims are sometimes denied or rejected, many times for errors the medical office made. Incorrect identification numbers, incorrect birth dates, missing diagnosis codes, and missing supporting documentation all delay payment of insurance claims. Attention to detail in the claim submission process saves time and effort in the end. A rejected claim is one that was not processed because the claim had incorrect information. These claims are returned to the provider for correction and resubmission.

A denied claim is one the carrier received and processed but did not make payment on due to problems with benefits or coverage. The reason for a denial may be that the patient's insurance coverage is no longer in effect, or that the patient does not have coverage for the service in question. When the provider receives a denial notice from an insurance company, the reason for the denial will be listed.

SENDING SUPPORTING DOCUMENTATION

Claims may be denied due to lack of proper information. This may be a copy of laboratory reports, x-rays, or a letter from the physician explaining why the patient needs the service. When such a denial is received, the medical office manager should determine what information the insurance company requires and then resubmit the claim with the appropriate information attached.

Critical Thinking 14.16 ?

In what ways can the medical office avoid having claims denied due to lack of proper information?

OFFICE OF THE INSURANCE COMMISSIONER

Each state has an Office of the Insurance Commissioner, a valuable resource for both the medical office and the patient. When medical office managers or patients believe claims were incorrectly processed and appeal attempts have been fruitless, office managers may file formal written complaints with the state's insurance commissioner. It is important to involve patients in this process because they are the consumer the insurance commissioner is charged with protecting from insurance abuse. Patients may be reluctant to appeal to the commissioner on their own because they are unfamiliar with the process. One good approach is for medical office managers to write a letter on behalf of the patient and ask the patient to sign it. Sometimes, the threat of complaint alone can inspire insurance carriers to review denied claims.

Case Study Questions

Refer to the case study presented at the beginning of this chapter to answer the following questions:

1. How would you suggest Roland set up a training plan for his new employees?
2. What important points about Medicare coverage should Roland ensure his staff understands and can explain to patients?

Chapter Review

Summary

- Health insurance has changed a great deal since its inception in the 1950s. Policies vary greatly from one to another. Premium costs are generally associated with coverage—the better the coverage, the higher the premium.

- Health insurance plans vary from the more restrictive HMOs to fee-for-service plans.

- COBRA coverage can be purchased by employees while they are between jobs. The premiums are generally high, but the individual is allowed to continue coverage, which may be very important if the patient has a chronic disease.

- Individual health insurance policies may be purchased by individuals, although the premiums are generally much higher than those of group policies.

- Flex spending and healthcare savings accounts are good options for patients to put pretaxed money away for medical expenses. Consumer-directed healthcare plans are those in which patients control their own healthcare costs by paying for them out of their premium account. These plans cause consumers to be far more aware of the amount being paid for medical expenses.

- Elective procedures are those that are not deemed medically necessary by the insurance carrier but are instead something the patient chooses to do, perhaps for aesthetic reasons. These procedures are not generally covered by insurance policies.

- Prescription drug coverage is part of most insurance plans today. The coverage varies according to the policy; however, generic drugs are typically covered and provided to patients at low cost.

- Medicare provides coverage to individuals over age 65, those with long-term disabilities, and those with end-stage renal disease. Medicare has multiple parts, with each part providing patients with different forms of coverage.

- Medicaid is insurance coverage for individuals who have low incomes. Medicaid funds are partly provided by the federal government and each state decides how funds will be allocated and what patients will be covered.

- TRICARE and CHAMPVA are insurance plans for active-duty military, retired military, or family members of military personnel.

- Patients who are injured due to an accident, such as an automobile accident, are typically covered under a liability policy for care related to the injury.

- Processing insurance claim forms follows steps assigned by CMS. If claims are not filled out accurately, denials or rejections may result.

- Health insurance claims are submitted on the CMS-1500 claim form. This form is accepted by all insurance carriers, including Medicare and Medicaid.

- Once payments, rejections, or denials have been received in the medical office, a reconciliation needs to take place to make sure the claim was paid appropriately. If additional information is required by the insurance carrier, the medical office manager should find out what is missing and submit it appropriately.

Multiple Choice

Choose the letter that best answers each question or completes each statement.

1. The Advance Beneficiary Notice is used for patients covered by which insurance?
   a. Medicaid
   b. Premera Blue Cross
   c. Aetna U.S. Health Care
   d. Medicare

2. Money in a flexible spending account must be spent by what date in the following year?
   a. January 15
   b. February 15
   c. March 15
   d. April 15

3. Jim Noonan has to pay $15 every time he sees his primary care provider. This is an example of which of the following?
   a. Copayment
   b. Deductible
   c. Coinsurance
   d. Stop loss

4. Which of the following plans pays providers a set per-member dollar amount each month, whether the patient seeks care with the physician or not?
   a. HMO
   b. PPO
   c. EPO
   d. Capitated plan

5. Which of the following types of insurance plans is rarely seen today?
   a. HMOs
   b. Fee-for-service plans
   c. EPOs
   d. PPOs

6. Which of the following describes a preexisting condition?
   a. A condition the patient had before beginning coverage with a new insurance carrier
   b. Any chronic illness the patient has ever been diagnosed with
   c. A new diagnosis of a long-term disease
   d. A life-limiting condition

7. Providers who do not participate with MCOs are called:
   a. uncooperative.
   b. nonparticipating providers.
   c. participating providers.
   d. None of the above

8. Which of the following tend to be the most expensive type of insurance policy?
   a. HMO
   b. PPO
   c. Individual policy
   d. Employer-provided policy

9. Hospital insurance coverage began in what year?
   a. 1919
   b. 1929
   c. 1939
   d. 1949

10. Which is the newest type of insurance plan?
    a. Managed care
    b. HMOs
    c. Consumer directed
    d. PPOs

True/False

Determine if each of the following statements is true or false.

_____ 1. Medicare claims submitted more than 365 days after the date of service are subject to a 10 percent penalty.

_____ 2. As of 2008, nearly 50 percent of all Medicare beneficiaries had prescription drug coverage.

_____   3. Medigap is supplemental insurance for Medicare-covered patients.

_____   4. Medicare Part A is optional for Medicare patients.

_____   5. The federal government determines what patients are covered by Medicaid.

_____   6. All Medicaid funds come from within each individual state.

_____   7. The federal government reimburses states for 100 percent of all costs associated with providing healthcare in Indian Health Service facilities.

_____   8. COBRA coverage covers patients for up to 48 months after they leave their place of employment.

_____   9. CHAMPVA is a federal program that provides healthcare benefits to families of current and retired military personnel.

_____   10. Point-of-service plans are found within some HMOs.

Matching

Match the following terms with their definition.

a. balance billing

b. beneficiary

c. certificate of coverage

d. flexible spending account

e. fee-for-service

f. capitated plan

g. allowed amount

h. catastrophic

i. experimental

j. formulary

1. The dollar amount for a service that an insurance company considers acceptable and uses to determine benefit payments

2. Tiered list of drugs covered by an insurance company

3. Person who is eligible to receive benefits and services under an insurance policy

4. Billing a patient for the dollar difference between the provider's charge and the insurance-approved amount

5. Process in which insurance companies pay providers fees for each service provided to covered patients

6. A letter from the insurance company that provides proof of type and time frame of coverage when a patient terminates a health insurance policy

7. Healthcare plan in which providers are paid set fees per month per member patients

8. A service or procedure that has not been approved by the Food and Drug Administration

9. Large and usually unforeseen

10. Account into which employees place pretax earnings for projected medical expenses

Chapter Resources

American Dental Association: www.ada.org

American Medical Association: www.ama-assn.org/

CHAPTER 15

Procedural and Diagnostic Coding

CHAPTER OUTLINE

- History of Procedural Coding
- Current Procedural Terminology Codes
- Determining the Proper Procedure Code
- Evaluation and Management Codes
- Anesthesia Codes
- Surgery Codes
- Postoperative or Follow-Up Days
- Radiology Codes
- Pathology and Laboratory Codes

- Medicine Codes
- Healthcare Common Procedure Coding System
- Proper Documentation
- History of Diagnostic Coding
- ICD-10-CM Coding
- Using the ICD-9-CM Coding Manual
- Coding More Than One Diagnosis
- Late Effect Diagnoses
- Coding for Suspected Conditions

LEARNING OBJECTIVES

Upon completion of this chapter, you should be able to:

- Spell and define the key terms in this chapter.
- Discuss the history of procedural coding.
- Describe CPT codes and their use.
- Describe the organization of the CPT manual.
- List the steps used to determine the proper procedure code.
- Understand how to use Evaluation and Management codes.
- Understand how anesthesia codes are used.
- Describe how surgery codes are used.
- Understand how postoperative or follow-up days are considered.
- Understand the use of radiology codes.
- Discuss pathology and laboratory codes and their use.

The CPT-4 codes in this chapter are from the CPT-4 2012 code set. CPT® is a registered trademark of the American Medical Association.

ICD-9-CM codes in this chapter are from the ICD-9-CM 2012 code set from the Department of Health and Human Services, Centers for Disease Control and Prevention.

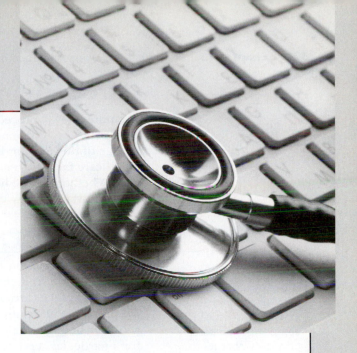

- Understand the use of medicine codes.
- Describe the Healthcare Common Procedure Coding System.
- Discuss the importance of proper documentation in reimbursement.
- Understand the history of diagnostic coding.
- Discuss the implementation of ICD-10-CM and the differences between ICD-9 and ICD-10 codes.
- Describe the contents and use of the ICD-9-CM and ICD-10-CM coding manuals.
- Understand how to find the correct diagnosis code.
- Describe coding for more than one diagnosis.
- Explain the use of late effect diagnosis codes.
- Explain when to code for a suspected condition.

KEY TERMS

abuse
E codes
eponym
etiology
Evaluation and Management (E&M) codes

fraud
global period
Healthcare Common Procedure Coding System (HCPCS)
modifier

tabular index
upcode
usual, customary, and reasonable (UCR)
V codes

Case Study

Take note of the following scenario and answer the case study questions that appear at the end of this chapter.

James McCollum is the medical office manager in a large multiple-specialty clinic. Part of his duties include overseeing the billing and coding staff in the clinic. After attending a medical office managers' conference on billing and coding, James returns to his clinic with information on how the coding process in his office could be improved.

Introduction

Accurate use of procedural and diagnostic coding is vital to the medical facility being paid in a timely manner by insurance carriers. The medical office manager may be in charge of this task, or he may delegate this task to others in the medical office. In larger healthcare facilities, entire departments may exist to perform the billing and coding function. Whether the medical office manager is performing this task or delegating to others, it is important to stay current with codes because they may change on a yearly basis.

History of Procedural Coding

usual, customary, and reasonable (UCR)
reimbursement method in which insurance companies compare providers' charges to other providers in the same geographic area

Before the mid-1960s, healthcare providers used the **usual, customary, and reasonable (UCR)** method to determine fair charges for their services. This system was devised by health insurance carriers to determine what the usual, customary, and reasonable fee was for providers of healthcare services. In other words, insurance companies would look at provider billing records to see what other providers in a geographic area were charging for a particular service. The average of these charges would determine the usual, customary, and reasonable fee that would be allowed.

To standardize medical fees and increase the accuracy of the coding process, in 1992 the U.S. Congress developed a system that assigned a relative value unit to every healthcare procedure or treatment.

Current Procedural Terminology Codes

The Current Procedural Terminology (CPT) manual includes all procedures approved by the U.S. Food and Drug Administration (FDA) (Figure ■ 15-1). When it was first published in 1966, the manual focused mainly on surgical procedures, with some codes covering

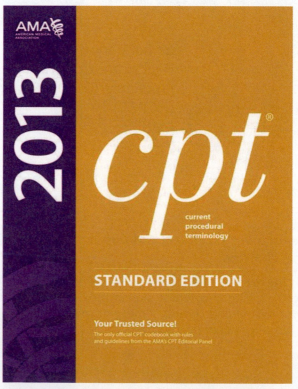

FIGURE ■ 15-1   2013 CPT manual. Reprinted with permission of the American Medical Association.
Source: This image was published in CPT 2013 Professional Edition 1, American Medical Association, Book Cover Image, Copyright American Medical Association (October 15, 2012).

radiology, laboratory, and pathology services. Although the manual is updated annually, the last major revision, the fourth, occurred in 1977.

In an effort to establish industry standards, in the 1980s the U.S. Congress began requiring providers to use CPT codes for all services rendered to Medicare patients. The codes, which are five digits long, must appear on the CMS-1500 insurance claim form. Procedures and services performed by physicians are reported using codes from the CPT-4 manual, which is published by the American Medical Association (AMA). The purpose of CPT codes is to provide a uniform language that will accurately describe medical, surgical, and diagnostic services so that those involved with health management and reimbursement will have an effective means of communication.

The challenge in procedural coding is to find the most appropriate and accurate code. Patient encounters for what is commonly referred to as an "office visit," for example, may be reported with any of 30 or more codes, depending on a number of circumstances surrounding the visit, but only one of these codes is correct in any given situation. Likewise, more than 50 codes exist for a patient receiving sutures for a wound, depending on the location, length, and depth of the wound. Medical office managers should be familiar with all of the criteria for coding the services offered by their office to be certain they select the most accurate code. When uncertain of the best code, it may be tempting to **upcode**, which is to code for a higher level of service than what was actually provided in order to gain a higher level of reimbursement. **Fraud** in billing and coding is to intentionally bill for services that were never given, which includes upcoding. **Abuse** in billing and coding is improper behavior and billing practices that result in financial gain but are not fraudulent. As in all areas of healthcare, ignorance is no excuse. If the medical office manager is unsure regarding a coding issue, she may consult with the physician, a colleague, or a professional organization.

The CPT lists over 8,800 procedural codes. They are updated every year and take effect on January 1. Medical office managers should use the edition of the CPT that was in effect on the date of service. In other words, if a patient was seen in December 2012, and the coding is taking place in January 2013, the 2012 version of the CPT manual should be consulted, not the new 2013 edition.

The organization of the 2013 CPT manual is shown in Figure ■ 15-2. The content and labeling of the many appendices sometimes change when the manual is updated. The inside of the front cover of the manual shows a list of commonly used symbols, modifiers, and place-of-service codes. The inside of the back cover lists commonly used medical abbreviations. The first material presented after the cover of the manual is a section of introductory matter, including the table of contents, instructions for use of the code manual, and other valuable information, depending on the publisher. Possible inclusions are a review of medical terminology and anatomical plates.

upcode
to code and bill for a higher level of service than what was actually provided

fraud
to intentionally bill for services that were never given, or to bill for a service that has a higher reimbursement than the service provided

abuse
improper behavior and billing practices that result in financial gain but are not fraudulent

Critical Thinking 15.1 ?

What do you think the benefit is to insurance companies of using standardization in procedural coding? What are the benefits to healthcare providers?

TABULAR INDEX

The CPT manual's **tabular index** is a numerical listing of all CPT codes, divided into three categories. Category I codes make up the vast majority of codes in the CPT manual. These are numbered 00100 to 99999. These codes describe all services and procedures that have been approved by the FDA and are organized into six sections (Figure ■ 15-3). While most of the codes in this section are in numeric order, the codes 99201 through 99499 appear in the first section. These codes are the Evaluation and Management codes. The manual is set up in this manner for ease of use; the Evaluation and Management codes are the ones that are used most often by medical providers of all specialties.

tabular index
the numerical listing of all CPT codes

Inside covers
Introductory matter
Tabular index
    Category I
    Category II
    Category III
Appendices
    A — Modifiers
    B — Summary of Additions, Deletions and Revisions
    C — Clinical Examples
    D — Summary of CPT Add-on Codes
    E — Summary of CPT Codes Exempt from Modifier 51
    F — Summary of CPT Codes Exempt from Modifier 63
    G — Summary of CPT Copes That Include Moderate (Conscious) Sedation
    H — Alphabetic Index of Performance Measures by Clinical Conditions or Topic
    I — Genetic Testing Code Modifiers
    J — Electrodiagnostic Medicine Listing of Sensory, Motor, and Mixed Nerves
    K — Product Pending FDA Approval
    L — Vascular Families
    M — Crosswalk to Deleted CPT Codes
Alphabetical index

FIGURE ■ 15-2 Organization of the CPT manual.

Section	Code Range
Evaluation and Management (E&M)	99201–99499
Anesthesiology	00100–01999
	99100–99140
Surgery	10021–69990
Radiology	70010–79999
Laboratory/Pathology	80048–89356
Medicine	90281–99199
	99500–99602

FIGURE ■ 15-3 Sections of the CPT-4 category codes.

Category II codes are supplemental tracking codes that can be used for performance measurement. The use of these codes is optional and they are not used to replace Category I codes. Category II codes are four numbers followed by the letter F, such as 1002F. These codes are not used very often.

Category III codes are temporary codes for data collection and tracking of the use of emerging technology, services, and procedures. The codes are four numbers in length, followed by the letter T, such as 0162T. If a Category III code is available, the medical office manager should use it in place of a Category I code. Category III technology and procedure codes may be items the AMA is considering adding to the Category I code list.

APPENDICES

The CPT manual has several appendices, each of which provides additional reference information.

Appendix A: Modifiers

modifier
two-digit numeric code appended to CPT or Level II HCPCS codes to further describe circumstances

Appendix A contains a list of **modifiers**. These are two-digit numeric codes used to further describe circumstances regarding the service performed. The proper use of modifiers allows the medical office manager to provide additional information to insurance payers, which can speed up the processing of claims and receipt of reimbursement. The following modifiers are the most commonly used:

- **22 Unusual Procedural Service**—This modifier is used when the service provided is higher than that usually required for the listed procedure. Typically, a report explaining the unusual service is submitted with the claim.

- **47 Anesthesia by Surgeon**—This modifier is used when regional or general anesthesia is provided by the surgeon, rather than an anesthesiologist. This does not include use of local anesthesia.

- **50 Bilateral Procedure**—This modifier is used when a procedure is performed on both sides of the body. This modifier is appropriate only when the bilateral procedures are performed during the same surgery.

- **51 Multiple Procedures**—This modifier is used when the same procedure is performed multiple times during the surgery. An example is the removal of skin tags. Use of the modifier alerts the insurance payer to the fact that more than one procedure was performed. If the medical office manager does not use this code, the insurance payer may believe the additional services were listed in duplicate on the claim form in error, and the additional services may be denied.

- **62 Two Surgeons**—This modifier is used when two surgeons are involved in a procedure, working together as primary surgeons.

- **80 Assistant Surgeon**—This modifier is used by the second surgeon when an assistant surgeon is needed for the procedure.

Appendix B: Summary of Additions, Deletions, and Revisions

Appendix B is helpful to the medical office manager at the beginning of each new year. All changes to codes, including newly added codes, are summarized in this appendix.

Appendix C: Clinical Examples

Appendix C provides examples of code scenarios for many medical specialties when using Evaluation and Management codes.

Appendix D: Summary of CPT Add-On Codes

This appendix includes code numbers for any code that cannot be used alone.

Appendix E: Summary of CPT Codes Exempt from Modifier 51

Some procedure codes do not require the use of modifier 51 (Multiple Procedures). This appendix lists a summary of those codes.

Appendix F: Summary of CPT Codes Exempt from Modifier 63

Modifier 63 pertains to procedures performed on infants weighing less than 4 kilograms. This appendix lists a summary of codes that do not require this modifier.

Appendix G: Summary of CPT Codes that Include Moderate Sedation

Another term for moderate sedation is conscious sedation. This appendix lists those procedure codes for which the moderate sedation service is included and cannot be billed separately.

Appendix H: Alphabetic Index of Performance Measures by Clinical Condition or Topic

This appendix contains a cross-reference between Category II codes and situations where these codes may be used. This is not a commonly used appendix by medical offices in the outpatient setting.

Appendix I: Genetic Testing Code Modifiers

This appendix lists the modifiers used for coding molecular laboratory procedures related to genetic testing. This appendix is used only in clinical settings where genetic testing is performed.

Appendix J: Electrodiagnostic Medicine Listing of Sensory, Motor, and Mixed Nerves

This appendix is used to accurately code nerve conduction studies.

Appendix K: Product Pending FDA Approval

This appendix contains codes for those procedures that are expected to be approved by the FDA.

Appendix L: Vascular Families

This appendix contains a list of first-, second-, and third-order vascular braches. This appendix is most commonly used by medical coders in coding for catheterization of the aorta.

Appendix M: Crosswalk to Deleted CPT Codes

Codes that were deleted from use from the previous year are listed in this appendix, along with the new code that should be used in its place.

Determining the Proper Procedure Code

The most important tool in determining the proper procedure code is the patient's medical record. It is important to code according to what is actually in the patient's record and not to assume any information that may be missing. If unsure, the medical office manager should check with the provider for clarification (Figure ■ 15-4).

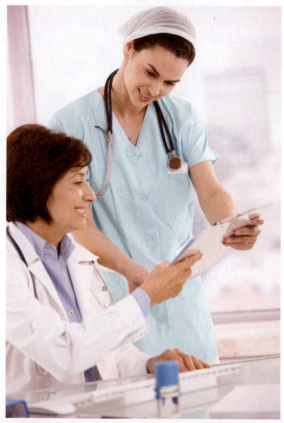

FIGURE ■ 15-4 When in doubt about coding, the physician who performed the procedure should be consulted.
Source: Nyul/Dreamstime.com.

Proper procedure coding involves 11 steps. Because proper coding results in prompt and accurate reimbursement, this process should be done paying great attention to detail.

1. Identify the primary and secondary services performed, as stated in the medical record. This information may be noted on the encounter form, or in the patient's record note for the day of the procedure. The primary procedure may be the examination, and secondary procedures may be laboratory tests ordered. After determining the primary and secondary services performed, the medical office manager must determine the quantity of each procedure so that these can be billed using modifiers, if appropriate. For any procedure that is billed according to the time spent performing the procedure, the medical office manager will need to determine where the time spent was listed in the medical record.

2. Locate the main term in the alphabetic index. The CPT index lists main terms used to locate procedure codes. The main term may be found by the name of the procedure or service, by the name of a condition, by the name of an organ or anatomical site, or by an **eponym**—a disease or condition named after an individual.

3. Review any modifying terms or instructional notes associated with the main term. Because main terms rarely provide the exact code needed, the medical office manager should review any descriptive words in the alphabetic index that further describe the service or procedure.

4. Identify the tentative code associated with the most appropriate modifying term. This step should be done for all codes associated with the visit.

5. Locate the tentative code in the tabular index. Every tentative code must be verified in the tabular index, where codes are arranged in alphabetical order.

6. Interpret the conventions used in the tabular index. The tabular index contains a list of conventions, which include formatting, punctuation, instructional notes, and symbols (Figure ■ 15-5).

7. Select the code with the highest level of specificity. This is where careful review of the medical record chart notes will help the medical office manager determine the appropriate coding level.

8. Review the code for appropriate bundling, add-on codes, and quantity. Attention to detail will help prevent coding errors.

9. Determine if modifiers are required. Use of modifiers alerts the insurance payer of any unusual circumstances.

10. Verify the final code against the documentation. After determining the proper code, refer back to the original documentation to determine if the coding has been done properly.

11. Assign the code. Write the final code in the chart, or enter it into the billing software.

eponym
a disease or condition named after an individual

⊙	Moderate sedation is automatically included in this code description.
⊘	This code is modifier 51 exempt.
+	Add-on code must be used with this code.
⁄	FDA approval is pending for this code.
( )	Parentheses are used to enclose synonyms, eponyms, or other descriptions that do not affect the code assignment.
●	New code in this edition of the CPT manual
▲	Revised code where the number is the same, only the descriptor has been updated.
▶◀	Contains new or revised text.

FIGURE ■ **15-5** Symbols in the CPT manual.

Critical Thinking 15.2 ?

What problems might arise if the wrong codes are used for procedural coding?

Evaluation and Management Codes

Evaluation and Management (E&M) codes describe patient encounters with a physician for the evaluation and management of a health problem. Although these codes begin with 99, they are located out of numerical sequence in the CPT manual, at the front of the manual in the first section. E&M codes are selected based on the category of service, which may be the location or the type of service provided.

The physician assigns the E&M code. Medical office managers should ensure that documentation in the medical record is consistent with the codes checked off on the encounter form or entered into the medical record. When coding for E&M services, it is important to first select the category of service. Categories may describe the location of service, such as office visit or hospital inpatient visit, or the type of service, such as consultation, critical care, or preventive care. When coding for E&M services, the medical office manager needs to determine if the patient is a new patient or an established patient.

ELEMENTS OF E&M CODES

The key components of E&M codes are based on the following guidelines, found in the CPT manual:

- History—to determine the proper level of history for the E&M code, the following descriptions are used:
  - Problem focused—the patient's problem is minor, he has only one chief complaint and gives a brief history of his present illness or problem.
  - Expanded problem focused—the patient's problem is mild to moderate, he has more than one chief complaint and/or a more extensive history of his present illness or problem.
  - Detailed—the patient's problem is moderate to severe and he has an extensive past, family, or social history that has direct relevance on his current problem.
  - Comprehensive—the patient's problem is moderate to severe, he has a more extensive history and requires a complete review of all additional body systems.
- Examination—to determine the proper level of examination for the E&M code, the following descriptions are used:
  - Problem focused—a limited examination of the affected body area is done.
  - Expanded problem focused—a limited examination of the affected body area is done along with other related organ systems.
  - Detailed—an extended examination of the affected body area and other related organ systems is performed.
  - Comprehensive—a general multisystem examination is performed.
- Medical decision making—to determine the proper level of medical decision making for the E&M codes, the medical office manager should consider the following:
  - The number of possible diagnoses the patient presents with
  - The amount or complexity of the medical records the provider must go through to treat the patient.
  - The risk of significant complications as a result of this treatment.

Critical Thinking 15.3 ?

Why do you think the level of decision making is important to determining the E&M code? Do you think it is more complicated to work with a patient who presents with multiple healthcare issues? Why or why not?

Anesthesia Codes

Anesthesia codes have their own section, which is located before the surgery section. Basic anesthesia administration services are those services provided by or under the responsible supervision of a physician (Figure ■ 15-6). These services include general and regional anesthesia, as well as supplementation of local anesthesia.

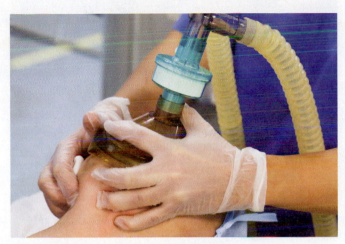

FIGURE ■ 15-6 A patient undergoing anesthesia.
Source: Beerkoff/Dreamstime.com.

Surgery Codes

The surgery section is the largest section of the CPT manual. The surgery section is broken down into the body systems, then further into anatomical sections within the body systems as follows:

- Head
- Neck and thorax
- Back and flank
- Spine
- Abdomen
- Shoulder
- Humerus
- Forearm and wrist
- Hand and fingers
- Pelvis and hip joints
- Femur and knee joints
- Legs and ankle joints
- Foot and toes
- Application of casts and strapping
- Endoscopy/arthroscopy.

Each surgical code is a bundled code. This is a single CPT code that is used to report a group of related procedures as in a surgical package. A surgical package includes the following services in addition to the surgical procedure itself:

- One E&M visit on the date immediately prior to or on the date of the procedure, subsequent to the decision for surgery (Figure ■ 15-7)
- Preparing the patient for surgery including local infiltration, topical anesthesia
- Performing the operation, including normal additional procedures, such as debridement

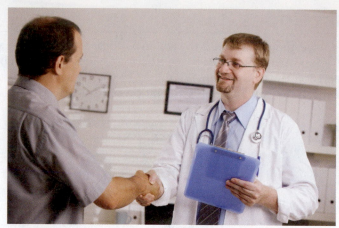

FIGURE ■ 15-7   For many surgical procedures, the physician will want to see the patient in the office prior to the day of surgery.
Source: Nyul/Dreamstime.com.

■ Immediate postoperative care, including dictating operative notes, talking with the family and other physicians

■ Writing orders

■ Evaluating the patient in the postanesthesia recovery area

■ Typical postoperative follow-up.

Critical Thinking 15.4 ?

What kinds of problems do you think could arise if the wrong site or surgery were coded for a patient?

Postoperative or Follow-Up Days

global period
the period of time, both before and after a surgical procedure, included in the surgical procedure fee

The typical postoperative care includes follow-up visits for normal, uncomplicated care. Each insurance company determines the number of days in which this follow-up care may take place. For this reason, it is important for the medical office manager to verify the number of days allowed for follow-up when certifying the procedure. This postoperative time is called the **global period**.

Critical Thinking 15.5 ?

Do you think a patient would have a copayment for a postoperative visit that occurs during the global period?

Radiology Codes

The codes in the radiology section are used to report radiological services performed by or supervised by a physician. Radiology codes may have two parts:

1. The technical component—this is the actual test or taking of the pictures or images (Figure ■ 15-8).

2. The professional component—this is the reading or interpretation of the test or study (Figure ■ 15-9).

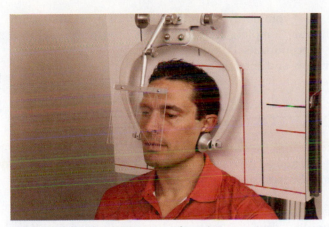

FIGURE ■ 15-8 A patient undergoing an x-ray.
Source: Rainerplendl/Dreamstime.com.

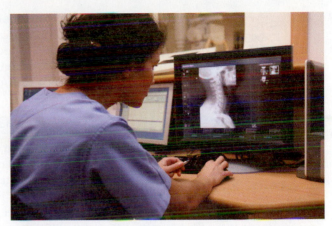

FIGURE ■ 15-9 A physician reading a digital x-ray.
Source: Aboltus/Dreamstime.com.

Pathology and Laboratory Codes

The codes in the pathology and laboratory section of the CPT manual cover services provided by physicians or by technicians under the supervision of a physician. A complete procedure includes ordering the test, taking and handling the sample, performing the actual test, and analyzing and reporting on the test results.

The 80000 services codes are used to report the performance of specific laboratory tests only and do not include the collection of the specimen via needlestick or other collection method.

Critical Thinking 15.6 ?

What do you think would be the best method for determining the proper pathology or laboratory code to use for your patient?

Medicine Codes

The medicine section of the CPT manual contains a variety of listings for reporting procedures and services provided by many different types of healthcare providers. In addition many services and procedures provided by nonphysician practitioners are found in the medicine section. Codes from the medicine section may be used with codes from any other section. Immunizations require two codes, one for administering the immunization and one for the particular vaccine that is given (Figure ■ 15-10).

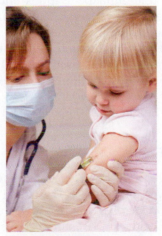

FIGURE ■ 15-10 A patient receiving a vaccination.
Source: Dmitry Naumov/Fotolia.com.

Cardiac catheterizations are the most commonly performed surgical procedure, with more than 1 million performed each year. Complete coding of these procedures includes at least three codes: a code for the procedure itself, a code for the injection procedure, and a code for the imaging supervision and interpretation. Each of these three codes includes both a professional and technical component.

Healthcare Common Procedure Coding System

Healthcare Common Procedure Coding System (HCPCS)
a set of codes developed and maintained by the Centers for Medicare and Medicaid Services

The **Healthcare Common Procedure Coding System (HCPCS)** is a set of codes developed and maintained by the Centers for Medicare and Medicaid Services (CMS) for the reporting of professional services, nonphysician services, supplies, durable medical equipment, and injectable drugs.

The HCPCS has three levels. Level I codes are CPT codes for professional services. Level II codes are those used for supplies, drugs, durable medical equipment, and non-physician services. When a CPT and an HCPCS code exist for the same service, the medical office manager should use the CPT code. Level III codes were developed by regional Medicare carriers, and are being phased out under HIPAA's administrative simplification mandate, which requires uniformity in coding.

Proper Documentation

The best method for receiving proper reimbursement in a timely manner is to have proper documentation of the services provided in the patient's medical record. The documentation must include a description of what was provided to the patient, along with any extenuating circumstances. For example, if an interpreter was needed for the visit, or if the patient had multiple complaints at the time of the visit or has an extensive health history, this should be documented in the medical record.

Critical Thinking 15.7 ?

Imagine you are coding a patient's visit and you cannot tell from the medical record exactly what procedure the physician performed. How would you go about obtaining this information?

History of Diagnostic Coding

Diagnostic coding has existed for more than a century, beginning in 1893 with French physician Jacques Bertillon. Dr. Bertillon composed the Bertillon Classification of Causes of Death, which the American Public Health Association (APHA) adopted in 1898. At the time, the classification contained an alphabetic index and a tabular list, and was quite small compared to coding references used today. The APHA recommended the classification be revised every 10 years to ensure it was current.

In 1901, the APHA published a coding manual called the International Classification of Diseases (ICD), Volume I. The ICD-1 was used until 1910, when the second revision, ICD-2, was published. Volume revisions continued to be published approximately every 10 years until the *International Classification of Diseases, Ninth Revision, Clinical Modification* (ICD-9-CM), was published in 1979 (Figure ■ 15-11).

ICD-10-CM Coding

ICD-10-CM was completed in 1999 and soon replaced the ICD-9-CM in all major countries except the United States. This version of the ICD manual was initially slated for implementation in the United States on October 1, 2013; however, at the time this text went to press, the U.S. Department of Health and Human Services (DHHS) announced its intent to delay the ICD-10-CM implementation date. Please refer to www.cms.gov/ICD10 for current requirements.

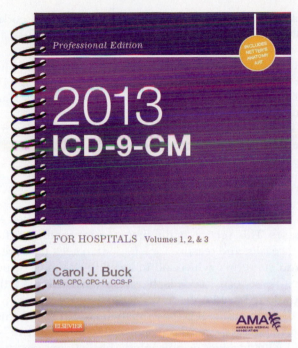

FIGURE ■ 15-11 2013 ICD-9-CM manual. Reprinted with permission of the American Medical Association.
Source: This image was published in 2013 ICD-9-CM for Hospitals, Volumes 1, 2 and 3 Professional Edition, 1e, Carol J. Buck MS CPC CPC-H CCS-P, Book Cover Image, Copyright American Medical Association/Elsevier (August 28, 2012).

The ICD-10-CM provides a revised and expanded code structure that incorporates updated terminology; makes it easier to add codes, such as for new technologies; allows for greater specificity and consistency; and complies with code set standards outlined by HIPAA. The ICD-10-CM far surpasses the ICD-9-CM in the number of codes included, with approximately 13,000 codes in the ICD-9-CM and 120,000 codes in the ICD-10-CM. This allows providers to code to a much higher level of specificity and for the government to better track diseases as well as causes of mortality in the United States.

The ICD-10-CM will replace ICD-9-CM Volumes I and II. The ICD-10-PCS will replace ICD-9-CM Volume III. Whereas in the ICD-9-CM, manual codes were three to five digits long, codes in the ICD-10-CM will be three to seven digits long.

Using the ICD-9-CM Coding Manual

As mentioned, the ICD-10-CM will not be implemented in the United States until further notice by DHHS. Until it is implemented, the ICD-9-CM manual is being used. It lists the codes to use for any diagnoses a provider assigns to a patient. The challenge is to find the most appropriate code to fit the condition with which the patient presents. Diagnostic codes describe the medical need of visits. If a patient presents in the office with a complaint of headache and sore throat and the physician orders a throat culture, the medical office manager must ensure that the claim form lists a diagnostic code that relates to a sore throat. If a sore throat diagnosis is not included, the insurance carrier may deny payment for the throat culture.

The ICD-9-CM manual lists about 13,000 diagnostic codes in three volumes. ICD-9-CM codes are updated annually and take effect on October 1 of each year. Medical office managers should always use the edition of the ICD-9-CM that was in effect on the date of service. For example, if a patient was seen on September 30, 2011, the 2011 coding manual should be used for assigning the code, even if the coding is not assigned until after the first of the following year.

The World Health Organization (WHO) has updated ICD codes since 1948. Code changes are published by the National Center for Health Statistics and the CMS, in conjunction with the WHO.

Each volume of the ICD-9-CM manual has a distinct purpose. Volume I is a tabular list of diseases, Volume II is an alphabetic index of diseases, and Volume III is a tabular list and alphabetic index of hospital procedures. Physicians use Volumes I and II of the manual; hospitals use all three volumes.

The ICD-9-CM manual is composed with Volume II appearing first, followed by Volume I, then Volume III. Many publishers print the manual with just the first two volumes for physician office use.

VOLUME II

Volume II of the ICD-9-CM manual contains two sections. The first section is the Alphabetic Index to Diseases. This section is the first step for medical office managers in coding. All conditions, diseases, and reasons for a patient to seek care are listed alphabetically by the main term and subterms, which aid in locating the most appropriate codes. After identifying the probable code, the code is then verified in Volume I, the Tabular List. Final code selection is not done based only on the index.

The second section of Volume II is the Alphabetic Index to External Causes of Adverse Effects of Drugs and Other Chemical Substances, Injuries and Poisonings. Any time a condition is caused by an accident or poisoning, this list contains the supplemental code used to describe the circumstances. The first part of this section is the Table of Drugs and Chemicals. This table contains an alphabetical list of drugs and other chemical substances, cross tabbed with a list of causes, to identify poisonings and external causes of drug-related adverse effects, such as drug-induced attempted suicide or an adverse reaction to penicillin. This is followed by an alphabetic index used to locate the external cause of any injury, such as a fall or motor vehicle accident.

VOLUME I

etiology
cause of a disease or an illness

After locating the diagnosis in the appropriate index in Volume II, it is verified by referencing the tabular list in Volume I. Volume I is a numerically sequenced list of all diagnosis codes, divided into 17 chapters based on cause, or **etiology**, of the disease or injury, as well as by location of the disease or injury on or in the body. Every chapter title describes the conditions within, followed by the range of three-digit codes within.

In addition to a title, each Volume I chapter has a subtitle in large print followed by a range of three-digit codes in that category. Each three-digit code combination describes a general disease; subsequent fourth and fifth digits add more specificity. Five-digit codes offer the highest level of definition. Volume I indicates the number of digits needed for coding: three, four, or five.

V CODES

V codes
codes used to classify the reason for care other than an active illness

At the end of the ICD-9-CM manual are two supplementary code chapters. The first of these contains a list of **V codes**. These codes start with the letter V and range from V01 to V83. Used to classify the reason for care other than an active illness, V codes are located through the alphabetical index in Volume II, Section 1.

E CODES

E codes
codes that classify causes of injury and poisoning

The second chapter of supplementary codes contains a list of **E codes**. These codes start with the letter E and range from E800 to E899. E codes classify causes of injury and poisoning and are located through the index in Volume I, Section 2.

ICD-9-CM APPENDICES

Volume I of the ICD-9-CM manual currently has four appendices. These are used as a reference to provide the user with a clinical picture or further information about the patient's diagnosis. The appendices are used to further define the diagnosis, to classify new drugs, or to reference the type and cause of on-the-job injury the patient has sustained.

Appendix A, *Morphology of Neoplasms*, provides M codes, which are used to describe how a neoplasm has morphed into another part of the patient's body. M codes are not used for billing; they are used only by tumor registries.

Appendix B, *Glossary of Mental Disorders*, was officially deleted from the ICD-9-CM manual in October 2004.

Appendix C is titled *Classification of Drugs by the American Hospital Formulary Service*. Each drug currently approved for use by the FDA is listed in this appendix. This appendix is used to code any adverse effects of drugs on patients.

Appendix D, *Classification of Industrial Accidents According to Agency*, describes on-the-job accidents. It provides codes for describing accidents according to the type or place of the accident.

Appendix E is titled *List of Three-Digit Categories*. All three-digit categories in the ICD-9-CM manual are listed here.

Critical Thinking 15.8 ?

What kinds of problems do you think might arise if the medical office manager does not appropriately code a patient's diagnosis?

VOLUME III

Because Volume III of the ICD-9-CM manual is used for inpatient procedure coding only, medical office managers will only use it if working in a hospital setting. Though medical office managers are commonly hired to manage hospital-owned physician practices, the majority of hospitals hire professional certified coders to code inpatient charts.

FINDING THE CORRECT CODE

Just as with procedural coding, diagnostic coding begins and ends with the patient's medical chart. Medical office managers obtain information from the medical record in order to code for services and determine the reasons why they were provided. Coding is done to the highest level of certainty, meaning that all relevant information in the chart should be coded, but missing information should not be assumed or coded. Only conditions, diseases, and symptoms documented in the medical record can be coded and billed. If the medical record is incomplete or inaccurate, it should be corrected or amended before attempting to code.

A number of the documents in a patient's medical record may contain needed information. When coding for office-based or other outpatient services, medical office managers should refer to the patient registration form, the encounter form, visit notes, lab and radiology reports, and operative reports for outpatient procedures. When coding for services physicians provide to inpatients, medical office managers should refer to the admitting history and physical (H&P), daily progress notes, operative reports, lab and radiology reports, and the discharge summary.

It is important to keep in mind that when performing diagnosis coding in order to bill for services, the diagnosis must describe the reasons the specific service was provided and related medical conditions that may affect the specific service. Diagnosis codes should not repeat a patient's entire problem list, which is a comprehensive list of all active conditions that often appears in the front of the medical record.

The following coding steps provide the practical details medical office managers need to patiently and accurately execute the coding process (Figure ■ 15-12):

1. Identify the first-listed diagnosis as stated in the medical record. Often the physician will indicate a diagnosis code on the encounter form, but it is wise to verify it against the medical record. Look for a definitive diagnostic statement by the physician for reason for the visit. The primary diagnosis is the reason chiefly responsible for the

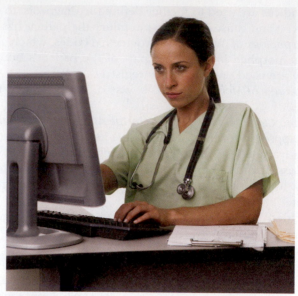

FIGURE ■ 15-12 The medical office manager may need to consult the patient's medical record to find the correct code.
Source: Imagez/Dreamstime.com.

patient's visit to the office for medical care. Additional conditions or complaints will become secondary diagnoses, which will be coded in the same way as the primary, but listed after them on the CMS-1500 billing form.

2. Locate the main term in the alphabetic index, Volume II. Identify the word from the first-listed diagnosis to be looked up under the main term in the index. It may be the name of a condition, such as "fracture"; a disease, such as "pneumonia"; or a reason for the visit, such as "screening." The main term may also be located by eponym, such as "Colles fracture"; an abbreviation, such as "AIDS"; or a nontechnical word, such as "broken" instead of "fracture."

3. Review any modifiers or subterms associated with the main term. Subterms are indented two spaces under the boldfaced main term and further describe the condition. Main terms may also have modifiers, which are words that appear in parentheses immediately after the main term.

4. Identify the tentative code associated with the most appropriate subterm. When the appropriate subterm is located, the tentative code is printed immediately to the right. Never use the index to make the final code selection.

5. Locate the tentative code in the tabular list of Volume I.

6. Interpret the Volume I conventions used with the category. Before verifying and finalizing the code, the medical office manager must interpret the conventions presented with the code and its category.

7. Select the code with the highest level of specificity.

8. Review the code for appropriate age, gender, and reimbursement edits. The bottom of the page in the ICD-9-CM manual contains symbols that indicate codes that should be used only with specific age groups and genders.

9. Verify the final code against the documentation.

10. Assign the code.

11. Repeat the process for any additional codes required.

Critical Thinking 15.9 ?

Imagine you work for a provider who tells you to quickly code the patients' diagnoses. How would you explain the importance of taking your time to make sure the coding is completely accurate?

Coding More Than One Diagnosis

Patients may be seen for more than one complaint at a visit. Up to four diagnosis codes may be entered on a CMS-1500 form. The main reason for the visit is the first-listed diagnosis.

Late Effect Diagnoses

There are many conditions for which patients are seen where the reason for the visit is related to a prior condition. Consider a patient who was treated for a broken arm. When the cast is removed, the patient has a rash that was caused by the cast (Figure ■ 15-13). Treatment of the rash is related to the broken arm, though it was a late effect of the original injury. These late effect codes are listed in the ICD-9-CM manual and should be used when the patient is seen for a condition that is related to a prior condition.

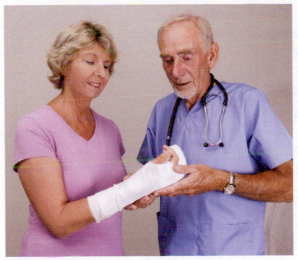

FIGURE ■ 15-13   Once the healing process is complete, the patient will be seen in the medical office to have her cast removed.
Source: Waxart/Dreamstime.com.

Critical Thinking 15.10 ❓

Aside from the example given in the paragraph above, what other late effect diagnoses can you think of?

Coding for Suspected Conditions

When a definitive diagnosis is not yet available, the medical office manager may assign a sign or symptom diagnosis code. This may be done when the physician suspects a certain diagnosis, but the verification will come when the final laboratory or x-ray results are in. Signs, symptoms, and ill-defined conditions are found in the ICD-9-CM manual under codes 780.56 to 781.1.

Case Study Questions

Refer to the case study presented at the beginning of this chapter to answer the following questions:

1. What steps should James take to implement the new coding information he learned at the medical office managers' conference?
2. What other members of the medical practice should James include in the process?
3. What members of the staff should be educated about the changes?

Chapter Review

Summary

- Procedural coding has a long history. The goal continues to be worldwide standardization of the codes used for coding procedures.

- CPT codes are those codes used to code physician visits and procedures.

- Care must be taken when determining the proper procedure code. The code used determines the level of reimbursement received for the service provided.

- Evaluation and Management codes, known as E&M codes, are used to code office visits with patients.

- Anesthesia codes are used to code anesthesia used for surgical cases. These codes do not include the use of local anesthetic for minor cases.

- Surgery codes are all of the codes used for any surgery performed, whether in the physician's office or in the hospital setting.

- Every surgery code has a set number of postoperative days assigned. When the patient is seen during this period for care related to the surgery, the visits are all included in the original surgery charge.

- Radiology codes include codes for any imaging done for the patient. This includes, for example, x-rays, MRIs, and CT scans.

- Pathology and laboratory codes are those codes used to describe the type of pathology or laboratory work done on tissue or body fluid samples taken from a patient.

- Medicine codes are those codes used for certain types of medical services provided to patients.

- The Healthcare Common Procedure Coding System (HCPCS) is a coding manual used for procedural coding.

- Like procedural coding, diagnostic coding has a lengthy history that has been defined by the goal of using standard definitions for diagnoses.

- The ICD-9-CM coding manual is used for coding all diagnoses related to patient care.

- The ICD-10-CM coding manual will be released in October 2013. This new manual will dramatically change the way coding is performed for medical services.

- When patients have more than one diagnosis assigned, the main reason for the visit, known as the chief complaint, is listed first on the insurance claim form.

- A late effect diagnosis is used for a condition that surfaces after a patient undergoes care for a medical reason. The late effect diagnosis is directly related to the original diagnosis.

- When coding for suspected conditions, the ICD-9-CM coding manual contains specific codes to indicate that the condition has not been verified, but that it was suspected at the time the diagnosis was assigned.

Multiple Choice

Choose the letter that best answers each question or completes each statement.

1. Which of the following best describes the usual, customary, and reasonable fee calculation method?
   a. Insurance carriers would determine this fee based on what similar providers in the area were charging for the same service.
   b. Providers would determine this fee based on what insurance carriers were paying for similar services.
   c. Patients would determine this fee based on what they expected to pay for a particular service.
   d. The insurance commissioner in each state determined this fee based on the prevailing rate statewide.

2. Which of the following affects reimbursement of healthcare claims?
   a. Proper documentation in the medical record
   b. Getting the patient into the office in a timely fashion
   c. Answering the office telephone within four rings
   d. Calculating the cost of goods and supplies

3. Which of the following best describes fraud in healthcare billing?
   a. Billing for services that were not rendered
   b. Neglecting to fully explain a procedure to a patient prior to the visit
   c. Quoting the patient the wrong coinsurance amount due at the time of service
   d. Leaving confidential patient information in sight of other patients

4. Evaluation and Management codes are used for what type of patient visit?
   a. Surgical services
   b. Laboratory services
   c. Office visits
   d. Emergency care

5. Which of the following is **not** part of determining the E&M code?
   a. Medical decision making
   b. History of the patient's condition
   c. Type of examination rendered
   d. Amount of time spent with the patient

6. What does it mean to upcode?
   a. To code a service at a lower level to avoid review of the medical chart
   b. To code a service at a higher level to receive a higher level of reimbursement
   c. To charge a higher fee for a service because the patient has medical insurance
   d. To ask the patient for payment up front for services rendered

7. The relative value unit was developed by which of the following?
   a. U.S. Congress
   b. FDA
   c. Medicaid
   d. State government

8. What is an eponym?
   a. A word that has two meanings
   b. A disease or condition named after an individual person
   c. An illness that is easily spread to others
   d. A medical facility that treats emergency patients

9. Which volume in the ICD-9-CM coding manual is used first?
   a. Volume I
   b. Volume II
   c. Volume III
   d. Appendices

10. In the CPT coding manual, a solid circle symbol means:
    a. a new code in this edition of the manual.
    b. a deleted code in this edition of the manual.
    c. an add-on code in this edition of the manual.
    d. none of the above.

True/False

Determine if each of the following statements is true or false.

_____ 1. The etiology of a disease is the cause of the disease.

_____ 2. Appendix M in the CPT code manual is for classification of neoplasms.

_____ 3. Proper documentation is important in coding for procedures but not as vital in coding for diagnoses.

_____ 4. Postoperative days are not billed separately to insurance carriers.

_____ 5. The ICD-10 coding manual has been used in the United States since 2008.

_____ 6. The most important component to choosing the proper E&M code is to determine the amount of time the physician spent with the patient.

_____ 7. When a CPT and an HCPCS code exist for the same service, one should use the CPT code.

_____ 8. There are four components to radiology codes.

_____ 9. The ICD-9 coding manual has 10 appendices.

_____ 10. The World Health Organization has updated ICD codes since 1948.

Matching

Match the following terms with their definition.

a. abuse

b. E codes

c. eponym

d. etiology

e. E&M codes

f. HCPCS

g. modifier

h. Tabular Index

i. upcode

j. V codes

1. Codes used to classify the reason for care other than an active illness

2. Improper behavior and billing practices that result in financial gain but are not fraudulent

3. Cause of a disease or an illness

4. Codes that indicate the external cause of an illness or condition

5. Codes that describe patient encounters with a physician for evaluation and management of a health problem

6. A disease or condition named after an individual

7. The numerical listing of all CPT codes

8. Two-digit numeric code appended to CPT or Level II codes to further describe circumstances

9. To code and bill for a higher level of service than what was actually provided

10. A set of codes developed and maintained by CMS for the reporting of professional services, nonphysician services, supplies, durable medical equipment, and injectable drugs

Chapter Resources

American Medical Association Coding Online: https://commerce.ama-assn.org/store/index.jsp

Centers for Disease Control and Prevention, Classification of Diseases: www.cdc.gov/nchs/icd.htm

ICD-10-CM coding resources: www.ahima.org

World Health Organization: www.who.int/en/

PEARSON
myhealthprofessionskit

Additional interactive resources for this chapter can be found at **www.myhealthprofessionskit. com.** Choose "Medical Assisting" from the discipline menu and then click on the book cover for *Medical Office Management*.

CHAPTER 16

Quality Improvement and Risk Management

CHAPTER OUTLINE

- Creating a Quality Improvement Program
- Avoiding Patient Injury
- Developing a Trusting Relationship with Your Patients
- Reporting Test Results Quickly
- Communicating Possible Outcomes
- Communicating with Other Team Members
- Recognizing Your Limitations and Scope of Practice
- Documenting Noncompliance

- Medication Errors
- Communicating After an Adverse Outcome
- Service Recovery
- Incident Reporting
- Decreasing the Likelihood of Mistakes
- Personal Accountability—Owning Our Mistakes
- Use of Protective Equipment
- Hazardous Waste Disposal
- Employee Safety

LEARNING OBJECTIVES

Upon completion of this chapter, you should be able to:

- Spell and define the key terms in this chapter.
- Describe ways to create a quality improvement program in the medical office, and list possible issues for quality improvement review.
- Understand how to avoid patient injury in the medical office.
- Understand how to develop a trusting relationship with patients.
- Discuss the importance of reporting test results to patients in a timely fashion.
- Describe the purpose of communicating possible outcomes to patients.
- Outline the importance of communicating well with other team members.
- Recognize the limits of scope of practice.
- Document noncompliance in the medical record.
- List common types of medication errors and the steps to avoid them.
- Understand how to communicate with a patient after an adverse outcome.
- Describe the use of service recovery.

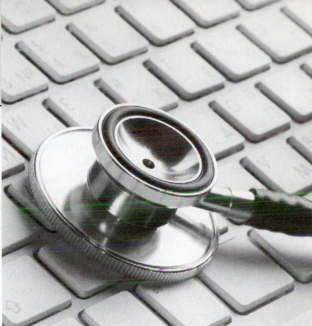

- List possible sentinel events in ambulatory care, and outline the steps for creating an incident report.

- Understand how to decrease the likelihood of mistakes.

- Describe personal accountability and how one owns their mistakes.

- Explain the proper use of protective equipment in the medical office, and describe the responsibilities of the medical office with regard to the equipment.

- Describe the different types of hazardous waste created by healthcare facilities, and how to properly dispose of hazardous waste in the medical office.

- Describe how employee safety is managed in the medical office.

KEY TERMS

quality improvement

risk management

Case Study

Take note of the following scenario and answer the case study questions that appear at the end of this chapter.

Saresh Mulumudi has recently been hired as the medical office manager in a multiple-specialty clinic. He soon discovers many opportunities for improvements in the office and he wants to get the staff and providers engaged in the improvement efforts.

Introduction

As healthcare consumers, patients face a wide array of choices. As in all other businesses, quality customer service is a crucial facet of medical offices' success. Patients who are treated respectfully and equitably communicate positive information about offices and will likely stay with those offices for the long term. Research has shown that patients rate their healthcare higher simply because they felt staff cared about them and took the time to listen to their concerns. Improving quality in the medical office includes looking for ways to improve the patient's experience in the medical office. This includes making sure patients do not wait long periods of time for their appointment, explaining charges to patients prior to services being performed, and maintaining patient confidentiality in all aspects of patient care.

Whereas **quality improvement** is the process of looking for ways to improve the patient experience in the medical office, **risk management** is the process of reducing or eliminating risks of injury to patients or employees. These two processes go hand in hand with efforts to reduce costs for the medical facility, as well as improve the quality of care.

Creating a Quality Improvement Program

Quality improvement programs that focus on patients' emotional and physical health are vital to the success of any healthcare practice. Such programs should be implemented whenever healthcare employees notice areas or situations that when improved would raise patient satisfaction or safety. When staff members notice broken chairs or hallway carpet that has begun to unravel, they should discuss the possible safety hazard with the appropriate parties. Table ■ 16-1 identifies other issues that could benefit from quality improvement.

Critical Thinking 16.1 ?

What other quality improvement areas in healthcare can you think of?

Healthcare staff should work as a team to solve problems immediately through quality improvement programs, which can be very simple. One common office problem is patient wait time. When office managers receive complaints about patient wait times, those managers should mobilize teams quickly to solve the problem by studying appointment times or discussing outcomes with physicians. When patient wait times are allowed to remain long, patients may find fault with the office or seek care elsewhere.

The medical office management team sets the tone for employees to feel comfortable about reporting possible problems in the clinic. Employees who feel secure about

TABLE ■ 16-1 Possible Issues for Quality Improvement Review

- Patient wait times
- Insurance company rejections of certain services or procedures
- Equipment needs
- Health Insurance Portability and Accountability Act (HIPAA) violations
- Collection practices
- Office remodeling
- Patient flow in the office
- Office waste
- Staffing
- Personal use of office telephones or computers

bringing ideas or problems to their manager will feel more empowered about creating and being a part of a culture of safety and improvement in the workplace. To accomplish this, managers should praise or even reward employees who bring forward ideas for quality improvement, or who report problems that may or have resulted in injury to a patient or employee (Figure ■ 16-1).

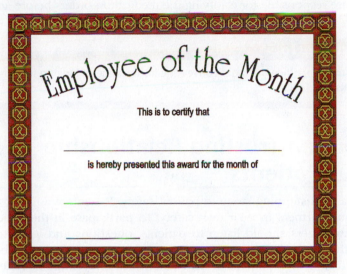

FIGURE ■ 16-1   Employees should be recognized and possibly even rewarded for submitting improvement ideas.
Source: Mehselltingle/Dreamstime.com.

Critical Thinking 16.2 ?

What type of reward or recognition program can you think of that might encourage employees to come forward with their quality improvement ideas?

One way to solicit improvement ideas is to provide employees with an anonymous method for submitting suggestions (Figure ■ 16-2). This method may work better in a clinic where the culture has not always been supportive of the employees' coming forward with ideas. By providing employees with a method for submitting suggestions, the manager shows employees that these suggestions are encouraged and valued.

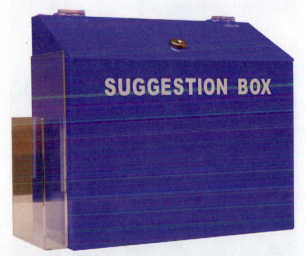

FIGURE ■ 16-2   A suggestion box is an anonymous method for employees to submit their quality improvement suggestions.
Source: Prestonia/Dreamstime.com.

Avoiding Patient Injury

Every member of the healthcare team is responsible for patient safety, which means any team member should speak up when she sees a potential risk factor. For example, when physicians order medications that medical assistants or nurses believe to be incorrect, those assistants or nurses are responsible for clarifying the medication orders before administration.

Critical Thinking 16.3 ?

How might the medical office manager convey the importance of looking for possible patient injury areas to his employees?

Developing a Trusting Relationship with Your Patients

Patient trust is a vital stepping stone to patient safety. Patients who trust their healthcare providers become partners in their own safety. To participate in the patient partnership, medical office managers should listen to patients' questions and learn to recognize the body language that alerts them to patients' unspoken messages. To make these tasks easier, managers should sit next to patients or their families whenever appropriate (Figure ■ 16-3) and try to anticipate patient questions. As much as possible, managers should provide the answers to commonly asked questions. It is also helpful for managers to use touch appropriately to show concern and to speak in patients' native languages when possible. To ensure communication is understood, medical office managers should ask patients and

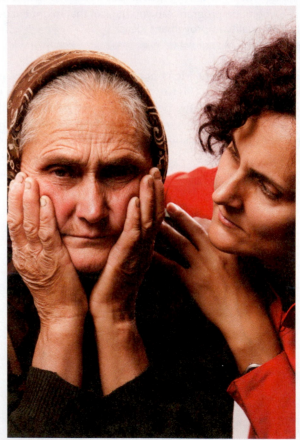

FIGURE ■ 16-3 Medical office managers can use touch appropriately to show concern.
Source: Xalanx/Dreamstime.com.

their families to repeat discussions in their own words. Respecting patients' decisions and maintaining patients' confidence are parts of advocating for patients in healthcare.

Critical Thinking 16.4 ?

In what ways would you work to develop a rapport and trust with the patient?

Reporting Test Results Quickly

A recent study performed by The Joint Commission found that medical facilities that report test results to patients in a timely manner have reduced errors and complications with patient care. Quick responses lead to patients undergoing needed care sooner, which can dramatically reduce the effects of disease and illness in many cases. One study performed by The Joint Commission found that faster responses to laboratory results could have prevented 4.1 percent of adverse events in a group of patients. Another study, this one performed in a hospital setting, found that a delay of more than 5 hours before communicating test results and starting patients on a prescribed treatment resulted in poor outcomes in 27 percent of the patients.

In the ambulatory setting, physicians and office managers must work together to devise a process for alerting patients to test results. With an electronic medical record, this process may be automated, with results coming to the nurse or physician. In many healthcare facilities today, patients are able to access a portion of their medical record online. A healthcare facility in Washington State uses a system called My Chart where the patients are alerted via e-mail of any test or study at the same time as the results are posted to the patients' medical records. This allows patients to be made aware of test outcomes at the same time the physician is notified, making communication of the results happen very quickly (Figure ■ 16-4)

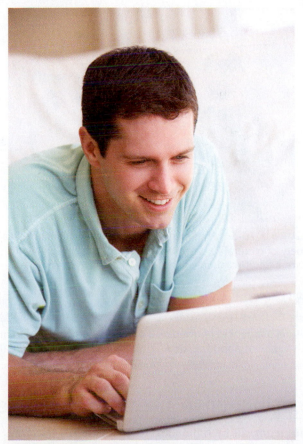

FIGURE ■ 16-4 Many patients today like to receive their results online.
Source: Monkeybusiness/Dreamstime.com.

Critical Thinking 16.5 ?

What kind of problems do you think might result from reporting medical tests or studies late? How might the medical office manager work to alleviate those situations?

Communicating Possible Outcomes

Good communication between the physician and the patient has many benefits. For patients, understanding the possible outcomes to treatment, or lack of treatment, is essential to making informed choices about their healthcare. As described in Chapter 8, communicating possible outcomes is part of the informed consent process. For the physician, good communication with the patient leads to better compliance with care suggestions, increased patient satisfaction, and lowered incidences of malpractice actions.

Patients need to be educated about possible outcomes prior to the prescribed course of treatment. Physicians can initiate this conversation effectively by showing empathy and respect to the patient. This conversation should take place in a quiet location where the patient feels unhurried and understands that the physician genuinely wants to answer any questions and ease the patient's fears. Physicians must answer questions honestly and involve the patient in the care choices. Knowing that patients have autonomy and can refuse care if they so choose, physicians must be careful to refrain from attempting to coerce the patient into choosing the option the physician feels is best. Part of the communication process includes paying attention to any cultural or ethnic issues that may affect the patient's understanding and decision making (Figure ■ 16-5). As with any conversation with the patient regarding care, conversations about possible care outcomes must be documented in the patient's chart.

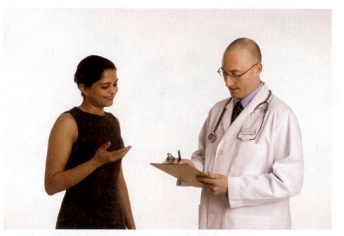

FIGURE ■ 16-5 Physicians will meet with patients from a variety of cultural backgrounds.
Source: lofoto/Dreamstime.com.

Critical Thinking 16.6 ?

Think about how cultural differences might play a part in how the physician or manager needs to communicate with a patient about possible outcomes. What ideas come to mind?

Communicating with Other Team Members

Within the healthcare team, all members are responsible for patient safety and quality of care. The most crucial part of this is accomplished with good communication among the team members. This communication takes many forms. For medical office managers who work in specialty practice settings, many of the patients will have been referred for care by their primary care physician. Proper communication includes sending a report of the visit, including any test results, from the specialist to the primary care physician. This fosters the co-treatment aspect of patient care that exists between primary care physicians and specialists.

Within the healthcare setting, communication among team members takes the form of the receptionist communicating any necessary information about the patient to the back-office staff, and the back-office staff communicating to the physician. After the patient's visit, the physician must properly communicate with her clinical team to make sure prescriptions are filled properly and any required tests, studies, and follow-up visits scheduled. With an electronic medical record, much of this communication can take place electronically. In the situation where a specialist sees a patient at the request of a primary care physician, the specialist is able to automatically fax her chart note about the patient's visit to the primary care physician. In large healthcare facilities, where the patient's primary care physician and specialists all share the same electronic medical record, the transfer of information is immediate.

Many clinics today provide patients with written instructions or information that summarizes the visit. These instructions may be called by a variety of names, but most will include information about the reason for the patient's visit, any instructions regarding medications or treatments, and information about the need for follow-up care. Patients report a higher level of satisfaction with their healthcare experience when they feel they better understand their instructions. These end-of-visit summaries provide the patient with that information. For patients who have been given extensive instructions, or who are having a hard time fully grasping the information or diagnosis given, these summaries offer the patient the ability to read through the information or to provide it to a family member after the visit (Figure ■ 16-6).

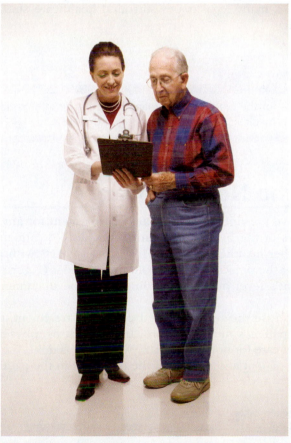

FIGURE ■ 16-6   A patient looks over his after-visit summary.
Source: lofoto/Dreamstime.com.

One of the most recognized issues surrounding communication among healthcare team members is the cultural deference given physicians, due to their advanced training and education, over other members of the healthcare team. In many malpractice cases, nurses, technicians, and medical assistants have repeatedly mentioned this barrier as the reason they did not speak up when they had a question about an order given by a physician. Though questioning the physician in front of patients is not advised, any member of the healthcare team who does not fully understand what he or she is being asked to do should take a moment to ask for clarification.

Critical Thinking 16.7 ?

What kinds of problems might come into play if the various members of the medical team do not communicate well with one another? What kinds of processes might be put into place to alleviate these concerns?

Recognizing Your Limitations and Scope of Practice

Each healthcare profession has a scope of practice, which is outlined in each states' medical practice laws. It is important for all members of the healthcare team to fully understand what is, and what is not, within their scope of practice. In some situations, a medical assistant may have been trained to perform a task while working in one state, but in another state that task is outside the scope of practice for medical assistants. As outlined in Chapter 3, many legal issues surround healthcare staff performing outside their scope of practice.

Critical Thinking 16.8 ?

Where is a good place for the medical office manager to go for information about scope of practice for the various medical professionals working in the office?

Documenting Noncompliance

Because patients have the right to refuse care or treatment for any reason, it is important for all members of the healthcare team to properly document when a patient is noncompliant with her healthcare needs. This process starts with proper education of the patient regarding the prescribed care from the provider (Figure ■ 16-7). This education, and the patient's level of understanding, must be documented in the patient's medical record.

When patients refuse the recommended course of treatment, that refusal must be documented in the patient's medical record. In some cases, physicians may choose to dismiss patients from care for noncompliance. When this is done, the physician must give proper notice to the patient and document the dismissal in the patient's chart.

Critical Thinking 16.9 ?

What problems might occur due to a patient being noncompliant with healthcare recommendations?

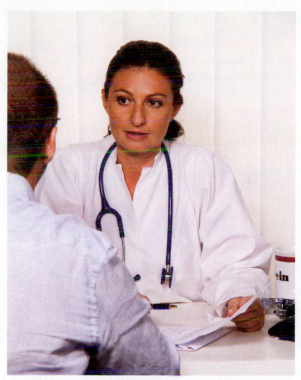

FIGURE ■ 16-7   Physicians will occasionally need to take extra time to go over treatment suggestions with patients.
Source: Ginasanders/Dreamstime.com.

Medication Errors

According to the U.S. Food and Drug Administration, a medication error is defined as any preventable event that may cause or lead to inappropriate medication use or patient harm while the medication is in the control of the healthcare professional, patient, or consumer.

The American Hospital Association (AHA) lists the following as the most common types of medication errors:

- *Incomplete gathering of patient information.* This error may happen when the healthcare professional does not know about patient allergies, other medications the patient is taking, previous diagnoses, or lab results.

- *Unavailable drug information.* This error may happen when the prescribing provider or pharmacist is unaware of up-to-date warnings about medications or contraindications.

- *Miscommunication of drug orders.* This type of error can occur with poor handwriting in the patient chart or on the prescription, confusion between drugs with similar names, misunderstanding of where zeroes and decimal points lie, confusion of metric with other dosing units, or use of inappropriate abbreviations.

- *Lack of appropriate labeling.* This error happens most commonly when drugs are prepared or drawn up.

- *Environmental factors.* Poor lighting, noise, interruptions, or other environmental factors that distract healthcare professionals can lead to this type of error.

Every medication error is preventable. Medical office managers should train staff to always follow the five rights of medication administration. These rights are:

1. Right patient
2. Right route
3. Right dose

4. Right time

5. Right medication.

No medication should be administered to a patient without the nurse, medical assistant, or provider first verifying that he has followed all of the five rights listed above (Figure ■ 16-8).

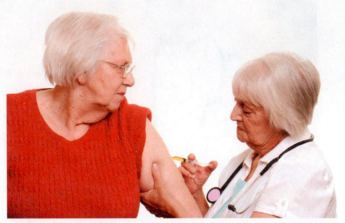

FIGURE ■ **16-8**   The nurse must verify that she has followed all of the five rights of medication administration prior to injecting the medication.
Source: Mg7/Dreamtime.com.

If a medication error occurs, the person responsible must immediately report the error to the medical office manager and the physician. If the patient requires care due to the error, that takes top priority. Once the patient has been cared for, or if the patient does not need care for the error, the person responsible for the error and the physician should explain to the patient what occurred. All questions from the patient must be answered honestly. After the discussion has been completed, the entire incident must be charted in the patient's medical record and a medication error report must be filled out. In many healthcare facilities, an investigation will occur to discover why the error occurred and what can be done to prohibit such an error from occurring in the future.

REPORTING NEAR MISSES/GOOD CATCHES

Two terms used interchangeably to discuss errors that are caught before they reach the patient are *near miss* and *good catch*. These terms apply when a healthcare provider realizes a possible medical error, such as a wrong medication, prior to it reaching the patient. It is very important for the medical office manager to implement a system for reporting these near misses/good catches so that an investigation may be started to determine how the error could have happened. Taking these investigative steps helps to eliminate future errors from happening at all.

Communicating After an Adverse Outcome

Historically, healthcare providers have been encouraged to stay close-mouthed after a patient experiences an adverse outcome. This line of thinking stems from the belief that patients will assign blame and file a lawsuit against the provider. During the past decade, however, many studies have shown that the majority of malpractice lawsuits are filed not because the patient wants to recover money but because the patient wants to know what happened. Healthcare facilities that have embraced a culture of openness after an adverse event has occurred and discussed with the patient and the family what has occurred have found they are involved in fewer malpractice lawsuits than those facilities that do not share information with the patient.

Through informed consent prior to a procedure, the patient is made aware of any possible side effects or problems that could occur as a result of the recommended procedure. Taking the time to thoroughly explain these things to the patient prior to the procedure saves providers from explaining problems to the patient when known side effects do occur.

Still, some adverse reactions or medical mistakes will happen. When they occur, it is important for the provider to be honest with the patient and explain, in layman's terms, what has happened. The *Journal of the American Academy of Physician Assistants* (JAAPA) published an article in 2010 that highlighted the benefits to healthcare providers, as well as patients, of honest disclosure of medical errors that harm patients. This article noted that nearly 100,000 people die annually in the United States due to a preventable medical error. This makes medical errors the eighth leading cause of death in this country. JAAPA, as well as many other professional organizations, has found that the healthcare provider may be just as traumatized by the medical error as the patient and family. Honest communication about the error, including how it happened, helps both sides heal when such an injury occurs. The Joint Commission has accreditation standards in place that require healthcare providers to inform patients about unanticipated outcomes.

If a medical error occurs, it is important to take care of the patient's needs first. Once the patient has been cared for, a conversation should take place with the patient and his family to discuss what has happened. This conversation may include the healthcare organization's risk manager or the medical office manager (Figure ■ 16-9). The patient's questions should be fully answered and documentation of the conversation should be made in the patient's medical record. If the error resulted in serious injury to the patient, the physician should contact her malpractice insurance carrier to alert them about the possibility of a claim.

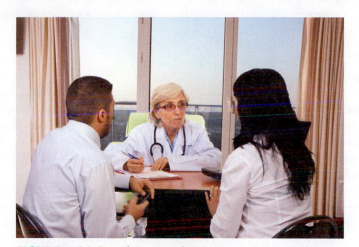

FIGURE ■ 16-9 When an unforeseen event occurs, the physician should meet with the patient or family to discuss what happened.
Source: Justmeyo/Dreamstime.com.

Service Recovery

The vast majority of the quality improvement or risk management events that occur in the medical office do not result in patient injury. Instead, these events may result in inconvenience to the patient. Examples include patients who were forgotten in an exam room, patients who were overlooked and left in the reception area for an extended period of time, or patients who arrived to find the physician was running an hour behind schedule. In these events, it is important for the medical office manager to acknowledge the patient's inconvenience and to offer some form of service recovery. A simple apology is often all that is needed to make the patient feel better about the inconvenience. Other times, a small gift card, for example to a local coffee vendor, may be in order. Patients who feel their concerns were addressed and acknowledged in a timely manner are typically put at ease and no further complaint will result (Figure ■ 16-10).

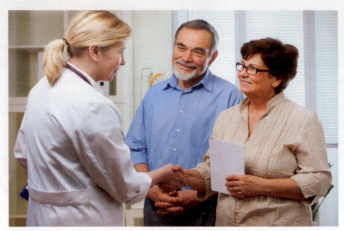

FIGURE ■ 16-10 When patients have been inconvenienced, the medical office manager should provide some form of service recovery.
Source: Alexraths/Dreamstime.com.

Critical Thinking 16.10 ?

What kind of items do you think would be best for service recovery in the medical office?

Incident Reporting

Adverse outcomes are events that were unexpected or that are the result of an error on the part of one or more persons on the healthcare team. Adverse outcomes that cause patient injury are called *sentinel events*. The Joint Commission describes sentinel events as ones in which injuries occurred, or could have occurred, in a medical setting. Table ■ 16-2 lists possible sentinel events in ambulatory care.

When sentinel events occur, medical office managers must document and report those events properly—not to blame or punish employees but to aid in prevention. Managers who strive to use errors as learning experiences rather than punishment tools promote cultures in which employees feel safe enough to self-report errors.

To report sentinel events, every manager should fully complete sentinel reporting forms or incident report forms, using a typed font or blue or black ink (Figure ■ 16-11). These reports may be purchased from medical office suppliers, or managers may create their own. No boxes should remain blank. When boxes do not apply, medical office managers should write "Not Applicable" or "NA" in them. Sentinel reports should reside in a

TABLE ■ 16-2 Possible Sentinel Events in Ambulatory Care

- Incorrect medication administration
- Patient falls in the office
- Missing prescription pads or medications
- Incorrect or absent patient instructions following procedures
- Needlestick injuries to staff
- Inappropriate handling of patient laboratory samples

INCIDENT REPORT

Name of injured party _____ Date _____

Address _____ Telephone _____

_____

The injured party was: ☐ Employee ☐ Patient ☐ Other _____

Date of accident/incident _____ Time of incident _____

Where did incident occur? _____

Names of witnesses (include titles):

_____   _____

_____   _____

What first aid/treatment was given at the time of the incident?

_____

_____

Who administered first aid? _____

Briefly describe the incident. _____

_____

_____

_____

Names of employees present at time of incident/injury:

_____

_____

Follow-up: What steps have been taken to prevent a similar accident? _____

_____

_____

Date _____   Employee's signature _____

Date _____   Supervisor's signature _____

FIGURE ■ 16-11   An example of a typical incident report.

master incident report file, but copies should not appear in employees' files or patients' medical records.

Decreasing the Likelihood of Mistakes

The most common type of medical mistake is a medication error. The Institute of Medicine (IOM) has determined that between 380,000 and 450,000 medication errors occur in the United States every year. Other mistakes include surgical and diagnostic errors, equipment failure, infections, and misinterpretation of medical orders.

The most effective method of reducing medical mistakes begins with communication among healthcare professionals. The IOM noted that most medical errors are related to systems errors, rather than negligence or misconduct. The key to reducing medical errors lies in focusing on improving the systems of delivering care and removing blame from individuals. Greater simplification of systems, such as instituting the use of bar codes in medication disbursement, and greater standardization of procedures and processes have shown to dramatically decrease preventable medical errors.

Because the IOM has determined that preventable medical errors cost approximately $37.6 billion in healthcare costs each year, this is an area that is well worth the focus of everyone who works in healthcare, including the medical office manager.

Personal Accountability—Owning Our Mistakes

Every medical office manager should work to create a culture of accountability in his or her organization. This includes encouraging employees to speak up when they see something that is not right, or admitting when they have been involved in a medical mistake. It is human nature to avoid admitting mistakes made; therefore, the medical office manager must devise a system to reward employees for admitting their mistakes, without fear of reprisal.

Critical Thinking 16.11 ?

Thinking about the culture of blame we currently have in society, how would you, as a medical office manager, encourage your employees to report problems without fear of reprisal?

Use of Protective Equipment

Most medical offices have equipment, or perform procedures, that require staff to use or wear personal protective equipment (Figure ■ 16-12). For example, whenever healthcare employees are exposed to patients' body fluids those employees must don gloves and possibly eye shields. Employees who x-ray patients must wear radiation badges to assess their possible x-ray exposure (Figure ■ 16-13). Employers must supply any needed protective equipment, as well as clean and dispose of it.

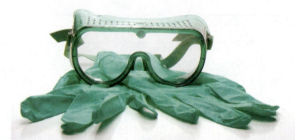

FIGURE ■ 16-12 Examples of protective equipment found in the medical clinic.
Source: Robeo/Dreamstime.com.

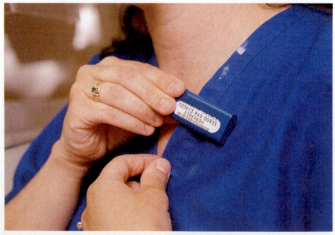

FIGURE ■ 16-13 A radiation exposure badge.
Source: Cliff Moore/Photo Researchers, Inc.

Hazardous Waste Disposal

Each year, healthcare facilities create 3.2 million tons of hazardous waste in the four following categories:

- **Solid**—Paper, cans, cups, and other garbage from nonclinical office areas.
- **Chemical**—Wasted drugs, cleaning solutions, and germicides. These items must be disposed of according to Occupational Safety and Health Administration (OSHA) guidelines.
- **Radioactive**—Any waste contaminated with radioactive material. Most common in oncology practices, this waste must be disposed of in containers clearly marked "Radioactive" and removed only by licensed facilities.
- **Infectious**—Any garbage exposed to body fluids or any laboratory cultures or blood products. These items must be separated from other waste items, placed in bags clearly labeled as "Biohazardous Waste," (Figure ■ 16-14), and removed by a licensed medical waste removal company.

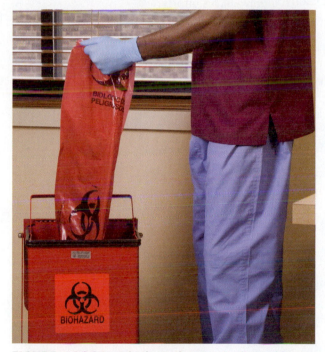

FIGURE ■ 16-14 A biohazardous waste disposal bag.
Source: Michal Heron/Pearson Education.

Though some hazardous waste may be disposed of through local garbage services, all must be disposed of according to federal and local law. On a federal level, medical offices must abide by OSHA guidelines when disposing of hazardous medical waste. These rules are in addition to any state or local laws the medical office must follow. OSHA requires medical offices to dispose of hazardous medical waste in the following manner:

- The waste must be placed into a container that is closable.
- The container must be designed to contain all of the contents. It must be closed prior to removal to prevent leakage of fluids during handling, storage, transport, or shipping.
- The container must be labeled or color coded noting that the contents are hazardous.
- If outside contamination occurs, the first container must be placed within a second container that meets all of the above listed standards.

Employee Safety

Just as patient safety demands constant attention in the medical office, so does employee safety. As a preventive step, all staff must remain vigilant to situations that may lead to employee error. For example, staff should keep current on the maintenance and repair of office equipment and ensure that all employees are properly trained in the equipment's use. Attention to proper lifting techniques and office ergonomics also helps avoid injuries and lost time in the workplace.

Case Study Questions

Refer to the case study presented at the beginning of this chapter to answer the following questions:

1. How would you suggest Saresh go about setting up a quality improvement program in his office?
2. Who should Saresh involve in his efforts?

Chapter Review

Summary

- A quality improvement program should involve all members of the healthcare team. The goal is to look for areas that, if improved, could reduce possible risks to the office staff and at the same time enhance the patients' experiences.

- Avoiding patient injury is the responsibility of all members of the healthcare team. It is important to properly investigate any possible errors in order to make certain those errors do not result in injury to patients or employees.

- By developing a trusting relationship and rapport with the patient, the medical office staff and providers will find patients are more likely to follow through with healthcare recommendations.

- Reporting test results in a timely manner has been proven to reduce unfavorable outcomes in patient care. Patients are able to obtain needed medical care sooner when results are communicated right away.

- Part of informed consent includes communicating possible adverse outcomes with patients. Once patients have all needed information about possible outcomes, the patient can make an informed decision regarding care.

- All members of the healthcare team must communicate well in order to safely and efficiently care for the patient. This includes communication within the facility as well as with outside healthcare providers.

- All healthcare professionals have a scope of practice dictated by the state. It is important for members of the team to follow this scope of practice in order to properly care for patients in a safe manner.

- Any time the patient chooses to go outside treatment recommendations, that choice should be properly documented in the patient's medical record.

- Medication errors are the most common medical error. Because all medication errors are avoidable, it is important for every member of the healthcare team to take the time to properly administer and document medications.

- When an unforeseen outcome occurs, medical providers and managers are responsible for communicating this information to the patient or patient's family. This communication should be open and honest and must be documented in the patient's medical record.

- Service recovery is the process of offering an apology or gift card to the patient after an event that causes the patient to be dissatisfied with his care.

- Incident reporting must be done any time a patient or employee is injured, or an event occurs that could have resulted in an injury. The purpose of the incident report is not to blame those involved but to make sure the process is examined so that the same problem cannot occur in the future.

- By concentrating on process improvement, the medical office manager can lead her team toward decreasing the likelihood of mistakes in patient care.

- Medical office managers must alter the culture in healthcare so that everyone feels safe to own their mistakes and look for ways to improve the systems.

- By using protective equipment, medical office personnel are able to avoid most avenues for infection from patients in the healthcare facility.

- Hazardous waste must be disposed of properly and according to the laws in the state where the medical practice is located.

- Employee safety is just as important as patient safety. The medical office manager must look for ways to keep employees safe.

Multiple Choice

Choose the letter that best answers each question or completes each statement.

1. Which organization published an article noting that nearly 100,000 people die annually in the United States due to a preventable medical error?
   a. AHA
   b. JAAPA
   c. The Joint Commission
   d. Centers for Medicare and Medicaid Services

2. Which of the following is true of dealing with a noncompliant patient?
   a. The healthcare provider should insist the patient follow the prescribed instructions.
   b. The healthcare provider should document the patient's noncompliance in the patient's medical record.
   c. The patient has the right to sue the provider if he does not wish to follow the prescribed course of treatment.
   d. The insurance company does not have to pay for care when the patient turns out to be noncompliant.

3. Which of the following best describes service recovery?
   a. A small gift or item given to the patient who has been mildly inconvenienced
   b. Money paid to the patient to avoid a lawsuit
   c. Return of funds paid by the insurance company when the patient is unhappy with care
   d. None of the above

4. One study performed by The Joint Commission found that faster responses to laboratory results could have prevented _____ percent of adverse events in a group of patients.
   a. 2.2
   b. 3.4
   c. 4.1
   d. 5.6

5. A patient comes in for a medical procedure. The physician asks the medical assistant to draw up medications to be administered to the patient. The medical assistant believes the order to be in error. Who is responsible for speaking up about the possible error?
   a. The physician   c. The patient's family member
   b. The patient   d. The medical assistant

6. What is meant by the concept that patients have autonomy in their healthcare choices?
   a. The patient can choose to refuse recommended care for any reason.
   b. The patient's family can choose to refuse recommended care for any reason.
   c. The provider can choose to refuse to provide care to the patient for any reason.
   d. The medical assistant can choose to refuse to participate in the patient's care for any reason.

7. Scope of practice is dictated by which of the following?
   a. The federal government
   b. The city government
   c. The state government
   d. The individual physician

8. Another term for a near miss is a (an) _____
   a. good catch   c. avoided lawsuit
   b. learning moment   d. missed failure

9. When patients refuse the recommended course of treatment, that refusal must be documented where?
   a. With the state Department of Health
   b. With the patient's insurance carrier
   c. With the physician's malpractice insurance company
   d. In the patient's medical record

10. What type of physicians typically refer to specialists?
    a. Primary care providers
    b. Other specialty providers
    c. Pediatricians
    d. Emergency department physicians

True/False

Determine if each of the following statements is true or false.

_____ 1. The Institute of Medicine determined that between 380,000 and 450,000 medication errors occur in the United States every year.

_____ 2. Patients who trust their healthcare providers become partners in their own safety.

_____ 3. One advantage to providing patients with timely information about test results is that the patients can access needed care sooner.

_____ 4. The nurse or medical assistant should never question the physician's orders regarding patient care.

_____ 5. The most common patient safety error involves medication errors.

_____ 6. Part of the communication process includes paying attention to any cultural or ethnic issues that may affect the patient's understanding and decision making.

_____ 7. If a medication error occurs, the first thing to take care of is to call the physician's malpractice insurer.

_____ 8. After any event in which a patient is injured, or could have been injured, an incident report must be filled out.

_____ 9. Each medical profession has its own medical scope of practice.

_____ 10. The person who fills out the incident report should be the person who was involved in the event.

Matching

Match each of the following terms with its definition.

a. One of the five rights to medication administration

b. Not one of the five rights to medication administration

1. Right patient
2. Right office
3. Right staff member
4. Right route
5. Right dose
6. Right time
7. Right appointment type
8. Right medication
9. Right medical record

Chapter Resources

American Hospital Association: www.aha.org

The Joint Commission: www.jointcommission.org

Journal of the American Academy of Physician Assistants (JAAPA): www.jaapa.com

myhealthprofessionskit

Additional interactive resources for this chapter can be found at **www.myhealthprofessionskit. com.** Choose "Medical Assisting" from the discipline menu and then click on the book cover for *Medical Office Management.*

CHAPTER 17

Marketing the Medical Office

CHAPTER OUTLINE

LEARNING OBJECTIVES

Upon completion of this chapter, you should be able to:

- Spell and define the key terms in this chapter.
- Describe the task of funding a marketing initiative.
- Understand how to market to a practice's demographic.
- Understand the importance of researching the strengths, weaknesses, and opportunities of a medical practice.
- Determine what to look for when researching the competition.
- Describe how the Internet can be used for marketing purposes.
- List the items available on a robust clinic website.
- Understand how direct mail advertising works.
- Describe the purchase of mailing lists as an advertising option for the medical office.
- Understand how the Welcome to the Neighborhood program works within communities.
- Describe the role of the medical office manager in setting up free or low-cost screenings.

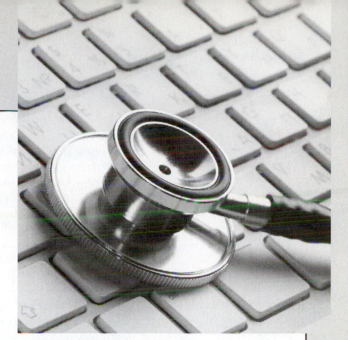

- List the steps involved at screening events.
- Explain how social media sites can be used in advertising.
- Define focus groups, and describe their use.
- Understand how local businesses might be targeted for marketing purposes.
- Describe possible venues for educational speaking engagements, and discuss the role of the medical office manager in planning for these events.
- Describe how to use telephone books as advertising sources.
- Describe on-hold messaging and explain how it is used.
- Discuss the use of surveys in determining patients' satisfaction with their health care.
- Explain how patients might be used as sources of advertising.
- Describe how writing articles for local newspapers or periodicals is a form of marketing, and list members of the medical team who may be involved in this advertising.
- Understand how to target local media for advertising.
- Describe the benefits of hiring a marketing consultant.

KEY TERMS

demographic
direct mail advertising
focus group
marketing budget
marketing firm

marketing plan
osteoporosis
prostate
return on investment
scoliosis

screenings
search engine optimization
social media sites

Case Study

Take note of the following scenario and answer the case study questions that appear at the end of this chapter.

Harold Price is the medical office manager with a large cardiology practice. The physicians in his clinic have asked Harold to put together a marketing plan and to present his ideas to them at the next department meeting.

Introduction

marketing plan
a plan for advertising a
business or product

Marketing any business takes time, money, and a good deal of preparation. Healthcare is no exception. The best preparation is a properly prepared **marketing plan**. A strong marketing plan helps the medical office manager stay on schedule and spend allocated funds appropriately. Any marketing initiative, whether designed to start a new practice or bring new business into an existing practice, should be undertaken only after investigation of a number of factors. The medical office manager should work in concert with the physicians or with the owners of the business, if not the physicians.

Funding a Marketing Initiative

marketing budget
the amount of money
allocated to a marketing
plan

marketing firm
a company that can be
hired for the purpose of
composing and carrying
out a marketing plan

return on investment
the amount of money
brought in after a
marketing initiative

The clinic's **marketing budget** outlines the costs of the marketing initiatives that are planned. These funds may be allocated to hiring a **marketing firm**, or they may be budgeted toward other in-house directed endeavors. Although the marketing budget should be determined before setting out to market the practice, no business should set this number in stone. The budgeted amount may need to be flexible as needs or opportunities arise.

To determine the return on investment for any marketing initiative, the medical office manager should perform a prospective view for the marketing plan. This should include the number of patients expected to be reached by the plan and the dollars those patients will bring in once they come in for care. This number will vary according to the type of practice and care offered. For example, a plastic surgeon may choose to market a particular product or service (Figure ■ 17-1). Knowing the amount of money the service brings in, the medical office manager will be able to determine how much money the marketing plan should return for the dollars invested in the marketing plan. This is called the **return on investment**. On the other hand, if it is a family practice physician who is marketing for new patients, the amount of money each patient brings in will vary according to the type of care each patient needs.

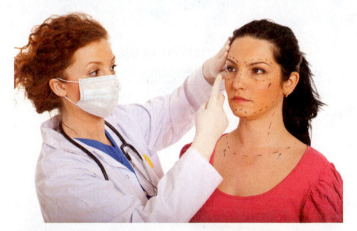

FIGURE ■ 17-1 A plastic surgeon may choose to market facial cosmetic surgery in a community where this service may be popular.
Source: Justmeyol/Dreamstime.com.

Critical Thinking 17.1 ?

What do you think the pros and cons are of hiring a marketing firm to prepare a clinic's marketing plans?

Understanding the Demographic

Before undertaking any marketing plan, the medical office manager should determine the targeted audience. If the clinic is located in an area where the main **demographic** is blue collar workers, the manager may think about marketing areas that are of interest to working families, such as sports physicals, or back-to-school exams (Figure ■ 17-2). In an area that is populated with a large number of patients over the age of 60, the medical office manager may wish to market in areas that are of interest to retired persons, such as **osteoporosis** or **prostate** screenings.

demographic
the makeup of a population, such as age and number of children

osteoporosis
a disorder in which the bones become increasingly porous, brittle, and subject to fracture

prostate
a gland in males that surrounds the neck of the bladder and urethra

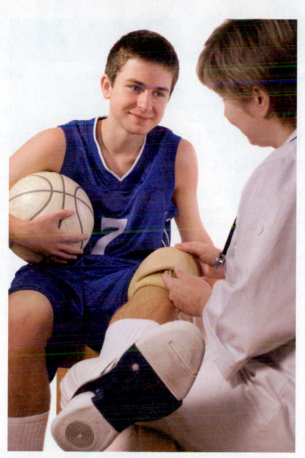

FIGURE ■ 17-2   The manager might consider marketing sports physicals in an area that is populated with families.
Source: Alexraths/Dreamstime.com.

The type and method of advertising should be considered along with the demographic of patients being targeted. For example, many young families are on the go and may be best reached by advertisements on the sides of buses or printed in school brochures. Elderly patients may be best reached with mailers sent directly to the home or via flyers placed in the local pharmacy or in local senior centers (Figure ■ 17-3).

Critical Thinking 17.2 ?

What problems might result if a marketing plan is put into place without consideration of the demographic in the clinic's area?

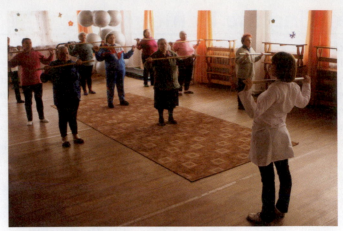

FIGURE ■ 17-3   Senior centers are a good place for medical offices to market their practice.
Source: Dimaberkut/Dreamstime.com.

Researching Your Strengths, Weaknesses, and Opportunities

The medical office manager will want to market those areas where the practice is doing well and is able to handle increased business. For example, if a family practice has recently lost one of its two pediatricians, and getting an appointment with the remaining pediatrician presents a challenge, this would not be the time to market care related to children. On the other hand, if the practice has just received a large shipment of influenza vaccine and has the staff available to administer the vaccine, this is the perfect time to advertise influenza vaccines to the community (Figure ■ 17-4).

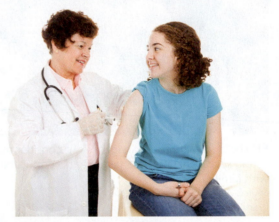

FIGURE ■ 17-4   The manager should market those areas where the practice is able to handle increased business, for example, advertising influenza vaccines.
Source: Lisafx/Dreamstime.com.

Researching the Competition

Part of researching the practice's strengths and weaknesses should include a broader look at the surrounding community. The medical practice manager should determine where the competition is strong and where their weaknesses lie. For example, if the only other family practice in town has a physician who is well known for his ability to work with children with behavioral issues, this might not be an area in which competing practices would want to market. Spending dollars on marketing in an area where the competition has a strong foothold is not typically a wise decision.

Using the Internet for Marketing

The Internet can be a strong tool for medical office advertising. Many practices manage their own websites and others purchase space on a community site. There are many places to purchase advertising on the Internet. The medical office manager should research the options and do a cost comparison to determine which one, if any, is appropriate for the practice and the marketing plan intended.

Search engine optimization is an option many businesses choose to pursue. This optimization process entails making changes to a company's individual website so that it will come up at the top of a results list during a search with an Internet search engine, such as Google. Businesses, including healthcare facilities, can also buy advertisements directly from Internet search engines. These advertisements appear on the main page of the search engine once certain terms are entered for a search. For example, if a potential patient is searching for a pediatrician in Portland, Oregon, she may go to an Internet search engine and type in "pediatrician in Portland, Oregon." A paid advertisement from a pediatrics practice in Portland, Oregon, will appear on the right side of the screen, bringing in potential new patients to the practice (Figure ■ 17-5).

search engine optimization
the process of making changes to a company's individual website so that the website will come up at the top of a results list during Internet searching

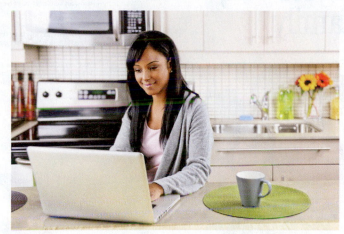

FIGURE ■ 17-5   Many patients today use the Internet to locate a new provider.
Source: Elanathewise/Dreamstime.com.

A Robust Website

Most businesses today have their own website on the Internet. These sites might be developed entirely by someone within the practice, such as the medical office manager or one of the physicians, or a company may be hired to design and manage the site. Many practices today have very robust websites, where patients are able to request or even schedule appointments, pay bills, and find answers to medical questions. Other items commonly found on a medical clinic's website include:

- Biographies of the individual physicians. This sometimes includes video segments of physicians discussing their care philosophies.
- Insurance information, including the types of insurance plans accepted.
- Locations and hours sites are open for care. This typically includes driving directions and parking information.
- A list of job opportunities available at the medical facility.

Critical Thinking 17.3 ❓

What other elements do you think a clinic's robust website should contain?

Direct Mail Advertising

direct mail advertising
a form of print advertising that is sent directly to individuals' homes

Direct mail advertising is any form of advertising that is sent via the mail directly to individuals' homes (Figure ■ 17-6). Marketing companies exist that provide direct mail services. Medical office managers may choose to contract with one of these companies to prepare a direct mail advertisement. Often, these advertisements are sent in an envelope along with other companies' advertisements. They are mailed to households in a desired zip code area, typically one that is within a certain driving distance to the business.

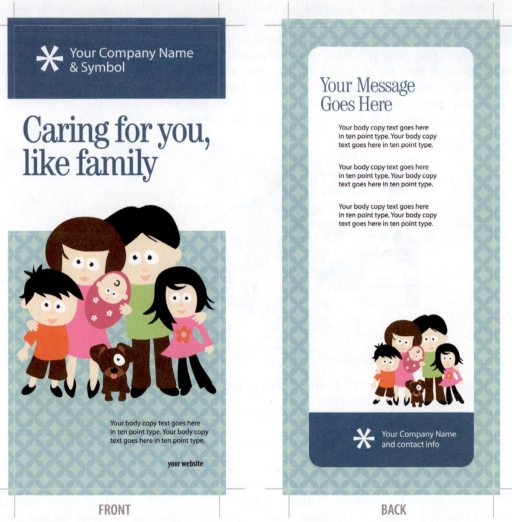

FRONT   BACK

FIGURE ■ 17-6 An example of a customizable marketing brochure that a medical office could purchase and have individualized for that practice.
Source: Wetnose1/Dreamstime.com.

Critical Thinking 17.4 ?

Think about any direct mail advertising you have received. Why have you looked through the advertisements? Or, why did you not look at them? Do you think this would be a successful way to market to someone like you? Why or why not?

Purchasing Mailing Lists

Some healthcare facilities may choose to send direct mail advertisements directly to households, rather than through a direct mail marketing firm. Mailing lists can be purchased from marketing firms. With this marketing option, the medical office manager should work with the physicians to determine the type of advertisement desired and the demographic to be targeted. A budget should be compiled for the artwork and printing of the mailing piece. Postage amounts must be taken into consideration as well.

Welcome to the Neighborhood

Most communities have a city- or county-funded committee whose function it is to provide information to new members of the community. Often, this function lies with the Chamber of Commerce or other similar department within the community government. These committees typically provide materials to people who are buying a home in the area, or even to those who are newly renting their home. The materials usually include information on the locations of libraries and other public facilities. Within these "Welcome to the Neighborhood" packets, advertisement space is often sold to businesses in the community. Knowing that new residents will need to begin care with a physician or dentist, this can be an excellent opportunity to spend advertising dollars in an area that has a good return on the investment.

Offering Screenings

Many healthcare providers offer free **screenings** in their community as a way to bring in new patients. These screenings range from **scoliosis** (curvature of the spine) to vision, to blood pressure checks, and many more. When setting up free or even low-cost screenings, the medical office manager should determine the proper venue for the screening event. The event may take place in the clinic, but this may not be the best option for bringing in walk-up traffic. Often, screenings are planned in local malls, at fairs, or at other community events (Figure ■ 17-7). The medical office manager should arrange to rent the space and to have appropriate supplies available for use at the screenings.

screenings
performance of a health-related study to rule out a certain disease or illness

scoliosis
abnormal curvature of the spine

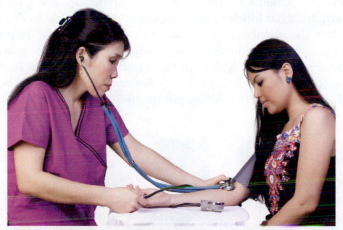

FIGURE ■ 17-7 Blood pressure testing is a common offering at health screenings.
Source: David10321/Dreamstime.com.

Some form of patient history form is filled out by the patient at a screening event. The purpose of the history form is not only to collect basic information about the patient, but also to gather contact information from the patient for future marketing endeavors. After the screening is done, the physician or other medical staff can offer additional services to the patient, if needed. The patient's mailing address can be added to a list of patients who will receive informational flyers or brochures in the future.

Critical Thinking 17.5 ?

What other ideas do you have for screenings? What demographic would you target for those screenings?

Social Media Sites

social media sites
Internet websites, such as Facebook, where individuals interact on a social level

Social media sites, such as Facebook, are becoming a popular method for medical offices to market their services. These sites offer the ability to set up a page at no cost, where marketing information about the business can be published. Articles written by providers or staff and news items about the clinic can be shared in this public format. These sites also offer paid advertising spots on the social media site's home page. When a user types in a certain word or phrase, the social media site's search engine will automatically bring up advertisements that appear to fit with the search item. For example, if a user types in the words "low back pain," a paid advertisement for a local chiropractor may appear on the user's screen.

Critical Thinking 17.6 ?

What other ideas do you have for using social media sites for advertising? What kind of advertising have you seen on these sites?

Using Focus Groups

focus group
a group of people gathered together to test product ideas

Focus groups are small groups of people who are used to survey satisfaction with a particular service (Figure ■ 17-8). In healthcare, these groups are typically one of two kinds. The first is a focus group of existing patients in the facility. These groups are asked to provide their opinions on types of care or to share their feelings about how physicians should interact with their patients. The second type of focus group consists of individuals who are not currently patients in the clinic. With this group, the goal is to survey the members to determine what kinds of services would be valuable to the group and what it would take to lure the members away from their current healthcare provider.

Use of focus groups is common in marketing other businesses, and the feedback gained is usually very valuable. Although this is not an expensive form of marketing, it does take time to set up the groups. Space for the meetings must be arranged, and the members are often given a thank-you gift for their attendance. Focus groups should

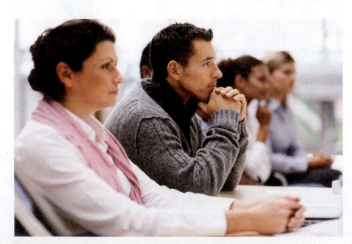

FIGURE ■ **17-8** Focus groups are commonly used to test new marketing ideas in a community.
Source: Yuri_arcurs/Dreamstime.com.

consist of a variety of people from the same demographic of people who live in the clinic's community. For example, if the clinic is located in a community that houses mostly elderly patients, a high percentage of the focus group members should be elderly patients. Having a focus group of young parents of young children would not provide the medical office with appropriate information about desired services if the clinic sees mostly elderly patients.

Critical Thinking 17.7 ?

What topics do you think you might want a focus group to discuss?

Targeting Local Businesses

Many healthcare providers reach out to market directly to local businesses in their community. This is a form of direct mail advertising in that advertisements may be sent to local businesses as an attempt to bring in new patients. Medical office managers may choose to use this method to contact local businesses about setting up private health screening events, or to make an offer to have one of the physicians give a presentation on workplace ergonomics. This type of advertising is very inexpensive in that the costs involved are confined to materials and postage and to the time required to follow up on offers to perform screenings or give educational talks (Figure ■ 17-9).

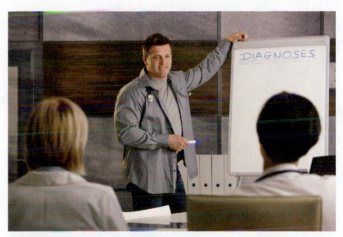

FIGURE ■ 17-9   Physicians often give presentations to other physicians.
Source: Nyul/Dreamstime.com.

Offering Educational Speaking Engagements

Many physicians offer to give educational speaking engagements in their communities. These engagements may be targeted to local businesses, as mentioned above, or they may be targeted toward local community groups. As an example, a physician might give an educational talk about exercising to elderly patients at a local senior center or one about proper nutrition at a local diet center.

Physicians have also offered their services at local colleges, especially in vocational programs, such as nursing or medical assisting. In these settings, physicians may speak about their particular profession, or on a particular subject matter, such as how to deal with noncompliant patients.

Another place where educational talks may be used are with other medical practices in the community. This is most commonly done in specialty practices, where the physicians wish to bring in referrals from primary care providers in the community.

The medical office manager working with a specialty practice can set these up by putting together a letter from the physicians in the practice with an offer to come and speak on an educational topic. Following up on the letters with a personal telephone call, either from the manager or one of the physicians, is one way to increase the likelihood of the offer being accepted.

Critical Thinking 17.8 ?

What educational topics can you think of that a physician might want to discuss at a public speaking engagement?

Telephone Books as Advertising Sources

With the popularity and ease of use of the Internet, many people today forego owning or using telephone books or directories (Figure ■ 17-10). This form of advertisement for the medical practice was one of the sole ways of reaching potential new patients prior to the advent of the Internet. Advertising in the telephone directory is still done by medical practices, though it is not recommended as a primary source of advertising. Just as with all forms of print advertising, the price is determined by the size of the advertisement and its placement.

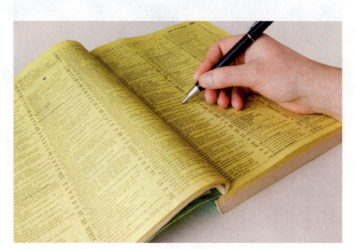

FIGURE ■ 17-10   Advertising in the Yellow Pages was one of the main ways of reaching new patients prior to the advent of the Internet.
Source: Artiomp/Dreamstime.com.

On-Hold Messaging

Medical clinics today frequently include advertising messages in their telephone systems. These messages are heard by callers who are placed on hold. On-hold messaging can be purchased from a vendor, or clinics can design and record their own. Because the caller is a captive audience during the hold time, this is a perfect opportunity to market items that may be of interest to the caller. New services in the clinic, the availability of a new provider, or expanded office hours are all examples of advertising information that may be included in the on-hold message (Figure ■ 17-11).

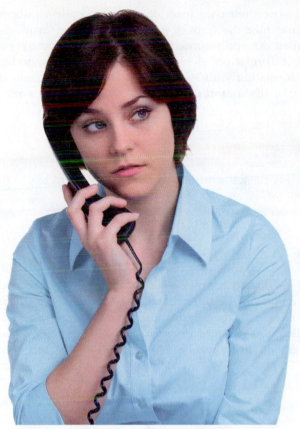

FIGURE ■ 17-11   The caller on hold may hear an advertising message.
Source: Rtimages/Dreamstime.com.

Offering Exceptional Customer Service to Keep Patients Satisfied

Patient satisfaction is looked at closely by most providers and clinics today. Patients are healthcare consumers and if they are not satisfied with all aspects of their care, they may choose to seek care elsewhere. Companies, such as Press Ganey, exist to provide services related to surveying patients on their satisfaction with care. These surveys are then compared to national averages to provide medical clinics with information on how well they are doing at providing satisfying care to their patients.

Because satisfied patients not only stay with their facility, but also refer new patients to it, this is an area that deserves focus and attention, regardless of the size of the clinic. Patient satisfaction concerns both the patient's clinical experience as well as how the patient was made to feel while she was in the office. The following questions are examples of those used to survey patients on their satisfaction with a particular medical visit. Patients are typically asked to rate areas such as these on a scale of 1 to 5, with 1 being very unhappy and 5 being extremely satisfied.

■ How do you feel about the amount of time you were on hold before your call was answered?

■ Do you feel you were greeted in a friendly manner by the receptionist?

■ How do you feel about the amount of time you waited to be taken back to the exam room after checking in?

■ Do you feel the medical assistant or nurse showed genuine concern for you?

■ How do you feel about the amount of time the physician spent in the exam room with you?

Many medical clinics use their own form of survey to collect information about patient satisfaction. These may take the form of postcards or other forms given to patients with a request they be filled out and returned to the clinic in a postage-paid envelope.

After gathering information about patient satisfaction, medical office managers should share the information with staff and providers. By sharing the information in a department meeting, a discussion can be started on how to work on areas that need improvement.

Critical Thinking 17.9 ?

What techniques do you think the medical office manager might talk to her staff about for raising patient satisfaction?

Patients as Advertising Tools

Patients who are very satisfied with their care will often refer their family and friends for care in the same facility. On the other hand, patients who are unhappy with their care will also discuss that fact with their family and friends, creating a negative effect on earning new business. Because patients are a form of advertisement—both good and bad—medical office managers should address patient concerns and complaints in a timely manner (Figure ■ 17-12).

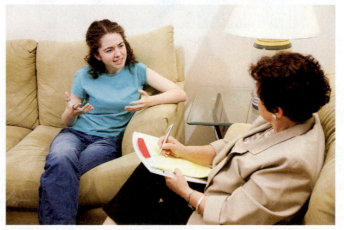

FIGURE ■ 17-12 The medical office manager will sometimes need to speak with patients who are upset.
Source: Lisafx/Dreamstime.com.

Writing Articles for Local Newspapers or Periodicals

Most communities have a local newspaper in which the news of the day is published. Many times, these periodicals are open to physicians writing informational articles to be published in the paper. This is a form of free advertisement in that it costs the office nothing in money to pursue this option; the only costs incurred are those of the physician's time in writing the article. These articles can be written on particular topics, or they can be written in a question-and-answer format. For the latter, the questions could be those the physician has answered in her own practice, or they could be questions submitted to the periodical for answers.

Other members of the medical team may be involved in this form of advertising, with nurses or medical assistants writing articles about caring for patients with particular illnesses, or the medical office manager writing an article about how patients may be more involved in their care.

Targeting the Local Media

Whenever a new development occurs in the medical practice, it provides a great opportunity to seek free advertisement with the local media. Examples include the addition of a new physician in the practice, a staff member who recently earned a new degree or certification, or the purchase of a new piece of equipment. These events may be submitted in the form of a press release to local newspapers or to the media as suggestions for news stories.

Hiring a Marketing Consultant

For clinics with larger budgets for advertising, a marketing consultant or marketing firm may be hired. These companies offer all of the services listed in this chapter, taking the work of researching products and competition, for example, off the shoulders of the medical office manager or physicians. If this method of setting up a marketing program is chosen, time should be spent first in researching the best firm. A company that has a good history of working with healthcare facilities, and one that freely provides contact information for some of their clients is a good place to start.

Case Study Questions

Refer to the case study presented at the beginning of this chapter to answer the following questions:

1. How would you suggest Harold begin putting together his marketing proposal for the practice?
2. As a specialty practice, what marketing areas might Harold look into that would not be of interest to a primary care office manager? How might Harold seize those opportunities?

Chapter Review

Summary

- Before beginning any marketing initiative, it is important to acknowledge the funds that will be allocated for this purpose. The amount may be fluid, but should not be surpassed without good reason.

- By understanding the demographic in the clinic's area, the medical office manager is better able to target the most effective advertising to the target audience.

- Spending time researching a practice's strengths, weaknesses, and opportunities in the community will save the practice money by targeting advertising dollars appropriately.

- By researching the competition in the local area, the medical practice is able to highlight areas where advancements may be made.

- Many practices today use the Internet as a marketing tool. This is done in a variety of ways, some of which are more expensive than others.

- Many practices today have a very robust website for marketing their practice. These websites offer the ability to make appointments and pay bills online.

- Direct mail advertising is the function of sending advertising pieces directly to the homes of the targeted audience.

- By purchasing mailing lists, medical practices are able to send their own direct mail pieces.

- Many medical offices use direct mail to target advertising to newcomers to the community.

- By offering screenings, medical practices are able to solicit new business from targeted audiences.

- Social media sites, such as Facebook, offer new marketing opportunities to medical practices.

- Focus groups may be used to understand how best to market products to a particular demographic in the practice's area.

- By targeting local businesses, medical practices may be able to garner new business.

- Offering educational speaking events to businesses or community centers is one way for the medical practice to attract new patients.

- Telephone books were once the only way to advertise to consumers. Today, this form of advertisement is not the only way to reach the public in the community.

- On-hold messaging can be used to advertise to patients as they hold the line when calling the medical office.

- By giving patients excellent customer service, medical offices are able to retain loyal patients, as well as build their practice base.

- Patients who have received excellent customer service are a good source of advertising. These patients will tell their family and friends about their care, bringing in new business to the medical office.

- Many physicians or other office staff write articles for local periodicals. This service to the community is often a good source of new business for the clinic.

- When new events occur in the medical practice, it is a good idea to notify the local media. Stories that run in the media about positive events are good advertising for the clinic.

- Some clinics choose to hire marketing consultants to assist with their marketing needs.

Multiple Choice

Choose the letter that best answers each question or completes each statement.

1. Which of the following best defines a *demographic*?
   a. The makeup of a population, such as age and number of children
   b. The number of physicians who work in an office
   c. The amount of time allotted for a particular healthcare service
   d. The medications prescribed for a certain condition

2. Welcome to the Neighborhood packets are typically sent to which of the following?
   a. Established residents who live close to the medical clinic
   b. Employees of the medical clinic
   c. Patients taking a certain medication
   d. Residents who have recently moved into the community

3. Which of the following would be appropriate for an educational speaking engagement?
   a. A senior's group
   b. The medical office staff
   c. Family of the physicians
   d. All of the above

4. Which of the following is the more expensive form of advertising?
   a. Speaking engagements
   b. Writing an article in the local newspaper
   c. Patients speaking to their friends
   d. Internet advertisements

5. Which of the following would be appropriate for free screenings?
   a. Blood pressure
   b. Physical exams
   c. Liver function testing
   d. Treadmill stress tests

6. Which of the following is appropriate for a focus group?
   a. Deciding on the name for a new clinic
   b. Determining a fee schedule for a new practice

   c. Choosing a candidate for a reception position
   d. Recruiting for a new physician

7. Which of the following stories might the local news media be interested in?
   a. New state-of-the-art equipment that no other medical practice in town has
   b. Newly hired receptionist
   c. Recently redone fee list
   d. New furniture in the medical practice

8. Which of the following is considered a social media site?
   a. Local newspaper
   b. Online message board for parents of small children
   c. Facebook
   d. Community bulletin board

9. Which of the following best describes the concept of *return on investment*?
   a. The amount of money spent on advertising
   b. The amount of money paid by patients for a particular service
   c. The amount of money paid to staff to work at a screening event
   d. The amount of money earned compared to the amount of money spent on a marketing initiative

10. What is the best reason for researching the competition before embarking on a marketing initiative?
    a. To make sure you are targeting an area where they are weak
    b. To give them competition in an area where they are strong
    c. To get an idea on how much money the competition is spending on marketing
    d. To understand how the competition's marketing plan is working for them

True/False

Determine if each of the following statements is true or false.

_____ 1. Once set, the marketing budget should never be adjusted.

_____ 2. The Internet can be a strong tool for medical office advertising.

_____ 3. The most lucrative form of advertising today is the telephone book advertisement.

_____ 4. Whenever a new development occurs in the medical practice, it is a great opportunity to seek free advertisement with the local media.

_____ 5. A strong marketing plan helps the medical office manager stay on schedule and spend allocated funds appropriately.

_____ 6. Patient satisfaction is looked at closely by most providers and clinics today.

_____ 7. Focus groups should only be made up of patients who are currently being treated in the clinic.

_____ 8. For clinics with large budgets for advertising, a marketing consultant or marketing firm may be hired.

_____ 9. The medical office manager will want to market those areas where the practice is doing well and is able to handle increased business.

_____ 10. Articles in the local newspaper do not have to be written by the physician; they may be written by other members of the office staff.

Matching

Match each of the following terms with its definition.

a. demographic

b. direct mail advertising

c. social media sites

d. return on investment

e. focus groups

f. marketing budget

g. marketing firm

h. marketing plan

i. screenings

j. search engine optimization

1. Internet websites, such as Facebook, where individuals interact on a social level

2. The amount of money allocated to a marketing plan

3. The amount of money brought in after a marketing initiative

4. A group of people gathered together to test product ideas

5. A form of print advertising that is sent directly to individuals' homes

6. A plan for advertising a business or product

7. Performance of a health-related study to rule out a certain disease or illness

8. A company that can be hired for the purpose of composing and carrying out a marketing plan

9. The makeup of a population, such as age and number of children

10. Making changes to a company's individual website in order to allow the website to come up at the top of the list during Internet searching

Chapter Resources

Marketing strategies for medical offices: www.physiciannews.com

Physician News Digest: www.physiciansnews.com/business/1001anwar.html

Physician web design and Internet marketing: www.doctorwebdesign.com

Internet Websites for Healthcare Professionals

American Association of Medical Assistants (www.aama-ntl.org)
This organization provides information about the medical assisting profession, including opportunities for becoming a certified medical assistant.

American College of Healthcare Executives (www.ache.org)
The ACHE provides information on healthcare legislation, diversity, and ethics in healthcare and publishes policy statements. This group provides educational opportunities for healthcare professionals and the opportunity to become a Fellow in the American College of Healthcare Executives.

Centers for Disease Control and Prevention (www.cdc.gov)
This government organization provides information on vaccinations, medications, and patient education. Information from this source may be used by the medical office manager to create informational pamphlets for patients.

Healthcare Providers Service Organization (www.hpso.com)
The HPSO provides information to healthcare professionals about medical malpractice insurance policies for every member of the healthcare team, from physicians to medical assistants and nurses.

Medical Group Management Association (www.mgma.com)
This association provides information on benchmarking, healthcare legislation, and regulation, as well as information on how to become certified as a medical practice executive.

Physician Office Managers Association of America (www.pomaa.net)
This group provides information about educational seminars on medical office management, as well as how to become certified as a practice manager.

Practice Management Institute (www.pmimd.com)
PMI provides the medical office manager with information on becoming certified in professional coding or insurance processing.

Professional Association of Health Care Office Management (www.pahcom.com)
This association provides information regarding the latest in medical office management. Joining this network of healthcare professionals provides the medical office manager with the ability to network with other managers across the country.

U.S. Department of Health and Human Services Flu Site (www.flu.gov)
This website is maintained by the federal government in order to provide healthcare professionals with the latest information on the seasonal flu virus.

U.S. National Library of Medicine (http://www.nlm.nih.gov/portals/healthcare.html)
This government library contains numerous links to medical websites that can act as important resources for the medical office manager. This site contains links to MEDLINE/PubMed; ClinicalTrials.gov; NIH MedlinePlus Magazine, PubMed Central, NLM Gateway, Toxicology and Environmental Health, DailyMed, MedlinePlus Consumer Health Information, Genetics Home Reference, and Trauma and Resilience: Mind, Body and Spirit.

Sample Medical Office Policy and Procedure Manual

Grace Pediatric Facility
Policy & Procedure Manual

Mission Statement:

All employees working towards a common goal, providing high quality care to all patients

Clinic Hierarchy

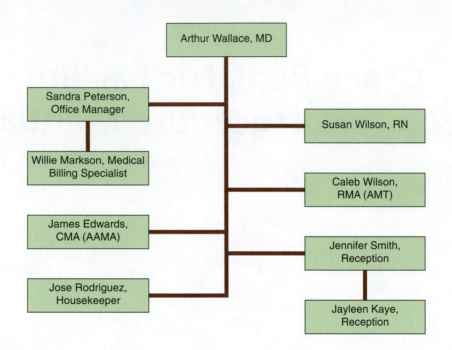

Table of Contents

Procedure: Opening and Closing

Purpose: Properly perform the duties and tasks necessary to maximize the efficiency of the clinic.

How to open:

— The clinic opens at 8:00 a.m. Monday–Friday and at 9:00 a.m. on the last Saturday of the month.

— All staff will arrive at 7:30 a.m. Monday–Friday and 8:30 a.m. on the last Saturday of the month to open the clinic for the day.

— All doors of the clinic will be locked upon arrival. Access to the clinic should be obtained with the employee-specific identification badges given upon hire; these I.D. cards act as keycards and will grant access into the clinic.

— Upon arrival, all employees should clock-in at the time clock located within the staff lounge.

— At the beginning of each day there are specific tasks that need to be completed:

  – All lights must be turned on.

  – Thermostat must be checked and is to stay at a constant 69 degree temperature.

  – Exam rooms need to be cleaned, supplies stocked, beds lined with paper, and equipment checked to ensure proper functioning.

  – Patient waiting rooms are to be cleaned and all supplies stocked (comment cards, face masks, hand sanitizer, magazines, etc.)

  – All voicemails need to be checked, although they may be taken care of throughout the day.

  – All employees need to be ready to work by 8:00 a.m.; patients will be waiting to be seen.

  – All tasks that are required to be completed for the opening of the clinic must be completed by 8:00 a.m.

How to close:

— The clinic closes at 5:00 p.m. Monday–Friday and at 5:00 p.m. on the last Saturday of the month.

— The last appointment of the day will be scheduled at 4:00 p.m. No patient is to be scheduled past this time unless staff is running behind or an urgent matter arises. Any appointment scheduled past 4:00 p.m. needs to be approved by a physician.

— After the last patient has been seen and has left the clinic, the doors are to be locked so that proper closing procedures can take place.

— At the end of each day there are specific tasks that need to be completed:

  – All work stations must be shut off.

  – All lights must be shut off.

  – Stock room supplies should be checked. If any supplies are low or needed soon, an order should be placed.

  – After all closing tasks have been completed, the last person to exit is to arm the clinic alarm. This task is completed by pressing the "ARM" button on the alarm system keypad located by the main entrance door. After arming the alarm, all persons must be out of the clinic within one minute. If anyone is in the clinic at that time, the alarm will sound.

  – By pressing the "ARM" button on the alarm system keypad, the clinic doors will automatically lock. To make sure that the doors were locked in the process, the main door must be checked.

Procedure: Job Postings

Purpose: Correctly and properly post job positions in a manner such that all employees and non-employees will be aware of open positions and to maximize the effectiveness of hiring procedures.

— Job openings, if any, will be posted on a weekly basis.

— Job openings will be posted on the clinic's external/internal website and in the employee break room.

— All postings will be available on Sunday by 9:30 a.m.

— It is the office manager's responsibility to post the open positions.

— Postings will include:

– Job title

– Job description

– Wages

– Hours

– Qualifications needed

– Requirements

– Contact information

— If there are any questions or comments about job postings, they must be directed to the office manager. The contact information is located on corresponding job posting.

Policy: Attendance and Tardiness

Purpose: To ensure the efficiency of the work environment by all employees reporting for their duties on their scheduled days and times.

— The hours are specific and each employee must arrive on time to ensure smooth operation.

— All employees must report to their designated workstations on time. Every employee has a five-minute grace period, in case of emergency but not by habit.

— Tardiness is unacceptable. Tardiness is defined as being more than five minutes late.

— A maximum of four tardies in a month period are allowed. If this number is exceeded there will be a write-up by the employee's supervisor.

— Three or more write-ups for the same offense is grounds for termination.

— If an employee is running late, the clinic needs to be notified as soon as possible. This ensures that the staff can make adjustments to ensure work efficiency.

— If for any reason an employee feels that he or she cannot make it to work (for example, illness, family emergency) the clinic needs to be notified as soon as possible. Advanced notice is preferred, if possible.

— A maximum of four absences per month is permitted. An excess of this will be reviewed and if absentness continues to happen, the employee will be written up.

— Three write-ups for the same offense is grounds for termination.

— Employees will not be penalized for illness, emergencies, and/or prior time-off authorization.

— It is the employee's responsibility to handle all elements related to time-off including informing office of time-off, filling out proper forms prior to leave or upon return from leave, and making sure that time-off is covered.

Procedure: Emergency Situation

Purpose: For all employees to know what to do in case an emergency arises.

— Remember, for any emergency situation call local emergency authorities at 911.
— For patient-related emergencies, the employee will need to state over the intercom:
  - The location of the emergency
  - The code name (e.g., "reception desk code red" means that there is a fire at the reception desk)
  - That patients need to evacuate via the nearest exit (for certain emergencies)
— The person experiencing the emergency should call the code and then call 911.
— Patients need to be evacuated for fire and/or bomb threats.
— Use the following emergency codes:
  - Code red-------------fire
  - Code black----------bomb threat
  - Code blue-----------heart/breathing stopped
  - Code orange--------child missing
  - Code silver-----------weapon
  - Code green----------dangerous patient
  - Code yellow---------natural disaster (to include type)

Policy: Phone Conduct

Purpose: For all employees to maintain professional phone relationships with everyone that they come into contact with.

— All phone calls should be limited to business use only.
— Personal calls can be taken in urgent situations and on breaks or during lunch.
— Our facility does not accept solicitations of any kind.
— All phone conversations should be professional and polite.
— When answering a call, employees should state:
  - The facility name
  - Employee's name
  - Ask caller if he/she can be helped
  - For example: "Grace Pediatric Facility. This is Martha. How can I help you?"
— When ending a call, employees must always thank the patient and ask if there is anything else that you can do for them.
— If someone calls into the clinic and asks for someone/something specifically, they must be transferred and/or if they are unavailable a message must be taken for the particular employee.

Policy: Computer and Internet Usage

Purpose: All employees must properly use the computer by following the policy to protect patient privacy.

— Computer/Internet usage should be limited to patient care or to assist in patient care.

— Computers and the Internet may be used for personal use during lunches and/or breaks.

— Certain sites and activities may not be viewed or done at any time:
  – Social networking sites
  – Explicit content
  – Streaming audio
  – Streaming video
  – Downloading content

— All computer/Internet usage is monitored.

— If there is any reason to suspect that there is inappropriate use of the clinic computers or Internet, disciplinary action will be taken.

— Each employee will have an individual username and password that will be required to log in to each workstation he or she may use.

  – Employees are prohibited from using another employee's username, password, and/or workstation that they are logged into.

Policy: Break and Meal Periods

Purpose: To ensure that every employee takes lunches and breaks as required by law.

— Each employee is entitled to a one-hour lunch.

— The lunch hour is 12:30–1:30 p.m.

— The clinic will be closed during the lunch hour.

— In addition to lunch, each employee is entitled to two 15-minute breaks (one before lunch and one after).

— It is each employee's responsibility to check with each staff member to ensure work duties are covered during break times.

— If an employee is outside of the clinic during the break and/or lunch period, the employee must act in a professional manner.

— It is each employee's responsibility to clean up after himself or herself to ensure cleanliness.

Policy: Appearance and Dress Code

Purpose: To represent the clinic in a professional way by following the required dress code.

— Always represent yourself professionally.
— No tattoos are allowed to show.
— Visible piercings are allowed only in the ears.
— Hair is to be of natural color.
— No inappropriate amount of skin is to be showing and must be covered at all times
— Dress pants, scrubs, and/or uniform required. No jeans allowed.
— Nice shirts only.
— All clothes are to be in good repair.
— Dress shoes, boots, and/or tennis shoes allowed. No flip-flops allowed.
— Name brands and/or logos on clothing should not show.
  – Identification and/or name badges should be worn at all times.

Procedure: Taking Inventory and Ordering Supplies

Purpose: To understand how to complete the tasks pertaining to supplies, so that supplies are stocked and the clinic runs smoothly.

— Supplies must be checked daily, before employees leave for the night.
— A schedule will be circulated every month, detailing whose responsibility it is to check the stock room. The schedule will also be posted on the stock room door.
— If supplies were delivered the previous day that need to be put away, that task needs to be done first. If this is not done first, too many supplies can be ordered, creating waste.
— Each supply is to be inventoried individually. The numbers below each supply on the shelf state how many of each supply there should be. If the amount posted is close to the number remaining, then the supply must be ordered.
— Write the name of each supply needed on the supply order list.
— The supply order list is to be sent to the supply company via fax. The fax number is in the supply room.
— After all tasks have been completed, it is the employee's responsibility to ensure the room is tidy and clean and to ensure that the door is locked.

Policy: Harassment

Purpose: To ensure a safe and positive work environment for all employees.

— Every employee is responsible for maintaining professional relationships with everyone in the clinic.
— Under no circumstance should anyone make rude comments, sexual comments or gestures, be violent, and/or make anyone feel incompetent.
— Any issues should be addressed with the immediate supervisor.
— Disciplinary action can and will be taken. Actions include such things as write-up, suspension, and/or termination.

Procedure: Patient Referral

Purpose: To properly manage patient care by understanding how to refer patients to outside physicians to receive treatment.

— To refer a patient, we must take all patient information into consideration.

— Locating a physician who can provide treatment, who is located as close as possible to the patient's home, and who is relatively cost effective is our goal.

— When sending a referral to another physician's office, send the referral along with the medical information necessary for treating the patient.

— It is our physician's responsibility to follow up with the care received from the other physician, by requesting the medical report.

— A follow-up visit is to be scheduled with the patient to be seen back with our clinic, to ensure the correct care has been received.

Policy: Patient Confidentiality

Purpose: To ensure that laws are followed in the care of all patients to guarantee patient confidentiality.

— All patient information is to be treated as confidential.

— HIPAA and privacy laws must be complied with by all employees.

— Violations will not be tolerated and must be reported.

— The confidentiality of minors is to be considered at all times. Certain medical information of patients between the ages of 13 and 17 (drug/alcohol use, sexual activity, STIs, reproductive treatment, and mental health treatment) is to be held to extreme confidentiality standards. Information of this type about these patients is not to be given without the consent of the patient to anyone, even to the parents.

Policy/Procedure: Release of Medical Information

Purpose: To correctly and accurately release patient's medical information, so as to comply with all state and federal laws.

— Patients, their parents, or legal guardian must consent in writing to release medical information.

— If a patient is between the ages of 13 and 17 and there is certain sensitive information in the patient's records, the patient must sign for the authorization of his or her own medical records.

— A patient's medical information is not to be discussed with anyone without consent.

— Records can be released without consent in certain situations, including for payment and treatment.

— Any accidental disclosure must be documented by the person who disclosed the information. The documentation is to be made on the Accidental Disclosure form. The date, the patient's name, the information disclosed, and the accidental recipient of the information is to be included.

— When a records request is received, the receptionist is responsible for processing that request within 15 business days.

— The employee handling the records request should correctly identify the patient, locate the records requested, and print the required information.

— After the records have been printed, the receptionist should place them in a security envelope, write the patient's name and date of birth on the front, and write the name of who will be picking up the records.

— When someone comes to pick up a patient's records, that person must show photo identification. If the person who picks up the records is not on the medical authorization or they do not have photo identification, they should not be allowed access to the records.

Policy: Medical Record Management

Purpose: To properly manage and maintain all patient files with HIPAA and privacy laws in mind.

— All patients' files will be maintained through the electronic health record system called EPIC.

— All employees have the responsibility to document all visits, telephone calls, patient correspondence, authorizations, and any other information pertinent to patient care.

— If something needs to be added to the patient file, it should be scanned into the system.

— All employees will have access to patient files, but should only access them on a need-to-know basis.

— Employees should not look up their family members, friends, coworkers, or any person that they know just because they are curious. The only acceptable reason for access is for patient care.

— Any errors or omissions in the medical record need to be corrected as soon as possible. The person who made the error is the person who must correct it. The previous version should always be available.

Procedure: Appointment Scheduling

Purpose: To ensure that all patients can be scheduled in a timely manner to address all of their health needs.

— Patients will be scheduled in the order in which they call to schedule appointments; the exception to this is if a patient needs to be seen urgently. If a patient needs to be seen urgently, then it is up to the physician to try to fit the patient in or send the patient to an emergency department.

— The person scheduling the appointment must verify all patient information including:
  – Name
  – Date of birth
  – Address
  – Phone number
  – Insurance information
  – Emergency contacts

— When an employee schedules the appointment, they must include:
  – Reason for visit
  – Duration of illness/injury
  – If it is a new visit or a recheck

— Patients must be informed to bring photo identification and insurance information to the appointment, to verify the identity of the patient.

— Patients must also be informed that if they wish to reschedule or cancel an appointment, they must give 24-hour notice if possible. There could be a charge for a missed appointment.

Procedure: Sorting and Sending Mail

Purpose: To ensure that all mail is sent, received, and delivered in a timely manner.

— All mail is to be picked up at the beginning of each business day. It is the receptionist's responsibility to sort and deliver mail to the addressee.

— If a piece of mail is marked confidential, it is to be delivered to the person it is addressed to without being opened.

— If mail is addressed to the clinic, it is to be opened and a determination made about who the mail is to be delivered to.

— All mail received and sent is to be kept out of patient view.

— Any mail to be sent is to be put in the outgoing mail box, located in the back office.

— The receptionist should weigh the mail, using a postage meter, to determine the correct amount of postage to apply.

— At the end of the business day, it is the receptionist's responsibility to place the outgoing mail in the locked post office box, located in back of the clinic.

Policy/Procedure: Drawing Blood

Purpose: To keep the patient safe by ensuring that all employees follow the proper procedures for drawing blood.

— Before the blood draw, the medical assistant will:
  - Grab the blood draw kit, which includes all necessary supplies.
  - Ask the patient to lie on an exam table (ask for assistance from another employee if needed).
  - Make sure that all supplies in kit are sterile before beginning.

— During the blood draw, the medical assistant will:
  - Clean the skin on the arm, where the blood is to be drawn.
  - Tie upper arm with a tourniquet.
  - Have patient squeeze a rubber ball with the hand of the arm that the blood is being drawn from.
  - Get sterile needle from kit.
  - Get the proper vials for blood draw.
  - Caution must be exhibited when inserting the needle.
  - Blood will be drawn into the proper vial.

— After the blood draw, the medical assistant will:
  - Have the patient release the rubber ball.
  - Remove the tourniquet from the patient's arm.
  - Remove the needle from the patient's vein.
  - Get a cotton ball and place it on blood draw site. Check to make sure bleeding has slowed before placing tape on the cotton ball.
  - Instruct patient to remove the tape in 15–20 minutes.
  - Ensure that the proper patient label has been placed on the blood vials.

— All contaminated blood draw supplies are to be disposed of in proper waste receptacles.

Procedure: Facility Maintenance

Purpose: To ensure that the clinic is well maintained and the clinic's appearance is upheld.

— Any facility maintenance that needs to be performed is to be documented on the Facility Maintenance List.

— The office manager is responsible for scheduling the necessary companies to perform the required maintenance on the facility.

— Employees should not perform maintenance themselves, to prevent injury. The only time an employee should perform maintenance is if a patient's health is at risk, only in emergencies.

Policy: Payroll

Purpose: To provide all employees with proper payment for the services that they provide to the clinic, in a timely manner.

— All employees will be paid every other week.

— Checks will be direct deposited or distributed on Friday.

— If there is a problem regarding payment, it should be directed to the office manager.

— All employees will receive holiday pay. Paid holidays are listed in the Office Closure policy/procedure.

Policy/Procedure: Office Closure

Purpose: To ensure that patients and staff are informed when the office will be closed.

— All patients will receive a letter at home when the office will be closed; days of closure need to be indicated.

— Closure should be scheduled at least six months in advance to guarantee that patients are aware.

— Office calls should be forwarded to another facility during the closure, so that patients can be transferred to other facilities for care if needed.

— The clinic will be closed for major holidays, including

– Christmas Eve and Christmas Day

– New Year's Day

– Memorial Day

– Labor Day

– Thanksgiving Day

Policy/Procedure: Withdrawal of Patient Care

Purpose: To ensure that patients receive the best care, by ensuring patients keep appointments and make payments on their accounts.

— Patients need to make sure that they make it to appointments when they are scheduled.

— If patients do not give notice when they cannot make it to appointments, after four no-shows, they will be given a Withdrawal of Care from our facility.

— For a Withdrawal of Care;

– A Withdrawal of Care letter will be sent to the patient's home, and they will be given the opportunity to stay a patient for 30 days while they locate another physician.

– Patients will be given a complete set of their records for free to take to another physician (one time only).

– If a patient disagrees with the Withdrawal of Care that he or she received, the patient can write a letter to the clinic, asking to have it rescinded. The clinic will deliberate and decide if the patient can come back for care.

— If the withdrawal is rescinded and the patient is allowed to come back, in the event another Withdrawal of Care situation arises, the patient will not be given the choice to come back.

Policy/Procedure: Staff Meetings

Purpose: To make sure that all employees attend staff meetings and gather all information necessary from those meetings.

— Staff meetings will be announced through clinic e-mail.

— All employees are required to attend.

— Any meeting agenda item that should be discussed should be sent to the office manager prior to the meeting.

— Anything discussed in the meeting will be summarized and sent to all employees after the meeting.

Policy/Procedure: Preventive Care

Purpose: To make sure that patients receive the best care possible by informing them of care that they need, before they actually need it.

— Yearly reminders will be sent to patients at home, to inform them of treatment that they may need. Such things could include:

– Immunizations

– Well-child checks

— All test results will be sent to patients' homes after they are complete

Receptionist Job Description

Posting Title: Office Receptionist

Shift: Day shift

Hours: Monday–Friday 7:30–5:00
　　　　Last Saturday of the month 9:00–5:00

Employment Status: Full-time

Wages: $15.15–16.75–18.25 per hour

Job Description:

— The receptionist is responsible for;
- Greeting all patients as they come in for their visits
- Checking patients in for their appointment
- Updating patient personal information
- Updating patient insurance information
- Calling patients to remind them of their appointment (giving 24-hour notice to patients)
- Sending letters to patients when they have missed appointments
- Releasing medical information

Minimum Requirements: High school diploma or GED. Previous experience will be considered.

Housekeeper Job Description

Posting Title: Housekeeper

Shift: Evening shift

Hours: Monday–Friday 6:30 p.m–3:00 a.m.
　　　　Last Saturday of the month 6:30 p.m. –3:00 a.m.

Employment Status: Full-time

Wages: $11.50–14.50–17.50 per hour

Job Description:

— The housekeeper is responsible for the cleanliness and neat appearance of the facility.
— Housekeeper responsibilities include:
- Cleaning and sanitizing of floors, countertops, door knobs, exam tables, bathrooms, waiting rooms, reception desks, and offices
- Emptying all garbage cans and taking out garbage to dumpster
- Refill all patients' supplies including hand sanitizer, gloves, masks, tissues, toilet paper, and paper towels
- Vacuuming all floors and shampoo carpets as needed. Once a month, an outside service will deep clean all carpets in the clinic.

Minimum Requirements: High school diploma or GED.

Medical Assistant Job Description

Posting Title: Medical Assistant

Shift: Day shift

Hours: Monday–Friday 7:30–5:00
       Last Saturday of the month 9:00–5:00

Employment Status: Full-time

Wages: $17.21–19.16–21.18 per hour

Job Description:

— The medical assistant is responsible for preparing patients to see the physician
— Medical assistant responsibilities include:
  – Taking vitals (temperature, weight, blood pressure, pulse, etc.)
  – Asking patients, and their families, if there are any concerns that they would like to address with their physician
  – After the visit, documenting the patient's vitals in the patient's chart
  – Checking the schedule to determine who is to check supply inventories and when to check them
  – Removing casts
  – Changing dressings
  – Administering injections and drawing blood
  – Stocking exam rooms
  – Assisting physician in exams

Minimum Requirements: High school diploma or GED, completion of a medical assistant program, and certification as a medical assistant.

Office Manager Job Description

Posting Title: Office Manager

Shift: Day shift

Hours: Monday–Friday 7:30–5:00
Last Saturday of the month 9:00–5:00

Employment Status: Full-time

Wages: $21.50-24.50-27.50 per hour

Job Description:

— The office manager is responsible for the management of all duties and tasks performed by employees of the clinic.
— Office manager responsibilities include:
  – Writing schedules
  – Processing time-off requests
  – Reviewing policies and procedures
  – Managing payroll
  – Managing health and safety in the office
  – Supervising inventory and supply purchasing
  – Hiring employees
  – Firing employees
  – Completing employee's yearly reviews

Minimum Requirements: High school diploma or GED, associate degree or higher in business, and accounting–associate in technical arts degree.

Registered Nurse Job Description

Posting Title: RN

Shift: Day shift

Hours: Monday–Friday 7:30–5:00
          Last Saturday of the month 9:00–5:00

Employment Status: Full-time

Wages: $21.15–32.15–43.15 per hour

Job Description:

— Nurses are responsible for the direct and indirect care of all patients seen at the facility
— Nurse responsibilities include:
  – Administering medication
  – Administering certain treatments
  – Conducting telephone triage
  – Processing patient paperwork
  – Entering and processing referrals
  – Assisting physician during certain procedures
  – Educating patients

Minimum requirements: High school diploma or GED, completion of RN program, RN licensure, and 1 year of clinical experience preferred.

Physician Job Description

Posting Title: Pediatric Care Physician

Shift: Day shift

Hours: Monday–Friday 7:30–5:30
          Last Saturday of the month 9–5

Employment Status: Full-time

Salary: Commensurate with experience

Job Description:

— The physician is responsible for the primary care of all patients who are treated at the clinic.
— Physician responsibilities include acting as the supervisor for all other employees who work in the facility.
— Must have current licenses.
— Benefits will be offered, including medical, dental, and vision.
— Any other questions regarding this position can be directed to the office manager.

Medical Office Billing Specialist Job Description

Job Title: Medical Office Billing Specialist

Shift: Day shift

Hours: Monday–Friday 7:30–5:30
Last Saturday of the month 9–5

Employment Status: Full-time

Wages: $16.50–18.50–20.50 per hour

Job Description:

— Medical billing specialists are responsible for applying proper record-keeping, billing, and coding techniques to ensure that healthcare providers and/or patients receive accurate and timely reimbursement from medical insurance companies.

— Medical office billing specialist responsibilities include:

  – Billing insurance companies for services rendered

  – Billing patients for services rendered after insurance company has been billed

Minimum Requirements: High school diploma or GED, medical billing specialist certificate, and medical coding certificate.

Guidelines for Documenting in the Medical Record to Ensure Proper Coding

To be paid appropriately for care rendered to a patient, the physician, physician-extender, or ancillary staff must be certain the following steps are followed:

- All portions of the medical record must be complete and legible. If the chart were to be reviewed by an insurance carrier, there should never be a question as to the accuracy or detail of the visit or service.

- All documentation made in the patient's chart must include all of the following:
  - The reason for the encounter and any relevant history
  - Details of the physical examination findings
  - Any prior diagnostic test results
  - The assessment and clinical diagnosis given to the patient for this visit or service
  - The plan for the patient's care for this diagnosis
  - The date of all visits or services, and the identity of the person who performed or recorded services in the patient's chart
  - The clinical reason for ordering any diagnostic studies or services, such as laboratory work or x-rays
  - Any past diagnoses this patient has had, and the care plans associated with each
  - Any applicable health risk factors known to this patient, such as chronic diseases or high-risk hobbies or behaviors practiced by the patient
  - Any medication allergies known to this patient
  - Any medications, both prescribed and over-the-counter, that the patient is taking, in addition to any supplements
  - Progress reports on the patient's condition or treatment for any ongoing conditions

Answers to Chapter Case Study Questions

Chapter 1: Today's Healthcare Environment

Steve Magnus has recently begun taking classes in healthcare management. He believes he would like working in the medical field and he wonders if this is a field that will be challenging to him. Steve enjoys working closely with others and he has always had a strong desire to help people. He has found that he does well at organizing tasks and supervising others.

1. After reading about the various members of the healthcare team, and the characteristics of the medical office manager, how do you think someone like Steve would do in this job?

   Because Steve enjoys working with and helping others, and because he has done well in the past at organizing tasks and supervising others, a career as a medical office manager will likely suit him well.

2. With Steve's desire to have a job that is challenging, do you believe this job would provide a challenge for him?

   Communicating in the workplace, both with his employees and patients, will provide Steve with challenging situations, particularly when situations happen without advance notice.

Chapter 2: Communications in the Medical Office

Sylvia Lang is the medical office manager of a busy orthopedic practice. She manages 25 people in the office and she uses various methods to communicate with her team. There are times when Sylvia communicates with an individual member, and times when she needs to communicate with the entire group. One challenge Sylvia faces is that the staff members work varying schedules, and their lunch and break times overlap. There is no single time of the day when all members of the department are available to meet in person.

1. What methods of communication would work best for Sylvia to communicate with her team?

   Sylvia may need to communicate with her teams in a department meeting, as well as communicate via memos or e-mails. With her team having different schedules on different days, Sylvia will find it difficult to reach everyone with an in-person meeting only.

2. How can Sylvia make sure her communications are being understood by her group?

   Sylvia can ask for feedback from her group. She can check in with them to be sure her message was understood and that no questions from staff go unanswered.

Chapter 3: Legal and Ethical Issues in Managing the Medical Office

Bobbi Schessler works as the medical office manager of a large, multispecialty clinic in the inner city. One of Bobbi's physicians tells Bobbi that she does not see the need for hiring a registered nurse for an open position in the office; she wants Bobbi to save money and hire a medical assistant instead.

1. How might Bobbi respond to the physician about hiring a medical assistant instead of a registered nurse?
    Bobbi should explain to the physician the difference between the scope of practice of a nurse versus that of a medical assistant. She should explain that there are many tasks a medical assistant cannot do that a nurse is able to perform.

2. How would you suggest Bobbi find out what the scope of practice is for a medical assistant, as well as a registered nurse, in the state where the practice resides?
    Bobbi can find this information through her state's department of health, in the medical practice acts.

3. What information should Bobbi collect before she discusses this with the physician?
    Bobbi should know the scope of practice and training for registered nurses and medical assistants, as well as the job description for the job she intends to fill. She might also have data available regarding the salary difference between the two professions.

Chapter 4: Personnel Management

Svetlana Pilat is the medical office manager in a busy family practice clinic. Her clinic is adding two new physicians and Svetlana needs to determine the appropriate support staff needed for the physicians. She is not sure if she will need to hire nurses or medical assistants and whether each physician will need his or her own staff or if the physicians can share. She also needs to determine if her current reception staff will be sufficient to cover the workload of two new physicians.

1. Once Svetlana has decided she needs to hire one medical assistant and a part-time receptionist, how should she go about finding those employees?
    Svetlana should post the positions in the local newspaper. She may also contact the local medical assistant training programs in her area to post the position for the medical assistant. Svetlana may also choose to work with an employment agency to recruit these new employees.

2. Would Svetlana use a different venue to advertise for the medical assistant than she would for the receptionist?
    She can post both positions in the newspaper, but she has other options for the medical assistant. For that position, she can contact local medical assistant training programs to see if any students just completing their training may be looking for work.

3. Who should Svetlana involve from her office in the interviewing process?
    Svetlana may want to involve one of the physicians in her practice, as well as other members of the team.

Chapter 5: Managing the Front Office

Roxanne Martin is the office manager in a busy pediatric office. She has had several issues of patients complaining about the comfort of the waiting area. The complaints involve the issues of trash being left on the tables and the lack of magazines to read.

In addition, patients have complained that they are not being kept aware of delays in their appointment times.

> In what ways might Roxanne address the patients' issues about garbage in the waiting area and the lack of reading materials?
>
> Roxanne should ask her reception staff to continually monitor the comfort of the waiting area. The reception staff should pick up any garbage or items left behind and straighten up the reception area and any magazines. Roxanne should also review the magazine subscriptions available in the office. She may need to have back-office staff bring magazines from the exam rooms out to the waiting area throughout the day. Receptionists should also keep all patients informed regarding any wait times. Roxanne may want to consider investing in a wait-time monitor for use in alerting patients to wait times.

Chapter 6: Appointment Scheduling

Tully West is a medical office manager working with a group of pediatric physicians. Each physician has a different schedule for clinic hours, and each physician has different requirements for how long they would like to see a particular type of patient.

1. How should Tully proceed in designing a system that will work with the pediatricians in this office?

    Tully should meet with each individual physician in order to understand the hours and time frames each physician wants.

2. Which of the tools presented in this chapter would be best suited to the task?

    Tully should look into creating a template for the schedules. This can be done with either a paper or electronic scheduling system.

Chapter 7: Medical Records Management

Corey Shephard is the medical office manager in a large multispecialty medical practice. The physicians have just purchased an electronic medical record program and are beginning the process of converting the paper medical records to electronic format.

1. How should Corey lead the group into the change from paper medical records to electronic?

    Corey should begin by putting together a schedule for how the process will work, which would include the types of files that will be transferred first, as well as the information in the paper medical records that will be transferred.

2. Would it be best to begin with the active patient files? Why or why not?

    Yes. The active patient files are likely to be needed sooner than inactive files.

3. What should Corey do with the paper medical records once the conversion has taken place?

    Once conversion has taken place, Corey can choose to either have the files shredded, or he can have them stored in a safe location, either on site or off site.

Chapter 8: Regulatory Compliance in the Healthcare Setting

Janeen Colbert is the HIPAA privacy officer in a large ambulatory healthcare center. As part of her job, she is responsible for the training of staff on HIPAA regulations and for responding to complaints about breach of privacy. Janeen has been faced with multiple complaints of breach of privacy during the past few months, most of them coming from patients who have been to a particular provider in the facility.

1. How should Janeen address the problem she is encountering with multiple complaints coming from patients who have seen a particular provider?
   Janeen should meet with the provider in person to discuss the complaints and to review the HIPAA guidelines with the provider.

2. What are some methods Janeen could use to keep these complaints from happening in the future?
   Janeen should enact a training session with this provider and, possibly, with his staff as well.

Chapter 9: Duties of the Medical Office Manager

Barb Totem has been managing a busy pediatric clinic for the past 10 years. She is friendly with her employees and considers many of them to be her friends. When conflict occurs in the workplace, Barb sometimes finds it difficult to separate her personal feelings for her employees from her job of disciplining them. Barb feels uncomfortable when she needs to speak to some employees about performance because she worries the employees will think she does not like them.

1. What type of management style do you think Barb falls under?
   Barb is a manager who leads with a very relaxed style. She likes to build consensus and she wants her employees to like her. This is similar to the humanistic style of management.

2. In what way do you think this style hampers Barb's ability with employees?
   This style of management is problematic if the manager is not comfortable disciplining her staff.

3. How does this style help Barb when interacting with employees?
   Employees working for this manager have a sense that their manager likes them as friends, on a personal level. This may cause employees to share personal information with their manager, and employees may be motivated to perform better.

Chapter 10: Use of Computers in the Medical Office

Nick Nowicki has just hired two new staff members into the family practice office he manages. One of the new hires has extensive experience in the use of computers in the medical office. The other new hire has been out of the medical field for several years and is new to the use of computers.

1. How might Nick make certain that each of his new employees receives the proper training on the computers and software used in the medical office?
   Nick will need to have his employees go through a training program when their employment starts. The training program should include as much training on the individual computer programs as each individual employee requires in order to be comfortable and competent when using the programs.

2. What should Nick do if the employee with extensive computer experience says she does not want to attend training classes?
   Nick should let the employee know that the training classes are mandatory for all new hires. He should remind her that there may be things about the programs used

in this particular office that the new employee may not be entirely familiar with, and therefore the training classes are likely to be beneficial.

Chapter 11: Office Policies and Procedures

Steve Croffut has recently obtained his first job as a medical office manager. On Steve's first day, he asks one of the physicians if there is a manual that outlines office procedures. The physician tells Steve that the previous office manager never took the time to compose a procedures manual. She asks Steve if he would be willing to take on such a task.

1. How would you suggest Steve begin to create a policy and procedure manual for his medical office?
    Steve should start by listing the types of policies he wants to create for the office. He might put the policies into categories and prioritize them to indicate the policies that should be done first.

2. Who should Steve speak to regarding the needed policies?
    Steve will want to consult each member of the office, starting with the physicians. Because Steve is new to the office, those who have been working there will be able to give him an idea of the policies that need to be created.

3. Where might Steve look for information on what should be included?
    Steve will want to look to other medical offices and ask other managers what is included in their policy and procedure manuals so he can get ideas for his own manual.

4. What type of policies would you suggest Steve begin with first?
    Steve should begin with emergency response policies first, then move on to policies that affect the daily operations of the medical office, such as opening and closing procedures.

Chapter 12: Accounting and Payroll in the Medical Office

Barb Rolette is the medical office manager in an internal medicine practice. The physicians in the practice would like to find out if adding a flu shot clinic will be profitable this upcoming flu season. Barb needs to find out if the cost of staffing the clinic and the cost of supplies weighed against the reimbursement from the flu clinic will be profitable to the clinic.

1. How should Barb begin her investigation into the profitability of the proposed flu shot clinic?
    Barb will need to know the cost of the vaccine and the cost of the staff to administer the vaccine. She will also need to come up with a realistic idea of how many patients her clinic would provide with flu shots.

2. What information will Barb need to gather?
    Barb will need to know the hourly rate for staffing, the cost of the vaccine, and the number of patients the flu clinic would expect to serve.

Chapter 13: Billing and Collections

Molly Garrison was recently hired as the medical office manager for Wayside Family Practice. As she is going through overdue patient accounts, Molly sees that there are several outstanding accounts that have not had any payments made on them in months.

1. How would you suggest Molly begin the task of collecting the overdue accounts she has discovered?

   Molly will need to go through all of the accounts to discover the ones that are past due.

2. What steps would you suggest Molly follow?

   Molly should call patients whose accounts are overdue and ask for payment. If the patient cannot be reached, Molly should send a letter to the patient reminding him of his past due balance and asking for payment by a specific date.

3. How would you suggest Molly document the work she is doing, as well as any conversations she has with patients?

   Molly should document any conversations with patients in the patient's financial record. This information should include the date and time of the conversation, the person she spoke with, and the commitment made for payment of the past due account.

Chapter 14: Health Insurance

Roland Rubowski works as the medical office manager in a cardiology practice. Many of the patients seen in his clinic are covered by Medicare as well as a supplemental insurance plan. Roland has just hired three new medical assistants and needs to train them on the basics of Medicare coverage, so that the medical assistants will be able to properly communicate coverage information to their patients.

1. How would you suggest Roland set up a training plan for his new employees?

   Roland should put together an outline of the information he wants his new employees to know. Once the outline is in place, Roland should put together the content in an easy-to-understand format.

2. What important points about Medicare coverage should Roland ensure his staff understands and can explain to patients?

   Roland should ensure that he covers the exclusions that exist in the Medicare plan, how Medicare coverage works with supplemental insurance coverage, and the various forms that may need to be signed by Medicare patients prior to receiving services.

Chapter 15: Procedural and Diagnostic Coding

James McCollum is the medical office manager in a large multiple-specialty clinic. Part of his duties include overseeing the billing and coding staff in the clinic. After attending a medical office managers' conference on billing and coding, James returns to his clinic with information on how the coding process in his office could be improved.

1. What steps should James take to implement the new coding information he learned at the medical office managers' conference?

   James should gather the appropriate staff together, perhaps in a department meeting, and go over the information he learned at the conference.

2. What other members of the medical practice should James include in the process?

   Any member of the staff who is involved in the coding process should be educated as to the changes. This will likely include the physicians, nurses, and medical assistants, as well as the staff who actually perform the billing and coding.

3. What members of the staff should be educated about the changes?

   Any staff member who is involved in the process of assigning codes or sending out the bills should be educated about the changes. In some cases, patients may need to be educated about the changes as well.

Chapter 16: Quality Improvement and Risk Management

Saresh Mulumudi has recently been hired as the medical office manager in a multiple-specialty clinic. He soon discovers many opportunities for improvements in the office and he wants to get the staff and providers engaged in the improvement efforts.

1. How would you suggest Saresh go about setting up a quality improvement program in his office?

   Saresh should begin by creating a list of the areas that he thinks would benefit from a quality improvement effort. After the list has been created, Saresh should put together teams to work on the various areas.

2. Who should Saresh involve in his efforts?

   Saresh should involve the staff members who actually perform the work in the areas where he would like to see improvement.

Chapter 17: Marketing the Medical Office

Harold Price is the medical office manager with a large cardiology practice. The physicians in his clinic have asked Harold to put together a marketing plan and to present his ideas to them at the next department meeting.

1. How would you suggest Harold begin putting together his marketing proposal for the practice?

   Harold should determine if any of the office's physicians have openings in their schedules, or if any of the physicians are skilled in a certain procedure or type of product that might be in demand in his area. Harold should look to see what other competing cardiology practices are offering and determine if there is a demand for Harold's physicians to offer similar services or product lines.

2. As a specialty practice, what marketing areas might Harold look into that would not be of interest to a primary care office manager? How might Harold seize those opportunities?

   Harold should consult cardiology group management associations to find out what other cardiology practices are offering to their patients. He may want to put together a focus group of patients in the community to find out what services or opportunities may be of interest to those patients.

Appendix E

Registered Medical Assistant (RMA) Task List

The various tasks that medical assistants perform include, but are not necessarily limited to, those on the following list.

The tasks presented in this inventory are considered by American Medical Technologists (AMT) to be representative of the medical assisting job role. This document should be considered dynamic, to reflect the medical assistant's evolving role with respect to contemporary health care. Therefore, tasks may be added, removed, or modified on an ongoing basis.

Medical assistants who meet AMT's qualifications and pass a certification examination are certified as a Registered Medical Assistant (RMA).

I. GENERAL MEDICAL ASSISTING KNOWLEDGE
  A. Anatomy and Physiology
    1. Body systems
    2. Disorders and diseases of the body
  B. Medical Terminology
    1. Word parts
    2. Medical terms
    3. Common abbreviations and symbols
    4. Spelling
  C. Medical Law
    1. Medical law
    2. Licensure, certification, and registration
  D. Medical Ethics
    1. Principles of medical ethics
    2. Ethical conduct
    3. Professional development
  E. Human Relations
    1. Patient relations
    2. Interpersonal skills
    3. Cultural diversity
  F. Patient Education
    1. Identify and apply proper communication methods in patient instruction
    2. Develop, assemble, and maintain patient resource materials

II. ADMINISTRATIVE MEDICAL ASSISTING
  A. Insurance
    1. Medical insurance terminology
    2. Various insurance plans
    3. Claim forms
    4. Electronic insurance claims
    5. ICD-9/CPT coding applications
    6. HIPAA-mandated coding systems
    7. Financial applications of medical insurance
  B. Financial Bookkeeping
    1. Medical finance terminology
    2. Patient billing procedures
    3. Collection procedures
    4. Fundamental medical office accounting procedures

5. Office banking procedures
6. Employee payroll
7. Financial calculations and accounting procedures

C. Medical Secretarial—Receptionist
1. Medical terminology associated with receptionist duties
2. General reception of patients and visitors
3. Appointment scheduling systems
4. Oral and written communications
5. Medical records management
6. Charting guidelines and regulations
7. Protect, store, and retain medical records according to HIPAA regulations
8. Release of protected health information adhering to HIPAA regulations
9. Transcription of dictation
10. Supplies and equipment management
11. Medical office computer applications
12. Compliance with OSHA guidelines and regulations of office safety

III. CLINICAL MEDICAL ASSISTING
A. Asepsis
1. Medical terminology
2. State/federal universal blood-borne pathogen/body fluid precautions
3. Medical/surgical asepsis procedure

B. Sterilization
1. Medical terminology associated with sterilization
2. Sanitization, disinfection, and sterilization procedures
3. Record-keeping procedures

C. Instruments
1. Specialty instruments and parts
2. Usage of common instruments
3. Care and handling of disposable and reusable instruments

D. Vital Signs/Mensurations
1. Blood pressure, pulse, respiration measurements
2. Height, weight, circumference measurements
3. Various temperature measurements
4. Recognize normal and abnormal measurement results

E. Physical Examinations
1. Patient history information
2. Proper charting procedures
3. Patient positions for examinations
4. Methods of examinations
5. Specialty examinations
6. Visual acuity/Ishihara (color blindness) measurements
7. Allergy testing procedures
8. Normal/abnormal results

F. Clinical Pharmacology
1. Medical terminology associated with pharmacology
2. Commonly used drugs and their categories
3. Various routes of medication administration
4. Parenteral administration of medications (subcutaneous, intramuscular, intradermal, Z-track)
5. Classes or drug schedules and legal prescription requirements for each
6. Drug Enforcement Agency regulations for ordering, dispensing, storage, and documentation of medication use
7. Drug reference books (*PDR, Pharmacopeia, Facts and Comparisons, Nurses' Handbook*)

G. Minor Surgery
1. Surgical supplies and instruments
2. Asepsis in surgical procedures

   3. Surgical tray preparation and sterile field respect
   4. Prevention of pathogen transmission
   5. Patient surgical preparation procedures
   6. Assisting physician with minor surgery including set-up
   7. Dressing and bandaging techniques
   8. Suture and staple removal
   9. Biohazard waste disposal procedures
   10. Instruct patient in presurgical and postsurgical care
H. Therapeutic Modalities
   1. Various standard therapeutic modalities
   2. Alternative/complementary therapies
   3. Instruct patient in assistive devices, body mechanics, and home care
I. Laboratory Procedures
   1. Medical laboratory terminology
   2. OSHA safety guidelines
   3. Quality control and assessment regulations
   4. Operate and maintain laboratory equipment
   5. CLIA-waived laboratory testing procedures
   6. Capillary, dermal, and venipuncture procedures
   7. Office specimen collection such as urine, throat, vaginal, wound cultures – stool, sputum, etc.
   8. Specimen handling and preparation
   9. Laboratory recording according to state and federal guidelines
   10. Adhere to the M A Scope of Practice in the laboratory
J. Electrocardiography
   1. Standard, 12-lead ECG testing
   2. Mounting techniques for permanent record
   3. Rhythm strip ECG monitoring on lead II
K. First Aid
   1. Emergencies and first-aid procedures
   2. Emergency crash cart supplies
   3. Legal responsibilities as a first responder

Reprinted with permission of American Medical Technologists, www.aamt1.com.

AAMA 2007-2008

Occupational Analysis of the CMA (AAMA)

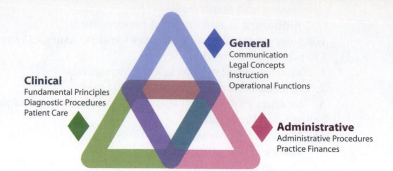

Clinical
Fundamental Principles
Diagnostic Procedures
Patient Care

General
Communication
Legal Concepts
Instruction
Operational Functions

Administrative
Administrative Procedures
Practice Finances

In furtherance of its leadership role in the profession, the American Association of Medical Assistants (AAMA) has completed the following *2007–2008 Occupational Analysis of the CMA (AAMA)*. In previous years, this document was titled *AAMA Role Delineation Study: Occupational Analysis of the Medical Assisting Profession*.

A Necessary Distinction

A professional's skills are largely determined by professional education. The CMA (AAMA) is the only credential that requires candidates to be graduates of a programmatically accredited medical assisting program. Therefore, it is appropriate and necessary that the qualifying language "of the CMA (AAMA)" be incorporated into this document's title.

About the Survey

A survey was sent to a random sample of CMAs (AAMA)—AAMA members and nonmembers. The CMA (AAMA) represents a medical assistant who has been credentialed by the Certifying Board of the AAMA. Of the 15,500 surveys distributed, 3,658 were collected and analyzed, resulting in a 95 percent confidence level. The results obtained from the sample are within ±1.6 percent of the results if all 15,500 individuals had responded.

Analysis Highlights

Today's CMA (AAMA) is expected not only to master the body of knowledge of the profession, but also to apply this knowledge in the complex and fast-paced world of ambulatory health care. Thus, critical thinking is emphasized in this *Occupational Analysis.*

Another dimension in the *Occupational Analysis* reflects the growing awareness that the CMA (AAMA) is uniquely qualified to "speak the patient's language" and serve as a "communication liaison" between the busy physician and patients. The roles of the CMA (AAMA) as "patient advocate" and "health coach," as well as "communication liaison," are given appropriate prominence in this document.

All health professionals have been expected to refine their knowledge and skills in responding to natural and man-made emergencies, and the vital roles of CMAs (AAMA) have come into increasing focus in recent years. In keeping with this priority, the *Occupational Analysis* includes emergency-related functions under Communication, Instruction, and Patient Care.

Uses of the Study

This document provides valuable data to the Certifying Board (CB) and the Continuing Education Board (CEB) of the AAMA, as well as to the Medical Assisting Education Review Board (MAERB). However, the *Occupational Analysis* should not be confused with the following documents:

- *Content Outline of the CMA (AAMA) Certification/Recertification Examination,* published by the CB

- *Advanced Practice of Medical Assisting,* published by the CEB

- *Standards and Guidelines for Medical Assisting Educational Programs,* published by CAAHEP

- *Curriculum Content and Competencies,* published by the MAERB

Legal Scope of Practice

This *Occupational Analysis* does not delineate the legal scope of medical assisting practice. Legally delegable responsibilities vary from state to state. Scope of practice questions should be directed to AAMA Executive Director and Legal Counsel Donald A. Balasa, JD, MBA, at dbalasa@aama-ntl.org.

Occupational Analysis Committee

Chair: Charlene Couch, CMA (AAMA)
K. Minchella, CMA (AAMA), PhD
Rebecca Walker, CMA (AAMA), CPC
Nina Watson, CMA (AAMA), CPC, COS

Ex officio
Linda Brown, 2007-2008 President
Kathryn Panagiotacos, CMA (AAMA), 2007-2008 Vice President
Donald A. Balasa, JD, MBA, Executive Director

AMERICAN ASSOCIATION OF MEDICAL ASSISTANTS
20 N. WACKER DR., STE. 1575
CHICAGO, ILLINOIS 60606
website: www.aama-ntl.org   800/228-2262

552 11/09

General, Clinical, and Administrative Skills* of the CMA (AAMA)

General Skills

Communication

- Recognize and respect cultural diversity
- Adapt communications to individual's understanding
- Employ professional telephone and interpersonal techniques
- Recognize and respond effectively to verbal, nonverbal, and written communications
- Utilize and apply medical terminology appropriately
- Receive, organize, prioritize, store, and maintain transmittable information utilizing electronic technology
- Serve as "communication liaison" between the physician and patient
- Serve as patient advocate professional and health coach in a team approach in health care
- Identify basics of office emergency preparedness

Legal Concepts

- Perform within legal (including federal and state statutes, regulations, opinions, and rulings) and ethical boundaries
- Document patient communication and clinical treatments accurately and appropriately
- Maintain medical records
- Follow employer's established policies dealing with the health care contract
- Comply with established risk management and safety procedures
- Recognize professional credentialing criteria
- Identify and respond to issues of confidentiality

Instruction

- Function as a health care advocate to meet individual's needs
- Educate individuals in office policies and procedures
- Educate the patient within the scope of practice and as directed by supervising physician in health maintenance, disease prevention, and compliance with patient's treatment plan
- Identify community resources for health maintenance and disease prevention to meet individual patient needs
- Maintain current list of community resources, including those for emergency preparedness and other patient care needs
- Collaborate with local community resources for emergency preparedness
- Educate patients in their responsibilities relating to third-party reimbursements

Operational Functions

- Perform inventory of supplies and equipment
- Perform routine maintenance of administrative and clinical equipment
- Apply computer and other electronic equipment techniques to support office operations
- Perform methods of quality control

Clinical Skills

Fundamental Principles

- Identify the roles and responsibilities of the medical assistant in the clinical setting
- Identify the roles and responsibilities of other team members in the medical office
- Apply principles of aseptic technique and infection control
- Practice Standard Precautions, including handwashing and disposal of biohazardous materials
- Perform sterilization techniques
- Comply with quality assurance practices

Diagnostic Procedures

- Collect and process specimens
- Perform CLIA-waived tests
- Perform electrocardiography and respiratory testing
- Perform phlebotomy, including venipuncture and capillary puncture
- Utilize knowledge of principles of radiology

Patient Care

- Perform initial-response screening following protocols approved by supervising physician
- Obtain, evaluate, and record patient history employing critical thinking skills
- Obtain vital signs
- Prepare and maintain examination and treatment areas
- Prepare patient for examinations, procedures and treatments
- Assist with examinations, procedures, and treatments
- Maintain examination/treatment rooms, including inventory of supplies and equipment
- Prepare and administer oral and parenteral (excluding IV) medications and immunizations (as directed by supervising physician and as permitted by state law)
- Utilize knowledge of principles of IV therapy
- Maintain medication and immunization records
- Screen and follow up test results
- Recognize and respond to emergencies

Administrative Skills

Administrative Procedures

- Schedule, coordinate, and monitor appointments
- Schedule inpatient/outpatient admissions and procedures
- Apply third-party and managed care policies, procedures, and guidelines
- Establish, organize, and maintain patient medical record
- File medical records appropriately

Practice Finances

- Perform procedural and diagnostic coding for reimbursement
- Perform billing and collection procedures
- Perform administrative functions, including bookkeeping and financial procedures
- Prepare submittable ("clean") insurance forms

*All skills require decision making based on critical thinking concepts.

Medical Terminology Word Parts

Medical terms are like individual jigsaw puzzles. Once you divide the terms into their component parts and learn the meaning of the individual parts, you can use that knowledge to understand many other new terms. Four basic component parts are used to create medical terms:

Root   The basic, or core, part that makes up the essential meaning of the term. The root usually, but not always, denotes a body part. Root words usually come from the Greek or Latin languages. For example, *bronch* is a root that means "the air passages in the lungs" or "bronchial tubes." *Cephal* means "head." An extensive list of root words is given on pages 420–423.

Prefix   One or more letters placed before the root to change its meaning. Prefixes usually, but not always, indicate location, time, number, or status. For example, the prefix *bi-* means "two" or "twice." When *bi* is placed before the root *lateral* ("side"), to form *bilateral*, the meaning is "having two sides." An extensive list of prefixes is given on page 420.

Suffix   One or more letters placed after the root to change its meaning. Suffixes usually, but not always, indicate the procedure, condition, disorder, or disease. For example, the suffix *-itis* means "inflammation," that is, damaged tissue that is red and painful. The medical term *bronchitis* means "inflammation of the bronchial tubes." Another example is the suffix *-ectomy,* which means "removal." Hence, *appendectomy* means "removal of the appendix." An extensive list of suffixes is given on pages 423–424.

Combining vowel   A letter used to combine roots with other word parts. The vowel is usually an *o,* but sometimes it is an *a* or *i*. When a combining vowel is added to a root, the result is called a combining form. For example, in the word encephalogram, the root is *cephal* ("head"), the prefix is *en-* ("inside"), and the suffix is *-gram* ("something recorded"). These word parts are joined by the combining vowel *o* to make a word more easy to pronounce. *Cephal/o* is the combining form. An *encephalogram* is an x-ray of the inside of the head.

Analyzing a Medical Term

You can often decipher the meaning of a medical term by breaking it down into its separate parts. Consider the following examples:

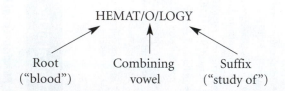

HEMAT/O/LOGY

Root ("blood")   Combining vowel   Suffix ("study of")

The term *hematology* is divided into three parts. When you analyze a medical term, begin at the end of the word. The ending is called the suffix. Almost all medical terms contain suffixes. The suffix in *hematology* is *-logy,* which means "study of." Now look at the beginning of the word. *Hemat* is the root word, which means "blood." The root word gives the essential meaning of the term.

The third part of this term, which is the letter *o,* has no meaning of its own, but is an important connector between the root (*hemat*) and the suffix (*logy*). It is the combining vowel. The letter *o* is the combining vowel usually found in medical terms.

Putting together the meanings of the suffix and the root, the term *hematology* means "the study of blood."

The combining vowel plus the root is called the combining form. A medical term can have more than one root word; therefore, there can be two combining forms. For example:

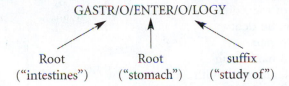

GASTR/O/ENTER/O/LOGY

Root	Root	suffix
("intestines")	("stomach")	("study of")

The two combining forms are *gastr/o* and *enter/o*. The entire term (reading from the suffix, back to the beginning of the term, and across) means "the study of the stomach and the intestines."

Keys to Success

Prefix Guideline

A prefix does not require a combining vowel. Do not place a combining vowel between a prefix and a root word.

Keys to Success

Word Part Guidelines

1. A single root word with a combining form cannot stand alone. A suffix must be added to complete the term.
2. The rules for the use of combining vowels apply when adding a suffix.
3. When a suffix begins with a consonant, a combining vowel such as *o*, is placed before the suffix.

Rules for Using Combining Vowels

1. A combining vowel is not used when the suffix begins with a vowel (*a-e-i-o-u*). For example, when *neur/o* (nerve) is joined with the suffix *-itis* (inflammation), the combining vowel is not used because *-itis* begins with a vowel. *Neuritis* (new-RYE-tis) is an inflammation of a nerve or nerves.

2. A combining vowel is used when the suffix begins with a consonant. For example, when *neur/o* (nerve) is joined with the suffix *-plasty* (surgical repair), the combining vowel *o* is used because *-plasty* begins with a consonant. *Neuroplasty* (NEW-roh-plas-tee) is the surgical repair of a nerve.

3. A combining vowel is always used when two or more root words are joined. As an example, when *gastr/o* (stomach) is joined with *enter/o* (small intestine), the combining vowel is used with *gastr/o*. *Gastroenteritis* (gas-troh-en-ter-EYE-tis) is an inflammation of the stomach and small intestine.

Suffixes and Medical Terms Related to Pathology

Pathology is the study of disease and the following suffixes describe specific disease conditions. (A more complete list of suffixes appears on pages 423–424.)

Suffix	Meaning
-algia	pain and suffering
-centesis	surgical puncture to remove fluid for diagnostic purposes or to remove excess fluid
-dynia	pain
-ectomy	excision or surgical removal
-gram	record or picture
-graphy	process of recording a picture or record
-necr/osis	death (tissue death)
-plasty	surgical repair
-scler/osis	abnormal hardening
-scopy	visual examination with an instrument
-sten/osis	abnormal narrowing

The Double RR Suffixes

The following suffixes are often referred to as the "double RR" suffixes:

* -rrhage and -rrhagia   Bursting form; an abnormal excessive discharge or bleeding. *Note: -rrhage* and *-rhagia* refer to the flow of blood.

* -rrhaphy   To suture or stitch.

* -rrhea   Abnormal flow or discharge; refers to the abnormal flow of most body fluids. *Note:* Although *-rrhea* and *-rrhage* both refer to abnormal flow, they are not used interchangeably.

* -rrhexis   Rupture.

Contrasting and Confusing Prefixes

The following contrasting prefixes can be confusing. Study this list to make sure you know the differences between the contrasting terms. (A more complete list of prefixes appears on page 420.)

ab- means "away from." *Abnormal* means not normal or away from normal.

ad- means "to" or "in the direction." *Addiction* means drawn toward or a strong dependence on a drug or substance.

dys- means "bad," "difficult," or "painful." *Dysfunctional* means an organ or body that is not working properly.

eu- means "good," "normal," "well," or "easy." Euthyroid (you-THIGH-roid) means a normally functioning thyroid gland.

hyper- means "excessive" or "increased." *Hypertension* (high-per-TEN-shun) is higher-than-normal blood pressure.

hypo- means "deficient" or "decreased." *Hypotension* (high-poh-TEN-shun) is lower-than-normal blood pressure.

inter- means "between" or "among." *Interstitial* (in-ter-STISH-al) means between, but not within, the parts of a tissue.

intra- means "within" or "into." *Intramuscular* (in-trah-MUS-kyou-lar) means within the muscle.

sub- means "under," "less," or "below." *Subcostal* (sub-KOS-tal) means below a rib or ribs.

supra- means "over" or "above." *Supracostal* (sue-prah-KOS-tal) means above or outside the ribs.

Singular and Plural Endings

Many medical terms have Greek or Latin origins. As a result of these different origins, the rules for changing a singular word into a plural form are unusual. Additionally, English endings have been adopted for some commonly used terms.

Keys to Success

Using a Medical Dictionary

Learning to use a medical dictionary is an important part of mastering the correct use of medical terms. Some dictionaries use categories such as "Diseases and Syndromes" to group disorders with these terms in the titles. For example:

- Venereal disease would be found under "disease, venereal."
- Fetal alcohol syndrome would be found under "syndrome, fetal alcohol."

When you come across a term and cannot find it listed by the first word, the next step is to look under the appropriate category.

GUIDELINES TO UNUSUAL PLURAL FORMS

	Guideline	Singular	Plural
1.	If the term ends in an *a*, the plural is usually formed by adding an *e*.	bursa vertebrae	bursae vertebra
2.	If the term ends in *ex* or *ix*, the plural is usually formed by changing the *ex* or *ix* to *ices*.	appendix index	appendices indices
3.	If the term ends in *is*, the plural is usually formed by changing the *is* to *es*.	diagnosis metastasis	diagnoses metastases
4.	If the term ends in *itis*, the plural is usually formed by changing the *is* to *ides*.	arthritis meningitis	arthritides meningitides
5.	If the term ends in *nx*, the plural is usually formed by changes the *x* to *ges*.	phalanx meninx	phalanges meninges
6.	If the term ends in *on*, the plural is usually formed by changing the *on* to *a*.	criterion ganglion	criteria ganglia
7.	If the term ends in *um*, the plural is usually formed by changing the um to *a*.	diverticulum ovum	diverticula ova
8.	If the term ends in *us*, the plural is usually formed by changing the *us* to *i*.	alveolus malleolus	alveoli malleoli

Basic Medical Terms

The following subsections discuss basic medical terms that are used to describe diseases and disease conditions, major body systems, and body direction.

Keys to Success

Accuracy in Spelling

Accuracy in spelling medical terms is extremely important! Changing just one or two letters can completely change the meaning of the word—and this difference could literally be a matter of life or death for the patient.

TERMS USED TO DESCRIBE DISEASES AND DISEASE CONDITIONS

The basic medical terms used to describe diseases and disease conditions are listed here.

- A *sign* is evidence of disease, such as fever, that can be observed by the patient and others. A sign is objective because it can be evaluated or measured by others.

- A *symptom,* such as pain or a headache, can only be experienced or defined by the patient. A symptom is subjective because it can be evaluated or measured only by the patient.

- A *syndrome* is a set of signs and symptoms that occur together as part of a specific disease process.

- *Diagnosis* is the identification of disease. To diagnose is the process of reaching a diagnosis.

- A *differential diagnosis* attempts to determine which of several diseases may be producing the symptoms.

- A *prognosis* is a forecast or prediction of the probable course and outcome of a disorder.

- An *acute* disease or symptom has a rapid onset, a severe course, and relatively short duration.

- A *chronic* symptom or disease has a long duration. Although chronic symptoms or diseases may be controlled, they are rarely cured.

- A *remission* is the partial or complete disappearance of the symptoms of a disease without having achieved a cure. A remission is usually temporary.

- Some diseases are named for the condition described. For example, *chronic fatigue syndrome* (CFS) is a persistent overwhelming fatigue that does not resolve with bed rest.

- An *eponym* is a disease, structure, operation, or procedure that is named for the person who discovered or described it first. For example, Alzheimer's disease is named for Alois Alzheimer, a German neurologist who lived from 1864 to 1915.

- An *acronym* is a word formed from the initial letter or letters of the major parts of a compound term. For example, the acronym AMA stands for American Medical Association.

TERMS USED TO DESCRIBE MAJOR BODY SYSTEMS

The following is a list of the major body systems and some common related combining forms used with each.

Major Structures and Body System	Related Roots with Combining Forms
Skeletal system	bones (oste/o)
	joints (arthr/o)
	cartilage (chondr/o)
Muscular system	muscles(my/o)
	ligaments (syndesm/o)
	tendons (ten/o, tend/o, tendin/o)

Cardiovascular system	heart (card/o, cardi/o)
	arteries (arteri/o)
	veins (phleb/o, ven/o)
	blood (hem/o, hemat/o)
Lymphatic and immune systems	lymph, lymph vessels, and lymph nodes (lymph/o, lymphangi/o)
	tonsils (tonsill/o)
	spleen (splen/o)
	thymus (thym/o)
Respiratory system	nose (nas/o, rhin/o)
	pharynx (pharyng/o)
	trachea (trache/o)
	larynx (laryng/o)
	lungs (pneum/o, pneumon/o)
Digestive system	mouth (or/o)
	esophagus (esophag/o)
	stomach (gastr/o)
	small intestines (enter/o)
	large intestines (col/o)
	liver (hepat/o)
	pancreas (pancreat/o)
Urinary system	kidneys (nephr/o, ren/o)
	ureters (ureter/o)
	urinary bladder (cyst/o, visic/o)
	urethra (urethr/o)
Integumentary system	glands (aden/o)
	skin (cutane/o, dermat/o, derm/o)
	sebaceous glands (seb/o)
	sweat glands (hidraden/o)
Nervous system	nerves (neur/o)
	brain (encephal/o)
	spinal cord (myel/o)
	eyes (ocul/o, ophthalm/o)
	ears (acoust/o, ot/o)
Endocrine system	adrenals (adren/o)
	pancreas (pancreat/o)
	pituitary (pituit/o)
	thyroid (thyr/o, thyroid/o)
	parathyroids (parathyroid/o)
	thymus (thym/o)
Reproductive system	*Male:*
	testicles (orch/o, orchid/o)
	Female:
	ovaries (oophor/o, ovari/o)
	uterus (hyster/o, metr/o, metri/o, uter/o)

TERMS USED TO DESCRIBE BODY DIRECTION

Certain terms are used to describe the location of body parts relative to the trunk or other parts of the anatomy. See Figure ■ G-1.

Ventral (VEN-tral) refers to the front or belly side of the body or organ (*ventr* means "belly side" of the body and *al* means "pertaining to").

Dorsal (DOR-sal) refers to the back of the body or organ (*dors* means "back of body" and *al* means "pertaining to").

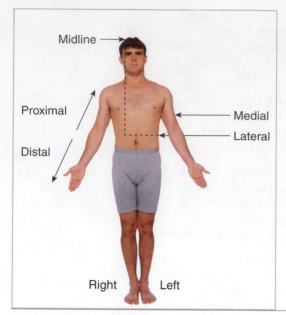 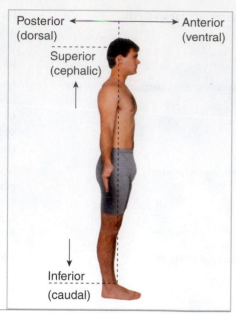

FIGURE ■ G-1 Directional anatomical terms.
Source: Richard Logan/Pearson Education.

Anterior (an-TEER-ee-or) means situated in the front. It also means on the forward part of an organ (*anter* means "front" or "before" and *ior* means "pertaining to"). For example, the stomach is located anterior to (in front of) the pancreas. *Anterior* is also used in reference to the ventral surface of the body.

Posterior (pos-TEER-ee-or) means situated in the back. It also means on the back portion of an organ (*poster* means "back" or "after" and *ior* means "pertaining to"). For example, the pancreas is located posterior to (behind) the stomach. Posterior is also used in reference to the dorsal surface of the body.

Superior means uppermost, above, or toward the head. For example, the lungs are superior to (above) the diaphragm.

Inferior means lowermost, below, or toward the feet. For example, the stomach is located inferior to (below) the diaphragm.

Cephalic (seh-FAL-ick) means toward the head (*cephal* means "head" and *ic* means "pertaining to").

Caudal (KAW-dal) means toward the lower part of the body (*caud* means "tail" or "lower part" of the body and *al* means "pertaining to").

Proximal (PROCK-sih-mal) means situated nearest the midline or beginning of a body structure. For example, the proximal end of the humerus (the bone of the upper arm) forms part of the shoulder. Or, it may be easier for you to think of it as "closer to the origin of the body part or the point of attachment of a limb to the body trunk."

Distal (DIS-tal) means situated farthest from the midline or beginning of a body structure. For example, the distal end of the humerus forms part of the elbow.

Medial means the direction toward or nearer the midline. For example, the medial ligament of the knee is near the inner surface of the leg.

Lateral means the direction toward or nearer the side and away from the midline. For example, the lateral ligament of the knee is near the side of the leg.

Bilateral means relating to, or having, two sides.

PLANES OF THE BODY

Medical professionals often refer to sections of the body in terms of anatomical planes (flat surfaces). These planes are imaginary lines—vertical or horizontal—drawn through an upright body. The following terms are used to describe a specific body part (see Figure ■ G-2):

- Coronal plane (frontal plane): A vertical plane running from side to side; divides the body or any of its parts into anterior and posterior portions.

- Sagittal plane (median plane): A vertical plane running from front to back; divides the body or any of its parts into right and left sides.

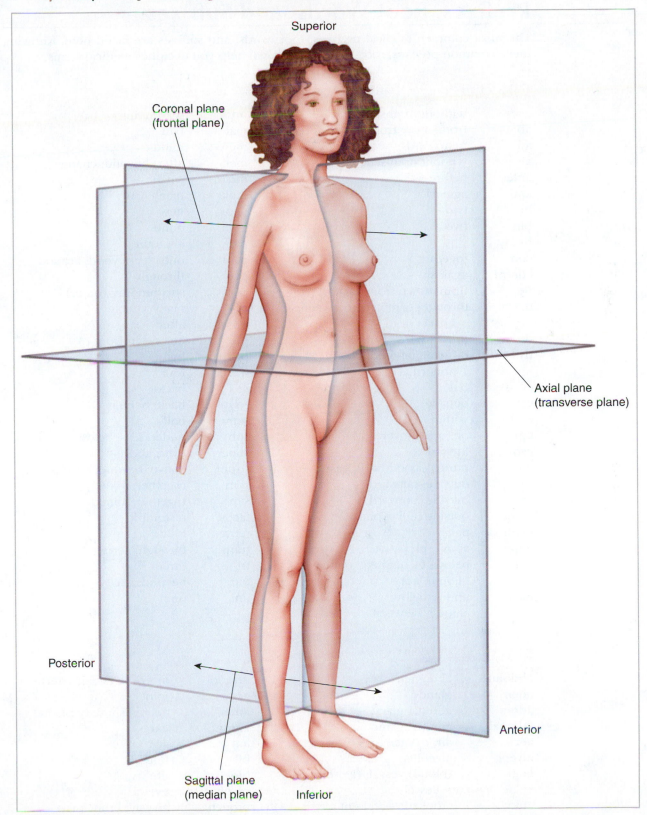

FIGURE ■ G-2 Anatomical planes.
Source: Richard Logan/Pearson Education.

- Axial plane (transverse plane): A horizontal plane; divides the body or any of its parts into upper and lower parts.

Prefixes, Root Words, and Suffixes

The most common medical prefixes, root words, and suffixes are listed here. Knowing these common prefixes, roots, and suffixes will help you decipher medical terms.

PREFIXES

a	without or absence of	intra	within; into
ab	from; away from	mal	bad
ad	to; toward	meso	middle
an	without or absence of	meta	after; beyond; change
ante	before	micro	small
anti	against	multi	many
bi	two	neo	new
bin	two	nulli	none
brady	slow	pan	all; total
con	together	para	outside; beyond; around
contra	against	per	through
de	from; down from; lack of	peri	surrounding (outer)
dia	through; complete; between; apart	poly	many; much
		post	after
dis	to undo; free from	pre	before; in front of
dys	difficult; labored; painful; abnormal	pro	before
		quadri	four
ec	out	re	back
ecto	outside	retro	back; behind
endo	within	semi	half
epi	on; upon; over	sub	under; less; below
eso	inward	super	over; above
eu	normal; good; well; easy	supra	above; beyond; on top
ex	outside; outward	sym	together; joined
exo	outside; outward	syn	together; joined
extra	outside of; beyond	tachy	fast; rapid
hemi	half	tetra	four
hyper	above; excessive	trans	through; across; beyond
hypo	below; incomplete; deficient	tri	three
in	in; into; not	ultra	beyond; excess
infra	under; below	uni	one
inter	among; between		

ROOT WORDS

abdomin	abdomen	arteriol	arteriole (small artery)
aden	gland	arthr	joint
adren	adrenal gland	ather	yellowish; fatty plaque
adrenal	adrenal gland	aur	ear
aer	air; oxygen; gas	aut	self
alveol	alveolus	bil	bile
angi	(blood) vessel; (lymph) vessel	bio	life
		blephar	eyelid
ankyl	crooked; stiff; bent	bronch	airway; bronchus
appendic	appendix	bronchiol	bronchiole
arteri, arter	artery	burs	bursa

carcin	cancer	gingiv	gums
cardi	heart	glauc	gray
caud	tail; toward lower part of the body	gloss	tongue
		gluc	sweetness; sugar
cephal	head	glyc	sugar; glucose
cerebell	cerebellum	glycos	sugar; glucose
cerebr	cerebrum; brain	gnos	knowledge; a knowing
cervic	neck; cervix	gonad	gonad; sex glands
cheil	lip	gyn	woman
chiro	hand	gynec	woman
cholangi	bile duct	gyr	turning; folding
chole	gall; bile	hem	blood
chondr	cartilage	hemat	blood
coccyg	coccyx; tailbone	hepat	liver
col	colon; large intestine	hidr	sweat
conjunctiv	conjunctiva	hist	tissue
corne	cornea	hom	same
coron	heart; crown of the head	home	sameness; unchanging
cost	rib	hydr	water
crani	cranium; skull	hyster	uterus
cutane	skin	ile	ileum
cyan	blue	ili	ilium
cyst	bladder; sac	immun	immune
cyt, cyte	cell	irid	iris
dacry	tears; tear duct	kerat	horny tissue; hard
dactyl	fingers or toes	kin	movement
dent	tooth	kinesi	movement; motion
derm	skin	labi	lips
dermat	skin	lacrim	tear duct; tear
dipl	two; double	lact	milk
diverticul	diverticulum	lapar	abdomen
dors	back (of the body)	laryng	larynx
duoden	duodenum	later	side
ectop	located away from usual place	lei	smooth
		leuk	white
edema	swelling	lingu	tongue
electr	electricity; electrical activity	lip	fat
		lith	stone; calculus
encephal	brain	lob	lobe
endocrin	endocrine	lymph	lymph
enter	intestines (usually small intestine)	macr	abnormal largeness
		mamm	breast
epiglott	epiglottis	mast	breast
epitheli	epithelium	meat	opening or passageway
erythr	red	melan	black
esophag	esophagus	men	menstruation
esthesi	sensation; feeling; sensitivity	mening	meninges
		ment	mind
eti	cause (of disease)	mes, meso	middle
exocrin	secrete out of	metr	uterus
faci	face	mon	one
fasci	fascia; fibrous band	morbid	disease; sickness
fract	break; broken	muc	mucus
galact	milk	my, myos	muscle
gastr	stomach	myc	fungus
ger	old age; aged	myel	bone marrow; spinal cord
geront	old age; aged	myelon	bone marrow

myring	eardrum	pylor	pylorus
narc	stupor; numbness	pyr	fever; heat
nas	nose	quadr	four
nat	birth	rect	rectum
necr	death (cells; body)	ren	kidney
nephr	kidney	retin	retina
neur	nerve	rhin	nose
noct	night	sacr	sacrum fallopian (uterine)
nyct	night	salping	tube
nyctal	night	sanit	soundness; health
ocul	eye	sarc	flesh; connective tissue
onc	tumor	scler	sclera; white of eye; hard
onych	nail	scoli	crooked; curved
oophor	ovary	seb	sebum; oil
ophthalm	eye	seps	infection
or	mouth	sept	infection; partition; septum
orth	straight	sial	saliva
oste	bone	sinus	inus
ot	ear	somat	body
ox	oxygen	somn	sleep
palpat	touch; feel; stroke	son	sound
pancreat	pancreas	sopor	sleep
par, part	bear; give birth to; labor	sperm	sperm, spermatazoa; seed
parathyroid	parathyroid	spermat	sperm, spermatazoa; seed
path	disease; suffering	spher	round; sphere; ball
pector	chest; muscle	sphygm	pulse
ped	child; foot	spin	spine; backbone to
pelv	pelvis; pelvic bone	spir	breathe
pen	penis	splen	spleen
perine	perineum	spondyl	vertebra; spinal or vertebral column
peritone	peritoneum		
petr	stone; portion of temporal bone	staphyl	grapelike clusters
		stern	(breastbone)
phac, phak	lens of the eye	steth	chest (muscles)
phag	eat; swallow	stoma	mouth; opening
phalang	finger or toe bone	stomat	mouth; opening
pharyng	pharynx, throat	strab	squint; squint-eyed
phas	speech	synovi	synovia; synovial membrane
phleb	vein		
phot	light	system	system
phren	mind	ten, tend	tendon
physi	nature	tendin	tendon
pleur	pleura	test	testis; testicle
pneum	lung; air	therm	heat
pneumat	lung; air	thorac	thorax; chest
pneumon	lung; air	thromb	clot
pod	foot	thym	thymus gland; soul
poli	gray matter	thyr	thyroid gland
polyp	polyp; small growth	thyroid	thyroid gland
poster	back (of body)	tom	cut; section
prim	first	ton	tension; pressure
proct	rectum	tone	to stretch
pseud	fake; false	tonsill	tonsils
psych	mind	top	place; position; location
pulmon	lung	tox, toxic	poison; poisonous
py	pus	trach, trache	trachea; windpipe
pyel	renal pelvis	trachel	neck; necklike

trich	hair	ven	vein
tubercul	little knot; swelling	versicul	seminal vesicles; blister
tympan	eardrum; middle ear	vertebr	vertebra; backbone
ulcer	sore; ulcer	vesic	urinary bladder
ungu	nail	vir	poison; virus
ur	urine; urinary tract	viril	masculine; manly
ureter	ureter	vis	seeing; sight
urethr	urethra	visc	sticky
uria	urination; urine	viscer	viscera; internal organs sternum
urin	urine or urinary organs		
uter	uterus	viscos	sticky
uvul	vula; little grape	vit	life
vagin	vagina	xanth	yellow
valv	valve	xen	strange; foreign
valvul	valve	xer	dry
vas	vessel; duct	zygot	joined together
vascul	blood vessel; little vessel		

ADDITIONAL ROOTWORDS

caus	burning sensation; capable of burning	genital	pertaining to birth
		lumb	lumbar; loin region
cusp	point; cusp	mediastin	mediastinum
flexion	bending	tens, tensi	pressure, force, stretching

Suffixes

SUFFIXES MEANING "PERTAINING TO"

ac		eal, ous	
al, ine		ial	
ar, ior		ic	
ary, ory		ical, tic	

SUFFIXES MEANING "ABNORMAL CONDITIONS"

ago	abnormal condition, disease	ion	condition
esis	abnormal condition, disease	ism	condition, state of abnormal condition
ia	abnormal condition, disease		
iasis	abnormal condition, disease	osis	disease

COMMON SUFFIXES USED IN MEDICAL TERMINOLOGY

algia	pain, suffering	crit	to separate
asthenia	weakness	cyte	cell
cele	hernia, protrusion	desis	fusion; to bind; tie together
centesis	surgical puncture to remove fluid	drome	run; running
		ductor	to lead or pull
cidal	killing	dynia	pain
clasia	break	ectasis	stretching out; dilation; expansion
clasis	break		
clast	break	ectomy	excision or surgical removal
clysis	irrigating; washing	ectopia	displacement
coccus	berry shaped (a form of bacterium)	emesis	vomiting
		emia	blood; blood condition
crine	separate; secrete	gen	producing, forming

genesis	producing; forming	plasm	growth; formation; substance
genic	producing, forming		
gnosis	a knowing	plasty	plastic or surgical repair
gram	record	plegia	paralysis; stroke
graph	instrument used to record	pnea	breathing
graphy	process of recording	porosis	lessening in density; porous condition
ictal	seizure; attack		
ism	state of	praxia	in front of; before
itis	inflammation	ptosis	drooping; sagging; prolapse
lepsy	seizure	ptysis	spitting
logist	specialist	rrhage	bursting forth, an abnormal excessive discharge or bleeding
logy	study of		
lysis	destruction; reduce; separation		
		rrhagia	bursting forth, an abnormal excessive discharge or bleeding
malacia	softening		
mania	madness; insane desire		
megaly	enlargement	rrhaphy	to suture or stitch
meter	instrument used to measure	rrhea	abnormal flow or discharge
		rrhexis	rupture
metry	measurement	schisis	split; fissure
morph	form; shape	sclerosis	hardening
necr/osis	death (tissue death)	scope	instrument used for visual exam
oid, ode	resembling		
oma	tumor; mass	scopic	visual exam
opia	vision (condition)	scopy	visual exam with an instrument
opsy	to view		
oxia	oxygen	sepsis	infection
paresis	slight paralysis	sis	state of
pathy	disease	spasm	sudden involuntary muscle contraction
penia	abnormal reduction in number; lack of		
		stalsis	contraction; constriction
peps, pepsia	digestion	stasis	control; stop; standing still
pexy	surgical fixation; suspension	stat	to stop
phagia	eating; swallowing	stenosis	narrowing; constriction
philia	love	stomy	new artificial opening
phily	love	therapy	treatment
phobia	abnormal fear of or adversion to specific objects or things	tome	instrument used to cut
		tomy	cutting into; surgical incision
phonia	sound or voice	tripsy	crushing
phoria	feeling	trophy	nourishment
physis	growth	ule	little
plasia	formation; development; a growth	uria	urine; urination

Source: Vines, Deborah, Braceland, Ann, Rollins, Elizabeth, and Miller, Susan Peterson. *Comprehensive Health Insurance: Billing, Coding, and Reimbursement.* © 2009. Reprinted and electronically reproduced by permission of Pearson Education, Inc., Upper Saddle River, New Jersey.

abuse—a practice that is inconsistent with sound fiscal, business, or medical practices, and results in unnecessary costs to the Medicaid or Medicare program or in reimbursement of services that are not medically necessary

accept assignment—when a physician agrees to accept the amount approved by the insurance company as payment in full for a given service

accounts receivable (AR)—money owed the medical practice

active listening—listening as well as observing behaviors during a conversation

active patient file—medical record for a patient who is actively treated in the medical office

administrative duties—clerical duties, such as answering the telephone and scheduling appointments

advance beneficiary notice (ABN)—a form patients sign agreeing to pay for services that may be denied by Medicare

advance directive—a legal document that outlines a patient's desire regarding life-sustaining treatment or names a guardian to speak for the patient

advanced care registered nurse practitioner (ARNP)—registered nurse who has pursued additional education beyond a nursing degree

agenda—a list of items to be discussed at a meeting

aging report—documentation of the money owed the medical office and how long accounts have been outstanding

allergist—physician who treats allergic conditions

allowed amount—the dollar amount for a service that an insurance company considers acceptable and uses to determine benefit payments

Americans with Disabilities Act—a federal law that outlines the legal rights of persons with disabilities

anesthesiologist—physician who performs and oversees anesthesia for surgical cases

appointment reminder cards—usually the size of a business card and contain the date, day, and time of the patient's next appointment, as well as the office's name and telephone number

assumption of risk—a defense to medical malpractice that physicians can use to prove they made the patients aware of the risks of their procedures

auditors—people who review personal or corporate bank or tax records on behalf of an agency like the Internal Revenue Service

authoritarian—a leadership style in which the manager is always in charge and control of the employees

autocratic—a management style wherein the manager makes all of the decisions without any input from others

autocratic leadership style—style where the leader makes all of the decisions for the group

automated system—a telephone answering system that automatically picks up a telephone call electronically

automatic dialer—a telephone feature that allows users to automatically redial a number until someone answers the line

automatic routing unit—a telephone system that electronically answers and routes telephone calls after receiving a prompt from the caller

autonomy—the ability to work with little oversight or help

background check—verification of any arrests or criminal convictions in an applicant's history

balance billing—billing a patient for the dollar difference between the provider's charge and the amount approved by the insurance agency

beneficiary—person who is eligible to receive benefits and services under an insurance policy

birthday rule—according to this rule, the parent with the birthday earlier in the year is the primary carrier for the children

bloodborne pathogens—any infectious material in blood that can cause disease in humans

body language—nonverbal communication, such as nodding the head, crossing the arms, and frowning

brochure—document containing information about a topic

budget—a list of planned expenses and revenues

buffer time—a scheduling system for leaving certain times of day open to accommodate situations such as patients calling for same-day appointments

call forwarding—a telephone feature that allows users to automatically forward calls to a different telephone number

capitated plan—healthcare plan in which providers are paid a set fee per month for each member patient

cardiologist—physician who treats conditions associated with the cardiovascular system

catalystic—a leadership style that consists of leading others by setting a fast pace for employees to follow

catastrophic—large and usually unforeseen

central processing unit (CPU)—the microchip inside the computer that processes the software program commands

certificate of coverage—a letter from an insurance company that provides proof of type and time frame of coverage when a patient terminates a health insurance policy

certified letter—postal service letter that the recipient must sign for

chain of command—a series of positions in which each position has authority over the position below

CHAMPVA—Civilian Health and Medical Program of the Department of Veterans Affairs; health insurance for spouses and children of veterans

charitable contributions—cash or other donations given to charitable organizations

chief complaint—the main reason the patient sought care today

chronologic—the order in which events occur in time, from oldest to newest

Circular E—yearly booklet published by the IRS that outlines the federal tax

claims-made policies—policies that protect policyholders from malpractice claims only when the insurance company insuring the policyholders at the time of the alleged malpractice is the same company at the time the claim is filed in court

clear—to the point and easily understood

clinical duties—back-office duties, including hands-on patient care

Clinical Laboratory Improvement Amendments (CLIA) Act—passed in 1988, this legislation guides policies and procedures for laboratories

closed patient file—medical record for a patient who has moved out of the area, is deceased, or has indicated that he will not be returning for care

cluster scheduling—a scheduling system in which several patients are booked around the same block of time

coaching—the process of giving advice to employees to help them find their own solutions to problems and encouraging employees to do their best

COBRA—Consolidated Omnibus Budget Reconciliation Act; this act gives workers and their families the ability to continue health insurance coverage for a limited period of time after loss of a job

coinsurance—percentage of medical charges patients are responsible for according to their insurance plan contracts

collection agency—company that pursues overdue accounts for a fee

community property laws—legislation that deems one spouse financially responsible for the other spouse's debts

comparative negligence—when both the physician and the patient are found to be responsible for an injury

compensatory award—money that is awarded to a patient or the patient's family to compensate for the cost of medical care, disability, mental suffering, any loss of income, and the loss of future income as a result of an injury

complete—containing all necessary information

computer virus—program designed to perform mischievous functions

concise—containing only the necessary information, nothing more

conference call—a telephone feature that allows numerous people to be on the same telephone call

consumer-directed healthcare plan—health insurance plans that place patients in charge of how their healthcare dollars are spent

continuing education—educational courses or seminars taken by professionals to further knowledge or skills

contributory negligence—a malpractice defense in which a physician may have been at fault for a patient's injury but can prove that the patient aggravated the injury or in some way worsened it

coordinating—the process of setting up separate functions so that a team is able to perform

copayment—set dollar fee per visit or service that patients are responsible for according to their insurance plan contracts

correct—accurate

cross-referencing—a process for locating files when a patient may go by one or more last names

Daily Management System (DMS)—a Lean concept used to share information with staff on a daily basis

damages—the actual costs associated with the injury sustained, such as medical care

deductible—monetary amount patients must pay to a provider for healthcare services before their health insurance benefits begin to pay

deductions—number of allowances to be withheld from an employee's wages

delegation—the process of taking one's tasks and giving them to another

democratic leadership style—a leadership style in which employee opinions are used in the decision-making process

demographic—the makeup of a population, such as age and number of children

dependent—a family member or other individual who qualifies for coverage on the insured's policy

dereliction of duty—physicians must meet standard of care guidelines for a healthcare provider with the same training, in the same location, under the same circumstances

dermatologist—physician who diagnoses and treats skin conditions

direct cause—a patient must prove that the physician's actions, or lack of actions, directly caused the patient's injuries

direct mail advertising—a form of print advertising that is sent directly to individuals' homes

direct reports—employee who reports directly to a particular manager

direct telephone line—a feature that allows callers to dial directly to the desk of a person in the office

discovery rule—the statute of limitations may begin from the date the injury was discovered or should have been discovered

double booking—when two or more patients are scheduled to see the same healthcare provider at the same time

duty—Physicians have a duty to care for patients once they have taken those patients on

E codes—codes that classify causes of injury and poisoning

e-billing—electronic transmission of medical claims to insurers

elective procedure—procedure that is generally considered not medically necessary

electronic billing—the process of sending medical claims to insurance carriers electronically

electronic signature—an electronic version of a person's signature, used in the electronic medical record

emergency physician—physician who has specialized training in emergency medicine

employment firm—agency that specializes in matching job applicants with employers

encrypt—to mathematically scramble information in a way that keeps unauthorized persons from viewing it

endorsement stamp—a method of endorsing a check so that the office's name and account number and the bank's name are listed on the back

eponym—a disease or condition named after an individual

ergonomic—designed to promoted good posture and limit physical injuries

established patient—a patient who has established care in the medical office

etiology—cause of a disease or an illness

Evaluation and Management (E&M) codes—codes that describe patient encounters with a physician for evaluation and management of a health problem

exclusions—procedures or services not covered under an insurance plan

exclusive provider organization (EPO)—a managed care contract with a small network of providers under which the employer agrees to not use any other networks in return for favorable pricing

experimental—a service or procedure that has not been approved by the U.S. Food and Drug Administration

Fair Debt Collection Practices Act—law that dictates how debts may be collected

Fair Labor Standards Act (FLSA)—law passed by the U.S. Congress in 1938 to address employment issues such as the federal minimum wage

false claim—billing for services that were not provided to the patient, billing for services that were different from what was actually rendered, and providing services to the patient that were not medically necessary

family practice physician—physician who treats patients of all ages for a variety of conditions

Federal Insurance Contributions Act (FICA)—law that addresses Social Security withholding taxes

Federal Unemployment Tax Act (FUTA)—law that addresses federal unemployment tax withholdings

fee schedule—list of services and their fees

feedback—opinions provided to an individual about what they have done or said

fee-for-service plan—plan in which insurance companies pay providers fees for each service provided to covered patients

financial accounting—the process of providing information to stockholders or creditors

financial information—items in the medical record pertaining to the patient's insurance coverage or account status

firewall—a software program or hardware device designed to work with the computer to add a layer of security between the data on the computer and the network to which it is connected

fixed appointment scheduling—a scheduling system in which each patient is given a specific appointment time

fixed costs—costs that remain the same no matter how many services are used or produced

flexible spending account (FSA)—account into which employees place pretax earnings for projected medical expenses

flowchart—chart used in the medical record to chart the progress of growth, such as child height, weight, and head circumference

focus groups—a group of people gathered together to test product ideas

form locators—the boxes on the CMS-1500 insurance claim form

formulary—tiered list of drugs covered by an insurance company

fraud—intentional deception or misrepresentation made by a person with the knowledge that the deception could result in a benefit to himself or another; for example, to intentionally bill for services that were never given, or to bill for a service that has a higher reimbursement than the service provided

front-line staff—employees who have direct contact with patients, such as a receptionist, medical assistant, or nurse

gastroenterologist—physician who specializes in the diagnosis and treatment of conditions associated with the digestive system

gatekeeper—physician responsible for determining when and if a patient needs specific types of healthcare

general partnership—a type of medical practice with more than one physician partnering to work together; also referred to as group practice

geographical practice cost index (GPCI)—Medicare system of adjusting fees based on the county in which the healthcare provider practices

gerontologist—physician who specializes in the treatment of conditions associated with aging

global period—the period of time, both before and after a surgical procedure, included in the surgical procedure fee

gross pay—amount earned before taxes or deductions are subtracted

group health insurance—a commercial insurance policy with rates based on a group of people; usually offered by an employer

gynecologist—physician who diagnoses and treats conditions associated with the female anatomy

hacker—person who illegally obtains access to a computer network

hands-free headset—a telephone answering system that allows the user to have his or her hands free while talking on the phone

hardship agreement—agreement a patient signs to indicate an inability to pay full healthcare costs due to financial hardship

Health Information Technology for Economic and Clinical Health (HITECH) Act—federal legislation that addresses the privacy and security concerns associated with the electronic transmission of health information

health insurance—insurance purchased to cover medical expenses

Health Insurance Portability and Accountability Act (HIPAA)—passed by Congress in 1996, this law addresses patient privacy and insurance carrier rules

health maintenance organization (HMO)—a group of physicians or medical centers that provide comprehensive services to members

Healthcare and Education Reconciliation Act of 2010—healthcare legislation produced to amend the Patient Protection and Affordable Care Act

Healthcare Common Procedure Coding System (HCPCS)—a set of codes developed and maintained by the Centers for Medicare and Medicaid Services for the reporting of professional services, nonphysician services, supplies, durable medical equipment, and injectable drugs

health-related calculators—Internet sites that provide calculators for determining pregnancy due dates, body mass index, and other numbers

hematologist—physician who diagnoses and treats conditions of the blood

hepatologist—physician who diagnoses and treats conditions of the liver

hold feature—a telephone feature that allows the receptionist to place the caller in a queue in order to take another call

holistic healthcare—natural, drug-free healthcare services

hospice—comfort care provided to patients who have six or fewer months to live

huddles—quick meetings in the medical office, most often done daily to share the important information for that day

humanistic—a leadership style in which employees are left alone to do their work as each employee believes is best

immunity—protection from being held responsible monetarily in a lawsuit

inactive patient file—patient file for a patient who has not been seen in a certain period of time, but who will likely return one day

indecipherable—unreadable

indemnity plan—plan in which insurance companies pay providers fees for each service provided to covered patients

individual health insurance—a commercial insurance policy with rates based on individual health criteria

infectious disease physician—physician who specializes in the treatment of infectious disease

informed consent—physicians must give patients all information about a procedure, including risks and alternatives to the procedure

insurance fraud—illegal act by a healthcare provider involving an insurance company

insured—the person who owns the insurance policy

Internet search engines—sites on the Internet used for locating needed information

internist—physician who treats conditions in adult patients

interview—the process of asking and answering questions of an applicant to determine suitability for hire

intimidate—to lead others through fear

The Joint Commission—Federal organization that bestows accreditation status to healthcare facilities after a thorough inspection and passage of safety and quality measures

laissez-faire—a management style wherein the manager allows others to make the decisions

laissez-faire leader—leader who sits back and allows others to make decisions within the group

last number redial—a telephone feature that allows the user to redial the last number by pressing one button, rather than redialing the entire telephone number

leading—the process of showing others how a task should be done; setting the vision or tone for the group

Lean process—modeled after the Toyota Production System; a tool used to streamline and standardize processes

liability insurance—type of insurance that covers injuries that occur on, in, or because of the insured's property

licensed practical nurse (LPN)—nurse who has less training than an RN. The scope of practice for an LPN is

generally more limited than that of an RN, and an LPN may be overseen by an RN

licensed vocational nurse (LVN)—nurse who has less training than an RN. The scope of practice is generally more limited than that of an RN

lifetime maximum benefits—monetary amount allowed by an insurance carrier for a member's covered expenses over the member's lifetime

limited liability partnership—type of practice where the physician partners have registered with their state in order to obtain limited liability for their partners

litigation—the act of filing a lawsuit against someone

maintenance medications—medications patients take on a long-term basis to treat a chronic condition such as high blood pressure, arthritis, or a heart condition

malfeasance—performing an incorrect treatment, such as operating on the wrong patient

malpractice—medical negligence that results in a patient being harmed in some way

malpractice insurance policy—liability insurance used to protect a physician in the event of a medical mistake or error

malware—software designed to destroy portions of a computer; more malicious than a computer virus

managed care—a system of healthcare delivery focused on reducing costs by transferring risk to the provider; may limit the type and frequency of care members may receive

managerial accounting—the function of collecting and applying financial information within an organization in order to make sound business decisions

marketing budget—the amount of money allocated to a marketing plan

marketing firm—a company that can be hired for the purpose of composing and carrying out a marketing plan

marketing plan—a plan for advertising a business or product

Material Safety Data Sheet (MSDS)—a sheet that outlines the potential risks associated with a chemical; required by OSHA for any potentially dangerous chemical

matrix—a system for mapping out the appointment times available in the medical office

Medicaid—a joint federal and state program that helps with medical costs for eligible people with low incomes and limited resources

medical assistant (MA)—allied healthcare professional who assists the physician or nurse, typically in the ambulatory clinic setting

medical information—information in the patient's medical record pertaining to his medical history or condition

medical management software—computer software used in the medical office to assist in tasks such as billing, coding, and payroll

medical record—a record of the patient's healthcare

medical research program—medical program geared toward researching a particular condition or treatment

Medicare—federal program that covers medical expenses for those ages 65 and over, those with end-stage kidney disease, and those with long-term disabilities

member—the person who owns the insurance policy

mentor—an established employee who is assigned to train a new employee

misfeasance—performing a treatment incorrectly, such as operating on a patient's arm and accidentally severing a nerve, leaving the patient without the use of the arm

mission statement—statement that describes a medical office's reason for existing

modified wave scheduling—a scheduling system in which two or three patients are scheduled at the beginning of each hour, followed by single patient appointments every 10 to 20 minutes for the rest of that hour

modifier—two-digit numeric code appended to CPT or Level II HCPCS codes to further describe circumstances

motivating—the process of encouraging others to perform well; recognizing employees for a job well-done

multitask—the ability to handle more than one task at the same time

narrative chart note—written description of a patient's visit; the oldest form of medical note taking

national conversion factor—number released by Medicare each year that determines fee schedules for all healthcare services

national provider identifier (NPI)—a unique, 10-digit number assigned to healthcare providers by the Centers for Medicare and Medicaid Services

national standard—point of reference for developing charges for healthcare services used throughout the United States

negotiate—the process of asking for a lower price or other benefits when purchasing an item or service

nephrologist—physician who specializes in the treatment of kidney disorders

net pay—amount of wages remaining after deductions and taxes have been subtracted

neurologist—physician who specializes in the treatment of conditions associated with the nervous system

new patient—any patient who has never been seen or has not been seen within the past 3 years by a provider in the facility

nominal award—small award or payment that is made when negligence is proven, but the damages are minimal

nonfeasance—delaying or failing to perform treatment

nonparticipating provider—healthcare provider who has not contracted with a particular health insurance carrier

nontherapeutic research—medical research that does not have therapeutic value to the patient

nutritionist—a healthcare professional who specializes in the field of nutrition

obliterated—completely marked out so that the original is unrecognizable

obstetrician—physician who treats women during pregnancy and childbirth

Occupational Safety and Health Act—legislation that affects safety for employees in all occupational settings

occurrence policies—policies that cover policyholders regardless of when claims are filed provided the policies were in effect at the time of the alleged malpractice events

Omnibus Budget Reconciliation Act (OBRA)—legislation passed by Congress in 1993 to calculate healthcare service fees by formula

oncologist—physician who treats cancerous conditions

open hours scheduling—a scheduling system in which patients are normally seen on a first-come, first-served basis, with no appointment necessary

ophthalmologist—physician who diagnoses and treats conditions of the eye

optometrist—healthcare professional who diagnoses and treats minor conditions of the eye

organizational chart—visual breakdown of the chain of command in a business

organizing—the process of gathering the necessary tools, staff, and resources to accomplish set goals

orientation—a period of time for training new employees

orthopedist—physician who specializes in treatment of the musculoskeletal system

osteoporosis—a disorder in which the bones become increasingly porous, brittle, and subject to fracture

otolaryngologist—physician who specializes in the treatment of conditions associated with the ears, nose, and throat

outsource—to send outside a business to another business for completion

overtime—wages paid beyond 40 hours in a workweek, usually at a rate that is 1.5 times the normal rate

participating provider—healthcare provider who has contracted with a particular health insurance carrier

participative—a management style in which the manager seeks out the opinions of those they manage

pathologist—physician who supervises the clinical laboratory and the tests performed there

patient billing statement—monthly statement sent to patients who have outstanding balances

Patient Protection and Affordable Care Act—healthcare legislation passed in 2010

payer number—the number that medical offices must include on an electronic claim to identify the insurance company to whom the claim is directed

payroll—process of calculating the amounts employees receive for their work

payroll taxes—monies withheld from wages for federal income, Social Security, and Medicare obligations

pediatrician—physician who limits care to that of children

performance evaluation—process by which a manager reviews job performance with an employee

personal information—information pertaining to the patient, such as address and telephone number

personnel file—set of employment-related documents for an employee; includes the original job application, résumé, credentials, licensing and insurance information, references, federal withholding requests, dates and copies of performance evaluations, and any information about disciplinary actions

personnel manual—a compilation of employment policies for an office; also called an employee handbook

petty cash—a small amount of money kept in the medical office to pay for unexpected items

phlebotomist—healthcare professional trained to draw blood for physician-ordered laboratory work

physiatrist—physician who specializes in the diagnosis of musculoskeletal conditions and their treatment by use of therapeutic means

physician assistant (PA)—healthcare provider who works under the supervision of a physician. In most states, PAs are able to prescribe medications and assist during surgeries

planning—the process of setting goals for a group

podiatrist—physician who specializes in the treatment of the feet

point-of-service option—an insurance offering in which a patient has access to multiple plans, such as an HMO and PPO

policy—statement of guidelines or rules on a given topic

policyholder—the person who owns an insurance policy

preauthorization—the process of obtaining approval from an insurance company for a patient's procedure

precertification—the process of obtaining approval from an insurance company for a patient's procedure

preexisting condition—condition for which a patient received treatment in a certain period before beginning coverage with a new insurance plan

preferred provider organization (PPO)—organization that contracts with independent providers to perform services for members at discounted rates

premium—dollar amount paid to an insurance company to have coverage in force

preventive care—healthcare designed to keep a person healthy

primary care practice—practice where providers offer services that are primary care in nature

privacy officer—an employee in a healthcare facility charged with the duty of educating others on HIPAA compliance

problem-oriented medical record (POMR) charting—a charting process that allows providers to assign a number to each medical problem and chart each item each time the patient is seen for care

procedure—steps used to perform a given task or project

products—supplies that the physician prescribes to the patient, such as a splint or crutches

professional corporation—a medical practice structure in which the physicians have filed paperwork with the state where the practice resides in order to obtain corporation status

professional courtesy—a discount offered to friends, colleagues, and family members of the physician

progress notes—the daily chart notes taken at the time of a patient's visit to a clinic

prostate—a gland in males that surrounds the neck of the bladder and urethra

protected health information (PHI)—any patient information that includes identifiers that could be used to identify the patient

psychiatrist—physician who specializes in the diagnosis and treatment of mental disorders

pulmonologist—physician who specializes in the diagnosis and treatment of lung conditions

punitive award—award made when judges or juries feel that a healthcare provider should be punished for his or her actions

purge—to go through files and remove the items or charts that are old or no longer needed

quality improvement—the process of looking for ways to improve the patient experience in the medical office

quarterly payroll reports—documents that specify the taxes withheld from wages quarterly

radiologist—physician who specializes in the diagnosis and treatment of patients via the use of x-rays, magnetic resonance imaging, computed tomography scans, and radioactive materials

Red Flags rule—government legislation requiring all healthcare facilities to implement a written Identity Theft Prevention Program designed to detect the warning signs of identity theft in their day-to-day operations

registered nurse (RN)—healthcare professional who provides direct patient care, including administering medications and treatments under a physician's orders

relative value unit (RVU)—numeric value assigned by Medicare to formulate fee schedules for healthcare providers

res ipsa loquitur—the Latin phrase for "the thing speaks for itself"

res judicata—the Latin phrase for "the thing has been decided"

respite care—care provided in a skilled nursing facility on a short-term basis for patients who are otherwise treated at home

respondeat superior—the Latin phrase for "let the master answer"

résumé—a job applicant's list of educational and work experience, including skills and talents

retail clinic—healthcare setting where providers offer services in a retail setting

return on investment—the amount of money brought in after a marketing initiative

rheumatologist—physician who specializes in the treatment of conditions associated with arthritis

risk management—the process of reducing or eliminating risks of injury to patients or employees

salary—wages for the job performed

scoliosis—abnormal curvature of the spine

scope of practice—the skills practiced by a person who has received training in a particular profession

screenings—performance of a health-related study to rule out a certain disease or illness

search engine optimization—the process of making changes to a company's individual website so that the website will come up at the top of a results list during Internet searching

security envelope—an envelope that does not allow for the contents to be viewed without opening the envelope

self-insure—insurance program in which an employer sets aside funds to pay for employee health expenses

sentinel event—any incident in a healthcare facility in which a patient is injured or could have been injured

service contract—a contract for maintenance and repair of equipment

services—things that are provided to the patient in the form of an activity, such as an examination or a surgical procedure

settled—a case is considered to be settled when the two sides in a lawsuit agree on a financial award to the injured patient

shadow—to watch another person perform his or her job in order to learn how to do that job

shingling—the process of taping small pieces of paper to a full size sheet of paper so that small items are not lost in the chart

skilled nursing facility—a facility for long-term care or other care facility where the patient must be monitored by nursing staff on a regular basis

slack time—a system for leaving certain times of day open to accommodate situations such as patients who call for same-day appointments

slander—the act of harming another person's reputation by stating something untruthful

sleep medicine physician—physician who specializes in treating conditions associated with sleep disorders

sliding fee scale—a provider's fee schedule that charges varying fees for a service based on a patient's financial ability to pay

SOAP note charting—subjective, objective, assessment, and plan; a common form of charting in the medical record where clinicians chart information in an easy-to-find format

social information—information in a patient's chart relating to his social status, such as smoking or participating in high-risk behaviors

social media sites—Internet websites, such as Facebook, where individuals interact on a social level

Social Security Act—law passed by the U.S. Congress in 1935 to provide workers and their families with financial security after retirement

sole proprietorship—physician who practices alone, with support staff, and is entirely responsible for all costs associated with maintaining his or her practice

speaker telephone—a type of telephone that allows multiple people in a room to participate in the phone conversation

specialty care practice—practice where providers offer care that is specialty related

staff meeting—meeting attended by members of a department or office

standard of care—the amount and type of care a reasonable and prudent person would provide, given the same training and circumstances

Children's Health Insurance Program (CHIP)—a program created to cover children who do not have another form of health insurance coverage

statute of limitations—the period of time provided by law for a patient to file a malpractice lawsuit from the date of the injury

stop loss—the maximum amount the patient must pay out of pocket for copayments and coinsurance

subpoena—a legal document that requires a medical office to release medical records or provide court testimony

subscriber—the person who owns the insurance policy

superbill—form used in the medical office for indicating the services rendered to the patient, as well as the diagnosis for the service

supervisor—the person who oversees staff and their work

surgeon—physician who specializes in surgical interventions

tabular index—the numerical listing of all CPT codes

teletypewriter (TTY) system—a telephone system that allows for communication with a person who has a hearing impairment

Theory X—a management theory that states employees cannot be trusted to think for themselves

Theory Y—a management theory that states employees want to do well and will perform well if given the opportunity

therapeutic touch—use of touch to convey concern and compassion for another

tickler file—tool for tracking future events, such as patient appointments

time clock—piece of equipment that records employees' arrival and departure times for payroll purposes

tort—wrongful act that leads to damages sustained by another

triage—the process of determining the medical nature and urgency of a patient's condition

TRICARE—health insurance for active-duty military personnel, retired service personnel, and their eligible dependents

unbundling—billing for services (typically, lab services) separately, instead of as a bundled group

uncollectible account—account that will likely never be paid

unemployment insurance—program that pays employees who have lost their jobs

unique identifier—a unique number issued by Medicare to each individual provider

upcode—to code and bill for a higher level of service than what was actually provided

upcoding—choosing to use a higher level of service code than is appropriate for the actual level of service provided

urologist—physician who specializes in the treatment of conditions associated with the urinary system

usual, customary, and reasonable (UCR)—reimbursement method in which insurance companies compare providers' charges to other providers in the same geographic area

V codes—codes used to classify the reason for care other than an active illness

variable costs—costs that vary with the number of services or products produced

verbal communication—communication in spoken words

verbal warning—the process of giving notice of disciplinary action to an employee verbally

visionary—a leader who offers a vision for the future

voice messaging system—an automated system that allows callers to leave a voice message for the intended recipient

volunteer—to offer time to or perform services for an agency or organization without payment

W-2 form—U.S. federal form that annually documents the wages employees drew during the previous year

W-4 form—U.S. federal form that indicates employees' marital status and federal tax exemptions

wages—monies paid for work performed

waiting period—period after a new health insurance plan begins during which certain services are not covered

waiver—a form patients sign agreeing to pay for services that may be denied by Medicare

warranty—the period of time within which the manufacturer is responsible for any repairs to equipment

wave scheduling—a scheduling system in which patients are scheduled only for the first half of each hour

withholding allowances—number of exemptions declared on federal tax forms

workers' compensation—insurance coverage for job-related illness or injury provided by employers

working supervisors—supervisors who spend a portion of their time working in the same role as the employees they supervise

write off—to remove a balance from a patient account

written communication—communication in written form

written warning—the process of giving notice of disciplinary action to an employee in written form; typically more severe than a verbal warning

Index

R

Radiologists, 14
Reception areas, maintaining, 109
Recommendations/references, providing, 88–89
Red Flags rule, 172, 266
References, checking employee, 80–81
Referrals, 310–311
Registered medical assistant (RMA) task list, 407–409
Registered nurses (RNs), 16–17
Regulatory compliance
  See also Health Insurance Portability and Accountability Act
  Clinical Laboratory Improvement Amendments Act, 178–179
  corporate compliance plan, 173
  fraud and abuse, 180–181
  Health Information Technology for Economic and Clinical Health Act, 173
  Joint Commission, 173–174
  OSHA, 174–178
  Red Flags rule, 172
Relative value unit (RVU), 262–263
Reminder cards, 125
Reportable conditions, 62, 154
Reporting incidents, 354–355
Research
  marketing, 366
  programs, 158
Res ipsa loquitur, 62
Res judicata, 62
Respite care, 299
Respondeat superior, 55–56
Résumés, screening, 77–78
Retail clinics, 5, 7–8
Retention of medical records, 147, 148
Return on investment, 364
Rheumatologists, 14
Risk management
  communicating after adverse outcomes, 352–353
  communicating possible outcomes, 348
  communicating with other team members, 348–350
  defined, 344
  hazardous waste disposal, 357
  incident reporting, 354–355
  limitations and scope of practice, recognizing, 350
  medication errors, 351–353, 355–356
  noncompliance, documenting, 350
  personal protective equipment, 177, 356
  procedures, 229–230
  service recovery, 353–354
Rolodex system, 106

S

Safety issues
  See also OSHA (Occupational Safety and Health Act)
  employee, 358
  hazardous waste disposal, 357
  personal protective equipment, 177, 356
Salary, 81
Scoliosis, 369
Scope of practice, 54

Screenings, marketing using, 369
Search engines
  Internet, 214
  optimization, 367
Security, computer, 212–213
Security envelopes, 253
Security rule, HIPAA, 169–170
Self-insure, 285
Sentinel events, 174, 354–355
Service contracts, 197–198
Service recovery, 353–354
Services, 236
Settled, 57
Sexual harassment, 88
Shadow, 80
Shingling, 144, 145
Signatures, on medical records, 140
Sixteenth Amendment, 238
Skilled nursing facility, 299
Slack time, 124
Slander, 88
Sleep medicine physicians, 14
Sliding fee scale, 285
Small claims court, 276–277
SOAP note charting, 141
Social information, 136
Social media sites, 370
Social Security Act (1935), 238–239
Software
  billing programs, 267
  coding, 211–212
  common features, 211
  defined, 206
  packages, 211
  payroll calculations, 252
  prescription management, 215
  training staff, 210
Sole proprietorships, 5–6
Speaker telephones, 97
Specialty care practices, 10–15
Staff meetings, 42–43, 195–196
Standard of care, 54, 140
State Children's Health Insurance Program (SCHIP), 304
Statute of limitations, 58–59, 60–61, 147
Stop loss, 289
Subpoenas, 66, 137, 153
Subscriber, 287
Superbill, 311, 312
Supervising employees, 83–84, 189
Supervisors, 189
Suppliers, contracting with, 196
Supplies, ordering and receiving, 196–197
Surgeons, 14

T

Tabular index, 323
Tax Equity and Fiscal Responsibility Act (TEFRA) (1982), 284, 290
Taxes, payroll, 238–239
Telecommunication relay systems, 108
Telephone books, marketing using, 372
Telephones
  answering services, using, 104
  automated system, 96
  automatic dialers, 98, 99
  automatic routing units, 98

callers, handling difficult, 103
callers, hard-to-understand, 103
call forwarding, 98
calls to other healthcare facilities, 105
collection calls, dos and don'ts for, 267
conference calls, 97
directing patient calls to physicians, 100
direct lines, 98
directories, using, 106
documenting calls from patients, 103–104
emergency calls, 102–103
etiquette, 99–100
hands-free headsets, 96–97
hold feature, 98
interviews by, 78
last number redial, 97
long-distance or toll-free calls, 107
messages, leaving, 105
messages, on-hold, 372
messages, taking, 104
music, for those on hold, 98
personal calls, making, 104–105
prescriptions and/or refills, calling in, 107
prioritizing calls, 102
screening calls, 100
speaker, 97
system features, 96–99
triage, 100–101
use of, 46
voicemail, 99
Teletypewriter (TTY) system, 108
Terminating employees, 87
Terminating relationship with patients, 63, 64
Test results, quickly reporting, 347
Theft, employee, 198
Theory X, 188
Theory Y, 188
Therapeutic touch, 40–41
Tickler files, 273
Time clocks, 248
Torts, 57
Training, for employees, 83, 210
Translation services, 107
Transportation for patients, arranging, 129
Triage
  defined, 73
  telephone, 100–101
TRICARE, 285, 304–305

U

Unbundling, 180
Uncollectible accounts, 275
Unemployment insurance, 239
Unique identifier, 170
U.S. Department of Health and Human Services, 332–333
Upcoding, 180, 323
Urologists, 15
Usual, customary, and reasonable (UCR), 322

V

Vaccine injuries, reporting, 62
Variable costs, 237
V codes, 334
Verbal communication, 26–27
Verbal warnings, 85–86
Visionary, 193